RELIGIOUS PERSPECTIVES IN BIOETHICS

The Annals of Bioethics

Religious Perspectives in Bioethics

Edited by

John F. Peppin
Director
Center for Bioethics, Pain Management & Medicine
Des Moines, Iowa

Mark J. Cherry
Department of Philosophy
Saint Edward's University
Austin, Texas

and

Ana Iltis
Center for Health Care Ethics
Saint Louis University
Saint Louis, Missouri

Taylor & Francis
Taylor & Francis Group
LONDON AND NEW YORK

Library of Congress Cataloging-in-Publication Data

A Catalogue record for this book is available from the Library of Congress

Typesetting: Charon Tec Pvt. Ltd, Chennai, India
Printed in the Netherlands by Krips, Meppel

Published by: Taylor & Francis, The Netherlands, Leiden
www.tandf.co.uk/books

ISBN 90 265 1967 2

Contents

ACKNOWLEDGEMENTS vii

Introduction: Text, Tradition, Authority, and Method in Religious Bioethics ix
B. Andrew Lustig

Roman Catholic Bioethics 1
Christopher Tollefsen and Joseph Boyle

Orthodox Christian Bioethics: Medical Morality in the Mind of the Fathers 21
H. Tristram Engelhardt, Jr.

Bioethics in the Episcopal Tradition 31
Cynthia B. Cohen and David H. Smith

Gospel Truth and Societal Consensus: Recent Bioethics Statements by the Protestant Church in Germany (EKD) 53
Corinna Delkeskamp-Hayes and Matthias Zierenberg

Reformed Perspectives in Bioethics 79
Ruth Groenhout

Southern Baptists and Bioethics 97
C. Ben Mitchell

Authority and Agency: Policies and Principles in Latter-day Saints Bioethics 109
Courtney S. Campbell

Jewish Bioethics 131
Harvey L. Gordon and Mark Washofsky

Jewish Perspectives on Embryo and Stem Cell Research 147
Aaron L. Mackler

Islamic Bioethics 153
Abdulaziz Sachedina

Buddhism and Bioethics 173
Damien Keown

Hindu Bioethics 189
Cromwell Crawford

Sikh Perspectives on Bioethics 211
Devinder Singh Chahal

Daoism and Bioethics: Daode Jin's Doctrine of Naturalness and the Principle of Non-Action 221
Jonathan Chan

NOTES ON CONTRIBUTORS 233

INDEX 235

Acknowledgments

This volume has benefited from the kind efforts of many. In particular, we would like to thank the members of the editorial board of the *Annals of Bioethics* for their ongoing assistance in reviewing and focusing the essays. Special thanks are owed to a number of individuals who contributed significant time and energy to preparing this volume: Joseph Boyle, H. Tristram Engelhardt, Jr., Ruth Groenhout, Henk ten Have, Kazumasa Hoshino, Loretta Kopelman, Anne M. Fagot-Largeault, José Alberto Mainetti, Maurizio Mori, Edmund D. Pellegrino, Ren-Zong Qiu, Hans-Martin Sass, W. David Solomon, Fabrice Jotterand, Matthew Lomanno, Jessica Lomanno, Lisa Rasmussen, and Jerome Schmelzer. In addition, H. Tristram Engelhardt, Jr. must be thanked for his tireless efforts and support of this project. We also wish to thank the contributors to this volume for giving their time and dedication to this endeavor.

We also wish to recognize the ongoing support of our universities and colleagues. We wish to thank Saint Edward's University, the School of Humanities, the Department of Philosophy, and the Center for Ethics and Leadership, especially Louis T. Brusatti, William J. Zanardi, and Phillip M. Thompson. We also wish to express our gratitude to Saint Louis University, the Center for Health Care Ethics, and the Graduate School.

John F. Peppin, Mark J. Cherry, and Ana Iltis

Introduction: Text, Tradition, Authority, and Method in Religious Bioethics

B. Andrew Lustig

Religious Perspectives in Bioethics surveys recent bioethics discussion in thirteen religious traditions. Christian contributions include chapters on Roman Catholicism, Orthodox Christianity, the Episcopal, German Protestant, and Baptist traditions, Reformed Christianity, and the Latter Day Saints. The volume also includes chapters on Judaism, Islam, Hinduism, Buddhism, Sikhism, and Daoism. While any one volume of the *Annals of Bioethics* is not encyclopedic, the series is committed to providing timely reports on recent religious discussions in bioethics as contributions become available. Over time, the *Annals* will therefore provide comprehensive coverage of both general themes and particular topics in religious bioethics, thereby providing an important resource for scholars and interested others.

The authors were asked to provide something of a uniform structure in their commentaries. Thus, most of the contributors set out, at least in summary fashion, the theological motifs and methodological principles at work in the traditions they survey, as well as commentary on many or all of the following topics: concerns with professionalism and the doctor-patient relationship; reproductive issues, including contraception, abortion, as well as issues raised by genetics and cloning; issues in death, dying, and end-of-life care; moral and political discussions concerning access to health care and the reform of health care delivery; procedural and substantive issues raised by the practice of ethics consultation and the functions of ethics committees; and other topics of current concern.

The theological themes at work in various religious traditions exhibit differences as well as commonalities. "Great religion" approaches have quite properly been criticized for their tendency to oversimplify much more complex theological dialectics within traditions and for their failure to attend to the rich pluralism of theological voices beyond the mainstream, especially ones that historically have been marginalized. While such cautions must be borne in mind, attentive readers will also identify certain commonalities across religious traditions, shared features that invite broadly ecumenical reflections on the ways that religious worldviews frame distinctive approaches to bioethical issues that may emerge in stark contrast to secular perspectives. Examples of such broadly shared themes include accounts of God's created purposes for humankind; accounts of God's providential care and its implications for human morality in response to the divine initiative; covenantal understandings that influence interpretations of the nature and scope of justice; and the imperative of good stewardship in relation to health care, both personally and societally.

At the same time, depending on how such themes are developed and applied, characteristic differences among religious traditions will be equally evident, even from traditions that draw on identical sources. Foundational texts, even when acknowledged as canonical within traditions, will be variously interpreted. Consider several examples. As Ruth Groenhout observes in her chapter on Reformed Christianity, an emphasis on continuing discernment is as much a feature of recent discussion as any given interpretation of relevant scriptural texts. While Cromwell Crawford highlights the importance of certain Hindu texts, especially the *Caraka Samhita*, in the tradition's discussion of the sanctity of life as a core principle, quite different arguments about the legitimacy of physician-assisted suicide can be offered, depending on how those texts are invoked. As Abdulaziz Sachedina notes in his discussion of Islam, the *Qur'an* and the *Sunna* are recognized as authoritative for Islam, but their status hardly leads to univocal interpretations of Qur'anic laws and prophetic traditions. And while Buddhism, in Damien Keown's judgment, lacks a clear hierarchy or locus of authority, Buddhist clergy provide moral guidance based on interpretations of texts that can be deemed canonical in the tradition as well, with different interpretations offered in various cultural settings.

As is evident, then, from the variety of textual interpretations both within and across religious traditions, judgments that certain texts are deemed canonical for and, in important respects, constitutive of the moral formation of believers, are not of themselves dispositive for settling questions about how such texts are to be invoked and applied, either to broad themes or to particular moral judgments. As Allen Verhey observes apropos the authority of Christian Scriptures, "To affirm the authority of scripture is to invoke the use of the Bible in moral discernment and judgment, but it is not to prescribe how the Bible is to be used" (Verhey, 1986, p. 57). Verhey's point may be suggestive for the variety of uses of foundational texts in non-Christian traditions as well. To appreciate the respective uses of canonical texts requires attention to a number of concerns. First, how shall authoritative writings be construed in the first instance, in their combination of divine perspectives uttered through diverse human authors? Second, what sorts of questions – primarily theological or moral – are appropriate to the use of canonical texts? Third, granting that canonical texts exert decisive moral influence, is that influence to be understood (at the personal level) as primarily addressed to questions of character or to deontological concerns with right and wrong actions? Finally, beyond the level of personal ethics, do such texts offer insights into larger questions of social and political ethics, and are they of obvious relevance to the modern context of political pluralism?

With regard to characteristic methods, one again finds commonalities and differences. Judaism and Roman Catholicism are both robustly casuistical in their methods; richly textured analyses of paradigmatic cases and their implications for novel or disputed issues invite a rich comparison between the two traditions. Other traditions, for example the Latter-day Saints (LDS), lack detailed commentary on many issues in bioethics. As Courtney Campbell underscores in his chapter, the LDS tradition often assumes a posture of ecclesiastical silence on conflicted issues. Thus, as a matter of theological and moral method, there are various levels at which different understandings of theological authority evince their theoretical and practical effects.

James Gustafson discusses four "base points" that are distinguishable in any comprehensive Christian ethic and, with appropriate cautions, one might be able to extend Gustafson's analysis to other religious traditions as well. Each of these fundamental points is related to the manner in which theological authority in ethics is understood and exercised. First is the way that God is interpreted – the doctrine of God and the understanding of God's relations with us. Second is the way that particular traditions understand and evaluate human history and experience, and the way that nature is interpreted as a source of moral insight. Third is the way that persons and/or communities are understood as moral agents, as well as an interpretation of human actions. Fourth, a comprehensive theological ethic will provide a more or less systematic account of the way that persons should proceed to make moral judgments and choices (Gustafson, 1986, p. 87).

By extension, a particular theological ethic will develop these base points by employing four distinguishable sources: (1) foundational or canonical texts and the accumulated insights of the interpretive tradition of theological reflection; (2) non-theological principles and methods (e.g., philosophical and legal); (3) science and other sources of knowledge about the world; and (4) "human experience" broadly conceived (Gustafson, p. 88). As a result, characteristic differences among perspectives in theological ethics and bioethics emerge from the ways that such base points are discussed and specific sources of ethical authority are weighted. As Gustafson observes about Christian perspectives:

> Discernible differences can be found in writings from various Christian traditions; great theologians or historical movements establish patterns that persist. Examples: the use of natural law in the Roman Catholic tradition; the distinction between law and gospel and between the heavenly and earthly realms in the Lutheran tradition; the emphasis on following Christ as he is portrayed in the Gospels and on rigorous obedience to his teachings in the Radical Reformation tradition; [and] the marked mystical aspects of ethics in the Eastern Orthodox tradition (Gustafson, p. 89).

The interpretation of God lies at the heart of much theological ethics and is integrally tied to the manner in which moral authority is legitimated and exercised. Apropos of Gustafson's second and third base points, differences in theological ethics may flow directly from the ways that human history and moral agency are understood. Again, employing a Christian example, while justification, as interpreted by Martin Luther, bestows an alien dignity upon redeemed persons, individual actions and the larger social order may be construed quite differently in Reformed understandings that stress the current efficacy of redemption in practices of sanctification. In addition, different interpretations of eschatology will frame and inform different interpretations of authority, especially in the emphasis on communal discernment as a current expression of God's continuing presence. A version of eschatology that stresses the fulfillment of God's good purposes in starkly discontinuous and future-oriented terms will generate an understanding of authority that differs markedly from a perspective that emphasizes a more realized eschatology, wherein God's kingdom is characterized as the fruition of, rather than the end to, human history.

At the same time, such comparison also underscores major differences between and among traditions regarding who speaks authoritatively on moral matters within the community. Indeed, considerations of authority are especially important in contextualizing the traditions of theological discourse represented by the contributions to this volume of the *Annals*. Any serious assessment of the particularities of different religious traditions in bioethics requires that we acknowledge the distinctive conceptions of teaching authority. Any discussion of authority in religious bioethics requires that attention be paid to the self-understandings of particular religious traditions vis-à-vis other religious traditions as well as secular understandings. Attending to different understandings of theological authority, in turn, will implicate (in mutually reinforcing fashion) other foundational issues – notions of what constitutes the licit structure and function of an authentic religious community, interpretations of the canonicity and bindingness of foundational texts, and judgments about who is empowered to speak in God's name.

One of the more intriguing aspects of reading the contributions to this Volume is to consider how ongoing debates *within*, as well as across, traditions have implications for particular issues. For example, as Christopher Tollefsen and Joseph Boyle emphasize, the role of natural law is central to Roman Catholic moral theology. Natural moral knowledge is, in principle, available to all individuals as the source of practical reason and, according to Tollefsen and Boyle, therefore provides an appropriate basis for recommendations by the Catholic hierarchy on matters of public policy. This stance is characteristically Catholic, but it raises a number of issues that have generated significant internal debates within that tradition. At the level of moral method, the Church has referred to the necessity to "clarify" the conclusions of natural reason by appeals to Revelation. However, on conflicted matters of bioethics, especially those involved in reproductive issues and issues at the end of life, the status of natural moral knowledge available to all persons of good will remains problematic. If epistemologically privileged claims are required to clarify conclusions in principle, but not apparently in fact, available to all, how are magisterial pronouncements on matters of public policy in the context of pluralism to be understood? Moreover, due to a lack of consensus on numerous reproductive issues between Catholics and their Christian fellows, much less between Catholic and secular minds, what implications follow for crafting appropriate public policy?

Or consider the different moral judgments that may emerge from traditions that seem to share at least strong family resemblances in their characteristic patterns of moral reasoning. For example, in considering the use of embryonic stem cells for research and potential clinical benefit, Catholicism draws on a rich casuistry to conclude that direct choices against basic goods, here the basic good of nascent personal life, is intrinsically wrong and illicit in all cases, regardless of the magnitude of potential benefits to others. By contrast, Aaron Mackler, in his thoughtful analysis of Jewish casuistic materials, draws characteristically different conclusions about the legitimacy of using embryonic stem cells, based on a different initial evaluation of the moral status of embryonic human life. Other traditions lack any recourse to casuistry. As noted above, the Latter-day Saints tradition, in response to novel developments in bioethics, often assumes an initial posture of ecclesiastical silence. To be sure, on some issues, such as abortion and euthanasia, clear judgments have been rendered, though as Courtney Campbell's discussion makes clear, the basis for such judgments has sometimes shifted over time. Indeed, in an interesting example of deeper engagement with a tradition that is officially more reserved, Campbell develops six categories to analyze LDS guidelines on ten bioethics topics, drawing out the plausible implications of positions that, in their various articulations, are often underdeveloped in explicitly religious terms. In this respect, Campbell's discussion exemplifies an enlargement upon the primary purpose of the *Annals* – not merely reportage and commentary from our contributors but also, when warranted, a creative and critical extension of a tradition's "first principles" in the interest of greater consistency and clarity on particular issues.

Given the vibrancy and variety of perspectives offered by our commentators, I am pleased to introduce this theological volume in the *Annals* series. Besides offering up-to-date summaries of recent discussion, our authors have also provided useful bibliographical references to a number of documents that would otherwise prove difficult for individual scholars to know about, much less to assemble. As noted above, readers will perceive characteristic similarities and differences among religious traditions in their characteristic moral methods and in their conclusions on specific issues. On the one hand, such similarities and differences may lead interested readers to muse about larger matters of fundamental theology to account for such agreement and divergence. Yet a word of caution is in order here. This volume, if successful, will achieve the important but limited purpose that its title implies. Each volume in the series is offered primarily as a summary and analysis of recent ethical discussion on specific topics. For scholars and others interested in more fundamental matters, the present volume may serve to exemplify basic theological themes and tendencies in concrete fashion, but it should not be misinterpreted as discussing issues of foundational theology (or ecclesiology) in a sustained or systematic way.

On the other hand, it is important to acknowledge again how bioethics discussions within and among religious communities reveal features that generally distinguish them from self-consciously secular approaches to bioethics. While it is to be expected that different interpretations of text, tradition, method, and authority often lead to different conclusions among religious traditions in their respective judgments on particular topics, it seems equally clear that religious understandings, although nuanced differently among various faith communities, often reveal broadly shared characteristics that stand in stark contrast to the moral minimalism at work in many secular approaches. Such similarities should not be that surprising. For the convictions at work in religious ethics often eventuate in a discernible consensus among traditions that nonetheless remain distinct in their understandings of ecclesiology, method, and authority. Theological arguments characteristically function in a richer, more robust fashion than the lowest-common denominator, procedurally driven arguments at work in secular perspectives. While that robustness of vision poses challenges to the development of a common morality workable at the level of policy, it also invites a broader conversation about, if not a prophetic challenge to, the assumptions that undergird much of the conventional wisdom in bioethics discussion.

Bibliography

Gustafson, J. 1986. Christian ethics. In: J. Childress & J. Macquarrie (Eds.), *The Westminster dictionary of Christian ethics* (2nd ed., pp. 87-90). Philadelphia: The Westminster Press.

Verhey, A. 1986. Bible in Christian Ethics. In: J. Childress & J. Macquarrie (Eds.). *The Westminster dictionary of Christian ethics* (2nd ed., pp. 57-61). Philadelphia: The Westminster Press.

Roman Catholic Bioethics

Christopher Tollefsen and Joseph Boyle

I. Introduction

Roman Catholic reflection on bioethical topics comprises a vast array of teachings, debates, and publications. This reflection embraces virtually all the topics of bioethics. It emerges from the rich tradition of moral theology and casuistic reasoning that is rooted in the works of St. Augustine, St. Thomas Aquinas, and the other great medieval theologians. Catholic bioethics is carried out in the scholarship and institutional work of Catholic theologians, philosophers, and Church officials around the world.

Catholics are significantly represented among the academics, physicians, and policy advisors who contribute to secular bioethics. Their work reflects more or less the influence of the Catholic moral tradition. Roman Catholic bioethics, however, is not usefully understood simply as bioethics carried out by Catholics. Some recognition of and deference to the authority of the Church defines moral reflection as Roman Catholic. That authority has several forms and is expressed in many ways. It exists in official writings from the Bible to the Fathers and Doctors of the Church. It exists in the preaching and teaching of the clergy and, most definitively, in the acts of bishops, especially the Pope, teaching alone and in collaboration with one another in synods and councils. There is considerable debate among Catholic scholars and Church leaders concerning the precise extent of the authority of the *magisterium*, or teaching office of the Church, but all Catholic scholars accord that authority some respect and must somehow take it into account in their bioethical and other moral reflections.

One major issue in the debate over the authority of the magesterium concerns the nature and extent of the authority of theologians. Pope John Paul II, who represents the magisterial view on this issue, regards moral theological research as a service to the Church and consequently as subordinate to the judgment of its leaders (Pope John Paul II, 1993, pp. 108-113).[1] This location of moral theology and other normative scholarship within the Church is not taken to imply either that the magisterium has answered all bioethical questions or that Catholic bioethicists lack discretion to pursue their inquiries.

Because magisterial teaching is central to Catholic moral life, the focus of this introduction to Catholic bioethics will be primarily on official Catholic teachings relevant to bioethics.[2] We will include enough references to the specifically scholarly literature to provide an entry into the fuller Catholic discussion.[3]

Roman Catholic work in bioethics is distinctive in several important ways. Two have been indicated already: (1) it is an extensive set of reflections covering virtually all the major concerns of bioethics, and (2) it includes an authoritative principle, the teaching of the Catholic Church as interpreted by the Pope and bishops. Catholic controversies about Church authority and the limits of its application to all the detailed issues of bioethics do not prevent this feature of Catholic bioethics and, more generally, moral thought from being perhaps its most visibly distinctive feature. The extensive teaching on moral matters generally and on bioethics specifically – especially by Vatican Council II, by the current and recent Popes, and by bishops and groups of bishops – comprises a body of religiously-based bioethics that is perhaps unique in the world today.

There are at least four other ways in which Catholic bioethics is distinctive. First, the characteristic methods of moral reasoning within the Catholic moral tradition and the Catholic conception of morality, as both rooted in the natural law and essential for God's plan for saving humanity, contribute to the distinctiveness of Catholic approaches to bioethics. More will be said on these matters below (in Section III.A.3).

Second, the content of Catholic teaching on bioethics is distinctive. This is most notable in the areas in which the tradition has specified moral absolutes, such as the prohibition of intentional killing of the innocent, other intentional harms to people, extramarital sexual activity, and lying. The application of these moral absolutes by casuistic reasoning has led to other distinctive Catholic positions (for example, the teaching regarding ordinary and extraordinary treatments). This teaching, which will be explained below (in Section III.D), holds that decisions to withhold or withdraw life-extending treatments are not necessarily choices to end life, and so are not always impermissible despite the prohibition of intentional killing.

Third, the Catholic approach to social organization and authority leads to a distinctive rationale concerning many of the social issues arising in health care. Catholic social teaching emphasizes the supporting function of social organizations, especially those with social authority. Such organizations are meant to help individuals live responsible lives. As we shall see below, these simple but basic ideas have implications for issues such as patient's rights, the right to health care, and the allocation scarce health care resources.

Fourth, there is a specifically political and cultural aspect to Roman Catholic bioethics whose wide extent is distinctive among religious approaches to bioethics. Beginning with Catholic opposition to legalized abortion, Catholic concerns with bioethical issues have not remained within the confessional, or narrowly within the bounds of evangelical preaching or individual spiritual direction. Catholic positions have been explicitly public and political. Consider the Roman Catholic contribution to pro-life politics, Pope John Paul II's appeal for a renewed "culture of life" (1995), and the efforts of many bishops and groups of bishops around the world to promote equity in the distribution of health care resources.

II. History

The history of Roman Catholic bioethics is completely intermingled with that of Catholic morality more generally. Although that morality continues to be expounded and developed by moralists working in the Roman Catholic tradition, its overall history is largely unwritten. There is, of course, a large body of established scholarly work on the great figures of Roman Catholic moral theory, especially on St. Thomas Aquinas and St. Augustine. There are also studies on the history of Catholic moral teaching on particular moral issues, including abortion (Connery, 1977), the distinction between ordinary and extraordinary treatments (Cronin, 1989), and contraception (Noonan, 1965). Finally, there are systematic treatments of Catholic bioethics (Ashley & O'Rourke, 1989). But there is no comprehensive study of the history of Catholic moral theology, much less the history of Catholic bioethics. In particular, little has been done to trace the development of Catholic moral thought in the period most essential for the development of distinctive Roman Catholic positions in bioethics – that is, the period from the sixteenth century Spanish scholastics to the dominance of the moral manuals in the half century before Vatican Council II.[4]

Several factors are relevant to the explanation of the development of Roman Catholic bioethics, and many of these are primarily explanations of the general Roman Catholic approach to moral life and thought. Catholics understand the moral life to be integral to the life of Christian faith. Living in accordance with all the requirements of morality and repenting one's failures is held to be an essential element of a life of faith.

This conviction, together with the Church's natural law conviction that the general outline and details of morality are not simply a matter of individual preference, social choice, or custom, but are derived from the natural law and can be known through the use of common human reason, led to the Catholic effort systematically to bring moral norms to bear on the details of the range of possible human lives. This effort to codify Christian morality as articulated especially by St. Augustine is manifest in the writings of medieval canonists, theologians, and bishops, as well as in the writings of the post-medieval casuists who applied this body of moral doctrine to the more complicated circumstances of early modern life.

These efforts have focussed primarily on those areas of the moral life in which mortal sin (sin incompatible with divine life) is possible. These include killing, sexual and procreative matters, and harming the vulnerable – central areas of bioethical perplexity. Furthermore, the social and political implications of Catholicism's natural law ethics has led to a Catholic concern (1) for social justice, including in the area of health care, and (2) for the proper allocation of authority and responsibility within the many communities and institutions in which humans participate.

There is an institutional explanation for the development of bioethics within Roman Catholic moral thought. Catholics, especially those in religious orders, have been institutionally involved in health care throughout its technological and institutional development. This is especially true of Catholic involvement in hospitals over the last 150 years, the period in which health care developed into its present institutional form (Kaufmann, 1999). The moral questions raised in the institutional context of Catholic health care, especially those involving difficult cases related to sexual morality, pregnancy, and the end of life issues, provoked a pedagogical literature directed at nurses, physicians, and others.[5] That literature is clearly continuous with, and an ancestor of, modern secular bioethics. Moreover, the institutional focus continues, for example, in the American bishops' *Ethical and Religious Directives for Catholic Health Care Services* (National Conference of Catholic Bishops, 1994 and 2001).

III. Topics

A. Bioethics in General

A.1. Important Institutions

The single most important institution in Roman Catholic bioethics is the Vatican. Papal teaching, whether from the Pope directly (in the form of addresses, instructions, and encyclicals) or indirectly (through decrees of Vatican offices which are approved by the Pope) is the most authoritative teaching in the Catholic Church. Moreover, the Vatican sponsors a number of worldwide organizations, some of which address issues in bioethics. The Pontifical Academy *Pro Vita* deals with pro-life issues, primarily by bringing pro-life activists and scholars together for meetings at the Vatican, and the Pontifical Council *Cor Unum* addresses the moral and spiritual problems of health care providers.

Next in importance to the Vatican in Catholic bioethics are the conferences of bishops. These conferences often can mount resources unavailable to individual bishops, and some conferences, notably the National Conference of Catholic Bishops, have produced a substantial literature. Bishops' conferences and other groups of bishops have established a number of bioethics research centers. Two of these are especially influential in English-speaking bioethical discussions: the National Catholic Bioethics Center, sponsored by American bishops; and the Linacre Centre, sponsored by the Catholic bishops of England, Ireland, Scotland, and Wales.[6] Many Catholic universities around the world support bioethical research, either within established moral theology and philosophy programs or by specially established bioethics units, often associated with medical faculties and hospitals. The various organizations representing Catholic health care institutions, most notably the Catholic Health Association in the United States,[7] are another distinctive group within the Catholic community. These organizations have important concerns regarding bioethical issues and considerable resources for addressing them.

A.2. *Important Personalities*

Catholic bioethics is not essentially dependent on personalities. But in this, as in all areas of Catholic thought, Pope John Paul II is a dominant figure. Some well known Catholic moralists, such as Elizabeth Anscombe, Germain Grisez, and Richard McCormick, S.J., have also made important contributions to bioethics. Edmund Pellegrino has made an enormous contribution to bioethics, both institutionally in his work at Georgetown University and increasingly through his written work. Benedict Ashley, O.P., Kevin D. O'Rourke, O.P., and Joseph M. Boyle also continue to do important work in bioethics.

A.3. *Dominant Bioethical Theory*

The vocabulary and leading ideas of Catholic bioethics have developed out of the moral work of the great scholastic theologians, most notably from the moral analyses of St. Thomas Aquinas. This tradition of moral thought is often called "natural law theory" or the "natural law tradition" after a dominant component of Aquinas's moral approach, namely the conviction that moral principles are accessible to human reason and binding on all human beings, independently of any special divine revelation and prior to social agreements. This tradition of moral analysis has continued since Aquinas's time, with notable highlights in the work of the 16th century Spanish scholastics, the 17th century casuists, the 18th century synthesis of St. Alphonsus Ligouri, and the revival of Thomistic study in the late 19th and 20th centuries. The working method throughout this period has been a form of casuistry: new and difficult cases are compared and contrasted with clearer, paradigm cases to illuminate their morally important properties so as to allow their correct moral classification. This method is compatible with the absolutism that characterizes Catholic moral analysis: the morally important properties of actions, once revealed by casuistry, can justify the application of an absolute rule. For example, once casuistry shows that a certain form of intervention in pregnancy involves an intention to end or, more precisely, to shorten the life of the fetus, then the intervention is excluded by the exceptionless prohibition against intentionally killing the innocent.

If there is a single element within Catholic casuistry that characterizes its analyses, it is the doctrine of the double effect. This doctrine originates in Aquinas' claim that killing in self-defense need not involve the intent to end the assailant's life. Thus, killing in this case does not violate the prohibition of intentional killing. This doctrine can be applied to many issues in bioethics, including mutilations whose intent is not to destroy bodily function but to save the patient's life; terminations of pregnancy where there is no intent to kill or harm the fetus (or even precisely to end the pregnancy); decisions to withhold treatment whose intent was not to shorten life but to avoid other evils; and actions in which support is given to wrongdoing, but not for the sake of fostering wrongdoing. Recent analysis of the case of the conjoined twins of Malta, for example, makes use of the doctrine of double effect to determine whether the loss of one twin's life, in an operation to separate the two, was intended as a means, or accepted as a side effect.[8]

There has been much dispute about the doctrine of the double effect among Roman Catholic theologians since the debates over contraception began in the 1960s (Boyle, 1993, pp. 11-18). These are part of the larger controversy over moral norms and the conduct of Catholic casuistry, which has dominated Catholic moral theology for the last sixty years. The view of the Vatican on these matters has been stated in Pope John Paul II's *Veritatis Splendor* (1993, pp. 108-127).

B. *Professionalism: The Patient-Health Care Professional Relationship*

The Roman Catholic conception of social life ascribes rights and responsibilities to many identifiable groups of people and especially to groups organized as professions. As emphasized by Pope Pius XII and Pope John Paul II, the professions dedicated to responding to acute human need, such as those in the health care professions, are especially respected because of the great goods they serve and the mercy they show to the needy (O'Rourke & Boyle, 1999, pp. 245-255). Professions and groups of people with special competence are organized to serve the common good, but this does not imply that professionals are to be available simply to satisfy the desires of others. In addition to the requirements of their own professional integrity, professionals are, like everybody else, bound by general moral norms. The implication is that health care professionals are to assist those in need of health care in accord with their own legitimate professional standards and must not do anything they regard as morally wrong.

However, Catholic teaching rejects the appeal to considerations such as these to justify what is often called medical paternalism. As Pope Pius XII emphasized, doctors are private persons and as such are not ordinarily entitled to treat patients without permission from those having appropriate authority over those persons. In the case of competent persons, the patient is the one who has the appropriate authority (O'Rourke & Boyle, 1999, pp. 223-224). In the case of non-competent persons, the identity of the appropriate authority is not so easily established. However, the health care professional is not as such the appropriate authority, even if, for other reasons, he or she is best situated to have the authority (O'Rourke & Boyle, 1999, pp. 311-312). These claims about the proper sphere of authority are true even in situations of life and death (O'Rourke & Boyle, 1999, pp. 280-282, 310).

This element of Catholic bioethical teaching may appear to provide an endorsement from a surprising corner: the modern exaltation of patient autonomy. But this is no all-purpose endorsement of autonomy. Rather, it is an indication of who should make the final decision about whether a given treatment is to be provided. The teaching does not require health care professionals to provide services they think are wrong, such as physician-assisted suicide, nor does it imply that patient or family refusal, just as an exercise of autonomy, is morally correct, but only that they make the final decision (Boyle, 1989, pp. 86-91).

C. *Reproductive Ethics*

Much of reproductive ethics is concerned, both within the Catholic tradition and without, with issues surrounding abortion. Within the Catholic bioethics tradition, much attention has also been given to issues of contraception and the use of new reproductive technologies or assisted reproduction. Often, but not always, these discussions concern the taking of human life. The problem of abortion, the incidental effects of assisted reproduction vis-à-vis the disposal of "spare" embryos, and more recent questions about the creation or use of young embryos to extract stem cells have all been addressed by the Church in recent years in terms of the taking of human life. As a general principle, the Church has held that it is always wrong intentionally to kill an innocent human being. But there have been developments in the Church tradition in the grounding of this claim and in the understanding of the generation of the human being, especially in the papal encyclical *Evangelium Vitae* (1995) and the statement by the Sacred Congregation for the Doctrine of the Faith, *Donum Vitae* (1987). Moreover, the value (or good) of human life has also played a role in one family of arguments against contraception, even though there is no taking of life as such. So an understanding of the Church's views on the value of life, the injunction against intentional killing, and the beginnings of the human person are all essential to an understanding of one class of issues in reproductive ethics.

As the case of contraception indicates, however, not all issues of reproductive ethics are decided based upon the prohibition of killing the innocent. The encyclical *Humanae Vitae* (1968) presents at least two different families of arguments against contraception. One centers on the illicitness of a choice which is contrary to the good of life. The other centers on the two-fold nature of the conjugal act, with its unitive and procreative significance, and the mutual self-giving of spouses who maintain the integrity of the conjugal act. Obviously the two arguments are related, since procreation enters into both. But the second argument, which is continuous with the Church's understanding of the nature of marriage, concerning the two-fold nature of sexual intercourse, enters also into a discussion of various forms of non-sexual reproduction that make use of new forms of technology, such as *in vitro* fertilization and artificial insemination. The discussion of these issues in *Donum Vitae* thus builds upon the discussion of contraception in *Humanae Vitae*.

C.1. *The Sanctity of Human Life and Intentional Killing*

While the Catholic tradition has always held it to be impermissible to intentionally take an innocent human life, whether one's own or another's, there has been some development in the understanding of the argument for this view. In its classical formulation, the restriction is limited in two ways: it is the innocent, generally understood to be either those who pose no threat or those who have not been convicted of capital crimes, who are not to be intentionally killed. And the prohibition against *intentional* killing is held by many in the tradition to apply only to those who are not authorized to kill. It would be consistent with the first limitation that an aggressor could be intentionally killed, and it would be consistent with the second that the state intentionally kill. Pope John Paul II's encyclical, *Evangelium Vitae* (1995) implicitly challenges both limitations. In *Evangelium Vitae*, the Pope sets out an argument against killing that grounds this prohibition in the intrinsic dignity and worth of all human beings, a dignity that is violated by any intentional attack. The Pope continues to stress that it is the innocent who are absolutely not to be intentionally harmed. He allows that, in extreme and rare cases of defense of a state, a criminal might be put to death. Still, the focus on the sanctity and intrinsic dignity of the human being seems to some to indicate a movement in the Pope's work towards a view according to which all intentional killing of human beings is illicit (Keenan, 1997; Boyle, 1989 and 1997).

This great value of the human being is understood in *Evangelium Vitae* largely but not exclusively in light of revelation and Church teaching. There are three reasons given in *Evangelium Vitae* justifying the strong claim of intrinsic dignity. First, each human being is created by God, as were the first human beings, Adam and Eve. Second, each human being is made in the image of God. And third, each human being is called by God to his or her personal destiny with God, a destiny – eternal life – made possible by Jesus Christ's supreme sacrifice of His own life. So this sacredness of human life emerges most fully in the Pope's distinctly Christian meditation on God as the God of Life and on the Gospel as the Gospel of Life.

The Pope also, however, asserts that the truth of the intrinsic value of human life is available to natural reason. This truth is reflected in an increasing attention to the fundamental rights of human beings, even as it is rejected in our contemporary culture in various anti-life practices. But the Pope holds, with the Catholic tradition generally, that the intrinsic good of human life and the commandment against killing are both parts of the natural law and thus written on the hearts of all persons.

Just as the intrinsic value of human life is asserted by the Pope, so the commandment not to kill is reiterated by John Paul II as a moral absolute. The great gift of life which God has bestowed is not something over which human beings have dominion; rather, they have a positive responsibility to promote life in all its aspects, and never intentionally to take it. This negative restriction the Pope characterizes as "the extreme limit which can never be exceeded" (Pope John Paul II, 1995, p. 96). As mentioned above, the development in the Pope's thought and in the work of many working in the Catholic tradition indicates that neither innocence nor lack or presence of authority are necessary considerations. Rather, in his emphatic rejection of "direct" killing, the Pope seems to make intentional killing the form of action ruled out. In turn, this calls for the use of the principle of double effect in the analysis of legitimate uses of force. In the area of reproduction, double effect would be used, for example, in justifying the removal of a cancerous uterus that threatened the life of a pregnant woman.

C.2. *The Generation of the Human Being*

In order to apply the norm against intentional killing of human beings, it is necessary to establish the scope of the class "human being." Increasingly in secular bioethics, a separation is made between being a human and being a person. In some sense, the Catholic tradition acknowledges the difference, asserting that personhood requires the conferral by God of the spiritual soul. Recent documents have acknowledged that there is no empirical way to determine the presence of the soul, but, at the same time, these documents have demonstrated a commitment to the view that if something is a human being, it is therefore a human person: "how could a human individual not be a human person?" (Congregation for the Doctrine of the Faith, 1990, p. 12).

The question should thus be, when does a human being come to be? In consequence of insufficient biological information, Catholic thinkers have not always held that a human being begins at conception. St. Thomas, for example, thinking that the active power of the sperm required a moderate amount of time to make the inanimate menstrual matter into a human being, placed the date of humanity, and hence ensoulment, at 40 days for a male and 90 days for a female (Ford, 1988). The Congregation for the Doctrine of the Faith's *Declaration on Procured Abortion* (1974) and *Donum Vitae* (1987), and Pope John Paul II's *Evangelium Vitae* (1995), by contrast, have held that modern science shows us something quite different:

> From the time that the ovum is fertilized, a life is begun which is neither that of the father nor the mother; it is rather the life of a new human being with his own growth. It would never be made human if it were not human already. This has always been clear, and ... modern genetics offers clear confirmation. It has demonstrated that from the first instant there is established the programme of what this living being will be: a person, this individual person with his characteristic aspects already well determined. Right from fertilization the adventure of a human life begins (Congregation for the Doctrine of the Faith, 1974, p. 12; Pope John Paul II, 1996, p. 107).

The Pope clearly thinks that the evidence is convincing that a new human being, and hence a new human person, exists from conception. But even if there was only a "probability" that a new human being then existed, what is at stake is sufficiently important that the Church would continue to assert that, "The human being is to be respected and treated as a person form the moment of conception" (Congregation for the Doctrine of the Faith, 1990, p. 13; Pope John Paul II, 1995, p. 108).

C.3. *Consequences for Abortion,* In Vitro *Fertilization, and Stem Cell Technology*

The consequences of the norm against killing and the claim that the human being deserves unconditional respect from conception are obvious: any intervention into the life of the embryo that intentionally causes it harm is forbidden. Foremost among such interventions is abortion. John Paul II thus asserts forcefully: "all direct abortion, that is, abortion willed as an end or as a means, always constitutes a grave moral disorder, since it is the deliberate killing of an innocent human being" (Pope John Paul II, 1995, p. 62).

The implications extend to various forms of reproductive technology. As a routine aspect of *in vitro* fertilization, surplus or spare embryos are created. These are tested, and those judged to have the best chance of life and health are implanted. Some are destroyed by the tests performed on them. The remainder are often cryopreserved, to be destroyed or perhaps used at a later date. All such practices are condemned. Likewise, any harmful experimentation on embryos, including the creation of embryos for research purposes or for the removal of their stem cells (pluripotent cells taken from the inner cell mass of the developing embryo), which can be stimulated to develop into various tissues of the human body. Since the removal of these stem cells ends the life of the developing embryo, stem cell extraction must be considered illicit (Mirkes, 2001).

Finally, although not wrongful in itself, prenatal diagnosis is viewed by the Pope and the Congregation for the Doctrine of the Faith as constituting a serious temptation to abortion in the event that fetal abnormalities are discovered. If undertaken with the intention to abort in the event of such abnormalities, the use of prenatal diagnosis is wrong in the way that abortion is, even if no abnormalities are found (and thus abortion not pursued).

Many of the positions outlined above have been challenged by Catholic theologians and philosophers, not to mention non-Catholics. These criticisms will be discussed after the treatment of contraception and non-sexual reproductive technologies.

C.4. Contraception: First Argument

From the early days of the Church, contraception has been condemned and linked, in its wrongness, to abortion. *Humanae Vitae* does not deny this linkage, and, on one interpretation, gives voice to it, by its understanding of contraception as that which "impairs the capacity of bringing forth life" in sexual intercourse. "Acts that attempt to impede procreation" are later explicitly linked in the encyclical to abortion, as they are in, e.g., *Evangelium Vitae*. The "contraceptive morality" and the "abortion morality" are likewise linked both in *Humanae Vitae* and in the work of John Paul II.

This naturally leads to an understanding of the wrongness of contraception in the Catholic tradition as involving an "anti-life" will. The significance of this is even more greatly appreciated in light of John Paul II's work on the intrinsic value and dignity of human life. In contracepted intercourse, the couple chooses directly against the intrinsic good of human life by choosing to prevent a possible life from beginning (Grisez, Boyle, Finnis, & May, 1988). *Humanae Vitae* seems to express the prohibition against such acts in a famous formula: "each and every marriage act must remain open to the transmission of life" (Pope Paul VI, 1968/93, p. 11).

C.5. Contraception: Second Argument

Two other well-known formulae from *Humanae Vitae* also enter into the Catholic discussion of contraception. One stresses the importance of spousal "mutual self-giving," which, John Paul II has stressed repeatedly, is violated by the use of contraception. The other asserts an "unbreakable connection between the unitive meaning and the procreative meaning of the conjugal act. ... This connection was established by God, and Man is not permitted to break it through his own volition" (Pope Paul VI, 1968/1993, p. 550).

An entire theology of marriage and sexuality would be necessary for a complete understanding of these claims. They are related, however, to the analysis of contraception as involving an anti-life will. For in true marriage, in the Church's view, the spouses enter into a communion of one flesh made possible by the organic unity of male and female in sexual reproduction. The love of the spouses is uniquely manifest in this unity, the natural fruit of which is the generation and rearing of children. So sexual intercourse which is severed from its procreative significance is seen by the Church as a failure of the spouses to give of themselves sufficiently to enter into a genuine one flesh union. That contraception intentionally effects this severance in an illicit way is made clear from the argument above concerning the anti-life attitude of contraception (Pope John Paul II, 1986; Smith, 1991).

These arguments, which represent the best of recent Catholic work on contraception, are not to be confused with an older, muddled argument, which no longer plays a role in Catholic thought. The argument that contraception is wrong because it violates the natural teleology of the reproductive organs is conveniently referred to on a regular basis by those who wish to argue against it, but the argument has few supporters. It is not mentioned in either *Casti Conubii* (1930) or *Humane Vitae* (1968). A charitable interpretation would have it that the underlying point of this fallacious argument is better expressed in the arguments above concerning the anti-life will in contraception.

C.6. *Reproductive Technologies*

If contraception severs the procreative from the unitive aspects of conjugal love, many forms of reproductive technology sever it in a different way. *In vitro* fertilization, artificial insemination (whether heterologous or homologous), cloning, surrogate motherhood (rarely accomplished without one of the other forms of reproductive technology) and, arguably, GIFT (gamete intrafallopian transfer) technologies all make reproduction possible without sexual intercourse.

As the previous section showed, the Catholic tradition holds that sexual intercourse is a unique expression and manifestation of marital love, and that children are the natural fruit of this love. When begotten in the context of such marital love, children thus come to be in a context of self-giving of spouses which extends, in its generosity, to the child, who is accepted and loved in his very generation. In *Donum Vitae*, it is asserted that it is a right of children to be conceived and begotten in such a context; an injustice is done to those who are conceived, as to those who are reared, in less than a fully loving context.

But, it is argued, not only is marital intercourse an especially suitable context for the procreation of children, it is the only suitable context. *Donum Vitae* provides the foundations for an argument for why, in particular, extra-sexual means of generation are substantially unjust to the children created by their means. After again discussing the "inseparable connection" of the unitive and procreative meanings of the conjugal act as well as the self-giving of spousal conjugal acts, *Donum Vitae* argues that non-sexual reproduction fails to show proper respect for the dignity of the child in virtue of its technological character. In a reproductive technology such as *in vitro* fertilization, the child must be seen as a

> product of an intervention of medical or biological techniques; that would be equivalent to reducing him to an object of scientific technology. No one may subject the coming of a child into the world to conditions of technical efficiency which are to be evaluated according to standards of control and dominion (Congregation for the Doctrine of the Faith, 1987, p. 26).

The key premises to this argument are two. First, non-sexual modes of reproduction are attempts to *make* a child, as if the new human life were an artifact to be brought about for human purposes. Second, in all acts of making, the material product is viewed as *subordinate* to those human purposes, and hence to the agents whose purposes they are. Artifacts are always treated as mere means. It is worth noting that this argument relies on no special premises of revelation. It is, in fact, rather Kantian in its structure and stands as an argument of natural reason, available for acknowledgement by all men and women of good will.

A final point concerning the Catholic Church's contribution to bioethical discussion in the past century. Because, as we have seen, the Church holds that most of the views articulated in the sections above are available to natural reason, and because many of the issues discussed involve potentially grave abuses against persons (as in abortion and many reproductive technologies), it is entirely legitimate – and in many cases obligatory – that these acts and techniques be subject to legislation. Contrary to current trends of liberal democracy, which hold that it is impermissible to legislate the morality of one group against another, the Pope has argued forcefully that it is the foundation of any legitimate democracy that it respect the basic rights of all persons (Pope John Paul II, 1995). If the Catholic positions articulated above are correct, many contemporary governments fail in precisely this regard, a failing which has led the Pope to warn of a "culture of death" prevalent in the Western world.

C.7. Some Disputed Issues

Clearly, much Catholic teaching in reproductive ethics is controversial. Among specifically Catholic authors, some areas of continued argument and analysis include, although they are not limited to, the following.

First, there is a continuing discussion of the nature of marriage, family, and sexuality, and how reproductive issues are to be understood in relation to these. For instance, some have argued that within the context of marital love and commitment, contraception, on the one hand, and non-sexual reproductive technologies, on the other, might be acceptable. Some such positions are defended by so-called proportionalists, who argue that the value overall to a marriage may be greater if contraception is allowed than if not. Proportionalists thus dispute the claim that the norm against contraception is absolute. Typically, proportionalists deny any absolute norms (McCormick, 1981; Grisez, 1983 and 1985). Pope John Paul II has vigorously denied that proportionalism is legitimate Catholic ethics (Pope John Paul II, 1993), but discussion continues, both at the level of moral theory and in terms of the discussion of reproductive ethics.

Second, while the Catholic tradition has condemned contraception, it has permitted non-contraceptive methods of regulating birth, such as natural family planning and the older "rhythm method". Arguments continue over how these methods differ from contraception, arguments which, of necessity, must make use of disputed positions in the philosophy of action (Grisez et al., 1988; Boyle, 1993).

The claim that the so called "Catholic position" on reproductive issues may be an appropriate subject of legislation is also called into question by some Catholics, both within the academic world and in the world of politics. Here, a wider context of dispute over political, legal, and ethical theory is relevant to an understanding and resolution of the arguments (Cuomo, 1984; Griffin, 1997; Alvare, 1997).

Finally, there have been recent attempts to argue that the Pope's and the Magisterium's increasingly firm assertion that the embryo is a human being from conception is scientifically or metaphysically misguided. Because of the possibility of twinning in the early days of the embryo's existence, some have argued that it is impossible for the embryo to be a "metaphysical individual" (for this argument, see Ford, 1988; Shannon & Wolter, 1990; Porter, 1995; for arguments to the contrary, Grisez, 1990; Johnson, 1995). If so, this would have consequences for the ethical evaluation of various forms of embryo creation and research. It is more than likely that the Church would still hold such activities to be wrong, but not homicidally wrong.

D. Death and Dying

In many ways, the discussion of the ethics of death and dying in the Catholic Church is continuous with the discussion of reproductive ethics. For just as a major part of reproductive ethics is given over to issues of killing, so a major part of the ethics of death and dying is concerned with killing. Euthanasia, both voluntary and involuntary, and suicide, assisted or not, all involve the intentional taking of human life. As the previous section has shown, the Church holds that it is impermissible intentionally to kill. Thus euthanasia and suicide are strongly condemned in Church writing.

Moreover, the Pope, for example, has argued that such practices are not only wrong in themselves, but are symptomatic of an abandonment of true compassion for the sick, suffering, and dying, and a misunderstanding of the nature and value of suffering. On the one hand, genuine compassion would involve sharing in the sufferings of the sick, rather than an attempt to eliminate the one who suffers. And on the other hand, suffering itself should be understood as a participation in the sufferings of Christ, "a sharing in his cross through which a victorious resurrection is to be achieved" (John Paul II, 1984). In the modern world, by contrast, we are increasingly

> faced with one of the more alarming symptoms of the "culture of death", which is advancing above all in prosperous societies, marked by an attitude of excessive preoccupation with efficiency and which sees the growing number of elderly and disabled people as intolerable and too burdensome (Pope John Paul II, 1995, p. 116).

There is also a concern for autonomy, unfettered by a concern for the truth of human life, which leads people to wish to take into their own hands the conditions of their death. Here again, the Pope's diagnosis of the cultural climate surrounding the rise of interest in euthanasia and assisted suicide mirrors his linkage of the "abortion mentality" to the "culture of death."

While the problems of euthanasia and suicide are among the gravest of the concerns of the Church, given their radically anti-life nature, the derivation of the norms forbidding them is relatively straightforward, granted the basic premises about life and intentional killing. More difficult, in certain ways, is the distinction between illicit killing, on the one hand, and, on the other, the withholding or withdrawal of medical treatment, or the administration of analgesics, when these will result in death. Many secular philosophers profess to see no difference between killing or letting die, intending death or allowing death, acting or omitting, and so on. Such philosophers argue that, if withholding treatment or administrating pain-killers is permissible, even when death will result, then euthanasia and suicide must likewise be permissible.

There is no doubt that some actions which might be called "withholdings" or "withdrawals" or "omissions" are indeed acts of killing. For it is possible to withhold or withdraw or omit what is necessary for life in order to bring about death. When it is one's intention to bring about death, then one is killing, whether "actively" or "passively." But a strict equivalence between intentionally killing and allowing to die as a foreseen side-effect is denied in the Catholic tradition (as, for instance, by Pope Pius XII in his 1957 "Address to the First International Congress of Anesthesiologists"). Man has a right and a duty, Pius XII wrote, in serious illness to take necessary treatment to preserve life and health. However,

> [N]ormally one is held to use only ordinary means – according to circumstances of persons, places, times and culture – that is to say, means that do not involve any grave burden for oneself or another. A more strict obligation would be too burdensome for most men and would render the attainment of the higher, more important goods too difficult. Life, health, all temporal activities are in fact subordinated to spiritual ends. On the other hand, one is not forbidden to take more than the strictly necessary steps to preserve life and health, as long as he does not fail in some more serious duty (Pope Pius XII, 1957, p. 212).

One is thus not required to do everything possible to prolong life. While life is a great and indeed an intrinsic good of human persons, it is not an ultimate good capable of trumping all other considerations. According to the "Address," extraordinary care may rightly be refused, if the intention is not to kill. "Ordinary" and "extraordinary" might seem in this context to mean simply "what is expected" versus "what goes beyond what is expected," but the emerging understanding of these terms does not conform to this descriptive approach. Rather, through the discussion of "ordinary" and "extraordinary" treatments, a normative standard has been developed: burdens disproportionate to the benefits of a treatment may give a patient reasons to refuse treatment without that refusal being a choice, strictly, to die. And while a choice to avoid proportionate burdens is wrong, it is not thereby a choice to end life.

Three points should be noted in this context. First, the right to refuse burdensome treatment is primarily a right of the patient, where the patient is able to understand the options and make a choice to accept or refuse treatment. The decision to refuse treatment must be made by the patient, not by the doctor or some third party. As is stated in the "Address," "The doctor, in fact, has no separate or independent right where the patient is concerned. In general, he can take action only if the patient explicitly or implicitly, directly or indirectly, gives him permission" (Pope Pius XII, 1957, p. 213).

Second, sometimes a patient might have a positive duty not to refuse treatment, for example, when the patient has some other responsibility that can only be met by accepting what might otherwise be a burdensome treatment.

Finally, the notion of "burdensome" is itself broad and in need of interpretation. The interpretation should not settle on one univocal feature of treatment that marks it off as burdensome. Rather, burdens may be relevantly disproportionate for a wide variety of different reasons, not reducible to some one type. Such burdens can include, for example, pains and sufferings incurred by the patient, costs and other burdens on the patient or on others, considerations of fairness in terms of resources used, or the relationship between acceptance or refusal and a patient's overall vocation. Moreover, it should be clear in all these cases that a burden which is proportionate for one patient may not be so for another; some patients have more resources, whether economic or spiritual, while others may have outstanding responsibilities. Even a personal but strong repugnance to some form of treatment might suffice to consider that treatment disproportionately burdensome. Still, patients should strive for the courage not to reject reasonable burdens. The refusal of treatment to avoid burdens that should reasonably be accepted is not, for that reason, intentional taking of life, but it is still a wrong to be avoided.

Clearly the patient is not capable in all cases of making these determinations, as when, for example, he or she is permanently unconscious. In such circumstances, it is the duty of the patient's family, when possible, both to make decisions regarding treatment and to do so in accordance with "the presumed will of the unconscious patient" (Pope Pius XII, 1957, p. 214). However, extreme burdens on the family can also constitute legitimate reasons for withholding or withdrawing treatment. If the burdens are too great, the family therefore can "lawfully insist that the doctor should discontinue" (Pope Pius XII, 1957, p. 214). What must be stressed is that the "burden" here cannot be the patient's life, or continued existence, itself. The life of the dying patient remains intrinsically good and may not be intentionally taken.

One area in which these questions have been disputed of late within the Catholic tradition involves the maintenance of nutrition and hydration for comatose patients or those in persistent vegetative states. Is such provision an extreme burden, as some have claimed? Or is withdrawal of nutrition often or always an instance of intentionally killing (Grisez, 1989; Bole, 1992)? Such discussions have been particularly prominent among theologians and clergy in the United States; precise Vatican guidance on these matters has not so far been given. For an example of the disagreement among bishops in the United states, see Pennsylvania Bishops (1992) and Texas Bishops (1990).

Also disputed are issues related again to the value of life. Although, as shown in the previous section on reproductive ethics, the Church seems to be moving to an account of human life as of intrinsic worth, some still argue for a more instrumentalist view of the good of life (Wildes, 1992). On such an account, the inability of a persistently vegetative patient to pursue any goods or share in a personal life would itself constitute such an extreme burden, or even loss of personhood as to justify removal of life support or nutrition. Against this, however, some hold that the patient's life is still a good, and that human solidarity with the patient can be promoted in some measure by continuing to care for the patient in his or her extremely debilitated state (Grisez, 1989; May et al., 1990).

A further issue concerns the provision of pain relief to dying patients. As with the removal of life support, in many cases, an amount of pain relief sufficient to relieve a patient's suffering will also have the consequence that the patient's death is hastened, sometimes significantly. Does this constitute a form of euthanasia?

The Catholic view of this is complex. For, it must be recalled, the Church does not view the relief of suffering as an unmitigated good, nor suffering itself as a total evil. Catholics are encouraged to accept all or some of their sufferings. Thus the Congregation for the Doctrine of the Faith suggests that "Christians [might] prefer to moderate their use of painkillers" (Congregation for the Doctrine of the Faith, 1980, p. 221). Further, since consciousness is necessary for the Christian patient to be able to pray, ask for reconciliation, receive the Eucharist, and "prepare ... for their definitive meeting with God," doctors are urged not to deprive patients of consciousness without significant reason. Death and dying are great evils, but can also be the context for important spiritual goods, and the Catholic tradition, thinking especially of Christ's death, is sensitive to this (Pope John Paul II, 1995).

Still, the Church recognizes that a full acceptance of suffering is heroic, and, as John Paul II writes, "cannot be considered the duty of everyone" (Pope John Paul II, 1995, p. 118). Thus, narcotics may be used to relieve pain "even when the result is decreased consciousness and a shortening of life" (Pope John Paul II, 1995, p. 118). Where the intention is to relieve pain, and death is foreseen and accepted as a side-effect, the principle of double effect may be applied: what it is unacceptable to intend (death) may in this instance be accepted as a side-effect of an otherwise good action (relief of pain).

There is, finally, a further parallel in the ethics of death and dying to the area of reproductive ethics regarding the scope of the class "human being." Just as at the beginning of life many secular bioethicists introduce a distinction between human being and person, thus removing from the realm of moral consideration "sub-personal" human beings such as embryos, fetuses, and neonates, so at the end of life do these same bioethicists distinguish between human beings and persons, asserting that a patient in a persistent vegetative state is the former but not the latter. As such, these non-persons would not be due the moral respect of persons.

As at the beginning of life, the Catholic Church holds that all human beings are due the respect of persons until they have died. So nothing may be done to a permanently unconscious human being which may not be done to a person as such. This includes, of course, intentionally killing, but also degrading forms of treatment, including sexual abuse and physical assault. Presumably, the removal of necessary organs from a still living human being would constitute a form of physical assault. Thus, it is crucial that there be a determination of the nature of death, since it is at death that the human being ceases to be (Pope Pius XII, 1957).

This determination has recently stirred some controversy in the Catholic Church. In an "Address to the International Congress on Transplants," Pope John Paul II accepted the recent "whole brain death" criterion as providing the necessary "moral certainty" for judgments regarding the permissible circumstances for removal of organs for transplantation (John Paul II, 2000). But some Catholic doctors and philosophers have recently questioned this criterion, arguing that a more "holistic" account of the integrated unity of the whole body is necessary for assessing life and death. According to this view, "the loss of no one organ, even the brain, is sufficient evidence of death" (Austriaco, Cole, & May, 2001, p. 11).

E. Access to Health Care

E.1. The Right to Health Care

The right to health care is an established part of Catholic social teaching. It was first explicitly announced by Pope John XXIII and has been reaffirmed in many magisterial teachings since then (O'Rourke & Boyle, 1999, pp. 365-368; Boyle, 1996, pp. 281-282). Bishops conferences have drawn policy implications from this affirmation, but the clarifications needed to answer conceptual questions about the right to health care are yet to be conducted. For example, who has the duty or set of duties which correspond to this right? How does the right relate to other welfare and liberty rights? What are its limits? These are questions for Catholic social teaching generally, and, although episcopal teaching and

Pope John Paul II's social encyclicals indicate broad normative directions, serious analytical work is needed.

E.2. Medical Delivery and Financing

The right to health care has not been understood as requiring a single, government-sponsored health care system which is supported by taxes. The right to health care is only indirectly a claim on political society, which has the subsidiary responsibility to help citizens carry out their prior responsibilities to their own health and to the health of their families and neighbors. So, the duty to which the right to health care responds is prior to political organization and exists whenever some have the capacity to help others in need. Consequently, bishops conferences have not ordinarily supported ideal solutions for remedying the inequities in health care, but rather have supported definite improvements which will make health care available to the poor. So, Catholic preference for a two-tier or a single-tier health care will be highly circumstantial. Which system is possible in a country? Which is most likely to guarantee the health care to which people have a right?

Since needed health care is not likely to be available for the poor without significant support from public revenues, taxation to support welfare rights is acceptable on Catholic moral principles. To those unwilling to give for such services, the response of Catholic social teaching is that these obligations are prior to politics and binding on the willing and the unwilling alike.

F. Ethics Committees

Catholic health care institutions ordinarily maintain ethics committees to serve a variety of educational and advisory functions. Relatively little has been said about ethics committees in magisterial teaching (National Conference of Catholic Bishops, 1994, directive 37) or in the scholarly literature. Still, the existence and function of such committees is easily justified by the general principles of social organizations and authority that have developed within the Catholic moral tradition. On this conception, such committees cannot replace the authority of patients concerning their own treatment, of health care professionals concerning what is good medicine, or of hospital administrators or relevant Church or public authorities over hospital policy. They can advise, educate, and seek to resolve disagreements, but they may not assume authority for the key decisions in health care.

G. Cooperation

During the period of high casuistry in the 17th century, the issue of a person's cooperation in the wrongdoing of others became a serious discussion. The issue arose when a person committed to a wrongful action had social or other power over another such that the person in the inferior position was significantly constrained to support the wrongdoing. The question was whether and under what conditions such cooperation was morally permissible. In the 18th century, St. Alphonsus Ligouri developed what has become the accepted Catholic response to perplexities of this kind. He provided a clear sense to the older, scholastic notions of formal and material cooperation. In formal cooperation, the helping person cooperates in a way that shares in the wrongdoer's intention. In material cooperation, the helper contributes to the wrongdoing, but does not intend precisely the wrongdoing or its successful completion. The former is always wrong; the latter can be permitted under certain circumstances (Boyle, 1999, pp. 187-199). This doctrine, itself an application of the doctrine of double effect, has important implications for health care professionals and politicians working in the modern context of radical moral disagreement (Pope John Paul II, 1995, p. 74). It also has great importance for the actions of Catholic institutions as they seek to cooperate with other facilities and individuals who do not share Catholic conviction on such things as abortion. This application to institutions is new, complex, and the subject of ongoing theological debate (National Conference of Catholic Bishops, 1994, Part 6, directives 67-70 and Appendix; Boyle, 1997, pp. 18-23).

IV. Conclusions

As we have seen, Roman Catholic bioethics is a conceptually and institutionally mature set of inquiries. It has deep historical roots within Catholic theology, doctrine, and canon law, and consequently a developed set of positions and methods of moral analysis. Although traditional authorities are accorded some respect by all engaged as Roman Catholics in bioethics, there are very significant disagreements among Catholic bioethicists. These disagreements reach so deeply into the fabric of moral life and thought that they suggest radical fissures within the Catholic community. These divisions of moral conviction would not be troubling if they were simply about new and difficult cases or about casuistical details; but, as the preceding summaries and citations indicate, they go to the heart of key norms themselves. The resolution of the most central of these disagreements is surely essential if the traditions of Catholic moralizing are to be effectively brought to bear on the bioethical perplexities facing the Roman Catholic community and others who may look to its riches for guidance.

Notes

1. Papal and other Vatican teachings are published in many languages and formats. These documents are divided into numbered paragraphs, which provide the accepted form of citation. This format is increasingly the norm in all magisterial publications. We will follow this method of citation. The titles of these documents are taken from the Latin version of the first words. The encyclical on which this note is attached is named Splendor Veritatis (in English, The Splendor of Truth).
2. Vatican Council II is perhaps the most important basis for current magisterial teaching on moral matters. There are several widely used editions (Vatican Council II, 1975). The complete texts of all papal and most North American episcopal teachings on bioethics since 1971 are available in English in Origins (Washington: National Catholic News Service). Catholic International (Worchester, MA: Assumption Communications) provides access in English to Catholic teachings from around the world since 1990. A useful, single-volume collection of Catholic teaching specifically concerned with bioethics (including some pre-Vatican II materials) is Medical Ethics: Sources of Catholic Teachings (O'Rourke & Boyle, 1999). The Catechism of the Catholic Church, first published in 1992 and available throughout the world in approved editions published by bishops' conferences, contains brief statements of all the major moral teachings of the

Church, including those relevant to bioethics. Papal and curial documents are available on the internet. See <http://www.ewtn.com>; <http://www.vatican.va>; <http://www.pauline.org>.

3. This literature is not limited to bioethical publications and appears in most of the venues in which Catholic theology and especially moral theology appear. *Theological Studies*, a quarterly published by the American Jesuits, has published surveys of moral theology, including bioethics, for the last sixty years. Boyle (1991; 1993; 1997) surveys Catholic bioethics from 1988 through 1994. Ashley and O'Rourke (1997) provide a useful, theologically oriented introduction to Catholic bioethics with ample bibliography.
4. Jonsen and Toulmin (1988) provide a glimpse of the rich texture of Catholic moral thought in the early modern period, but this work is not intended to be a strictly historical account of moral reasoning in this period. Entries in *The New Catholic Encyclopedia* (1965) provide useful introductions to historically important figures and issues. See also Mahoney (1987) and Kelly (1979) for useful starts on the needed research.
5. See H.T. Engelhardt, Jr. (2000, p. 52) for citations of examples of this literature.
6. The National Catholic Bioethics Center, 159 Washington Street, Boston, MA, 02135, (617-787-1900) <www.ncbcenter.org>, was formerly named the Pope John Center. It sponsors bishops' meetings; publishes the proceedings of these meetings and other timely books, a newsletter (for 26 years), *Ethics and Medics*; and has begun a scholarly journal, *The National Catholic Bioethics Quarterly*. The Linacre Centre for Healthcare Ethics, sponsors scholarly meetings and prepares position papers on public policy matters. See <www.linacre.org>.
7. The Catholic Health Association of the United States publishes *Health Progress*, a bimonthly journal, which over the years has addressed virtually all of the bioethical problems addressed by Catholics, especially those affecting Catholic health care institutions. See <www.chausa.org>.
8. See the contributions by Benedict Guevin, O.S.B., William E. May and Michel Therrien to the "Case Study: The Conjoined Twins of Malta," in *The National Catholic Bioethics Quarterly*, Vol. 1, No. 3, 2001, pp. 397-427.

Bibliography

Alvare, H. (1997). A response to Leslie Griffin. In: K. Wildes & A. Mitchell (Eds.), *Choosing life: a dialogue on Evangelium Vitae* (pp. 179-185). Washington, D.C.: Georgetown University Press.

Ashley, B. & O'Rourke, K. (1997). *Health care ethics: a theological analysis* (4th ed.). Washington, D.C.: Georgetown University Press.

Austriaco, N., Cole, B., & May, W. (2001). Reply to Fr. Ashley. *The National Catholic Bioethics Quarterly, 1*, 9-11.

Bole, T. (1992). Why almost any cost to others to preserve the life of the irreversibly comatose constitutes an extraordinary burden. In: K.W. Wildes, F. Abel, & J. Harvey (Eds.), *Birth, suffering, and death* (pp. 171-187). Dordrecht: Kluwer Academic Publishers.

Boyle, J. (1980). Contraception and natural family planning. In: J. Smith (Ed.), *Why Humanae Vitae was right: a reader* (pp. 407-417). San Francisco: Ignatius Press.

Boyle, J. (1981). The patient/physician relationship. In: D. McCarthy & A. Moracezewski (Eds.), *Moral responsibility in prolonging life decisions* (pp. 80-94). St. Louis: The Pope John Center.

Boyle, J. (1989). Sanctity of life and suicide: tensions and developments within common morality. In: B. Brody (Ed.), *Suicide and euthanasia* (pp. 221-250). Dordrecht: Kluwer Press.

Boyle, J. (1991). Who is entitled to double effect? *The Journal of Medicine and Philosophy, 16*, 475-494.

Boyle, J. (1991a). The Roman Catholic tradition and bioethics. In: A. Lustig (Ed.), *Bioethics yearbook: Volume 1: Theological developments in bioethics: 1988-1990* (pp. 2-22). Dordrecht: Kluwer Press.

Boyle, J. (1993). The Roman Catholic tradition and bioethics. In: A. Lustig (Ed.), *Bioethics yearbook: Volume 3: Theological developments in bioethics: 1990-1992* (pp. 19-42). Dordrecht: Kluwer Press.

Boyle, J. (1997). Sanctity of life and its implications: reflections of James Keenan's essay. In: K. Wildes & A. Mitchell (Eds.), *Choosing life: A dialogue on Evangelium Vitae* (pp. 71-76). Washington, D.C.: Georgetown University Press.

Boyle, J. (1997a). The Roman Catholic tradition and bioethics. In: A. Lustig (Ed.), *Bioethics yearbook: Volume 4: Theological developments in bioethics: 1992-1994* (pp. 11-32). Dordrecht: Kluwer Press.

Boyle, J. (1996). Catholic social justice and health care entitlement packages. *Christian Bioethics, 2*, 280-292.

Boyle, J. (1999). Collaboration and integrity: how to think clearly about moral problems of cooperation. In: L. Gormally (Ed.), *Issues for a Catholic bioethic* (pp. 187-199). London: The Linacre Centre.

Congregation for the Doctrine of the Faith (1974). *Declaration on procured abortion.* Boston: Daughters of St. Paul.

Connery, J. (1977). *Abortion: the development of the Roman Catholic perspective.* Chicago: Loyola University Press.

Cronin, D. (1989). *Conserving human life.* Braintree, MA: The Pope John Center.

Cuomo, M. (1984). Religious belief and public morality: A Catholic governor's perspective. *Notre Dame Journal of Law, Ethics and Public Policy, 1*, 13-31.

Engelhardt, Jr., H.T. (2000). *The foundations of christian bioethics.* Lisse: Swets & Zeitlinger.

Ford, N. (1988). *When did I begin? Conception of the human individual in history, philosophy, and science.* New York: Cambridge University Press.

Griffin, L.C. (1997). *Evangelium Vitae*: abortion. In: K. Wildes & A. Mitchell (Eds.), *Choosing life: a dialogue on Evangelium Vitae* (pp. 159-173). Washington, D.C.: Georgetown University Press.

Grisez, G., Boyle, J., Finnis, J., & May, W. (1988). "Every marital act ought to be open to new life": toward a clearer understanding. *The Thomist, 52*, 365-426.

Grisez, G. (1989). Should nutrition and hydration be provided to permanently unconscious and other mentally disabled persons? *Issues in Law and Medicine, 5*, 165-179.

Grisez, G. (1990). When do people begin? *Proceedings of the American Catholic Philosophical Association, 63*, 27-47.

Grisez, G. (1993). *The way of the Lord Jesus: Volume 2: Living a Christian life.* Chicago: Franciscan Press.

Howsepian, A.A. (1992). Who or what are we? *Review of Metaphysics, 45*, 483-502.

Johnson, M. (1995). *Questio Disputata* – delayed hominization: reflections on some recent Catholic claims for delayed hominization. *Theological Studies, 56*, 743-763.

Jonsen, A. & Toulmin, S. (1988). *The abuse of casuistry: A history of moral reasoning.* Berkeley: University of California Press.

Kauffman, C.J. (1999). Catholic health care in the United States: American pluralism and religious meanings. *Christian Bioethics, 5(1)*, 44-65.

Keenan, J.F. (1997). The moral argumentation of *Evangelium Vitae.* In: K. Wildes & A. Mitchell (Eds.), *Choosing life: A dialogue on Evangelium Vitae* (pp. 46-62). Washington, D.C.: Georgetown University Press.

Lee, P. (1996). *Abortion and unborn human life.* Washington, D.C.: The Catholic University of America Press.

Mahoney, J. (1987). *The making of moral theology.* Oxford: Oxford University Press.

May, W.E., et al. (1990). Criteria for withholding or withdrawing treatment. *Linacre Quarterly, 57*, 81-90.

May, W.E. (2000). *Catholic bioethics and the gift of life.* Huntington, IN: Our Sunday Visitor Press.

McCormick, R. (1981). *How brave a new world: Dilemmas in bioethics.* Garden City, N.J.: Doubleday.

Mirkes, R. (2001). NBAC and embryo ethics. *The National Catholic Bioethics Quarterly 1(2)*, 163-187.
National Conference of Catholic Bishops (1994). Ethical and religious directives for Catholic health care services. *Origins, 24*, 450-462.
National Conference of Catholic Bishops (2001). *Ethical and religious directives for Catholic health care services*. Washington, D.C.: National Conference of Catholic Bishops.
The new Catholic encyclopedia (1965). New York: Harper and Row.
Noonan, J. (1965). *Contraception: A history of its treatment by Catholic theologians and canonists*. Cambridge, MA: Harvard University Press.
O'Rourke, K. (1989). Should nutrition and hydration be provided to permanently unconscious or other mentally disabled persons? *Issues in Law and Medicine, 5*, 183-196.
O'Rourke, K. & Boyle, P. (1999). *Medical ethics: Sources of Catholic teachings* (3rd ed.). Washington, D.C.: Georgetown University Press.
Pennsylvania Bishops (30 January 1992). Nutrition and hydration: Moral considerations. *Origins, 21*, 541-553.
Pope John Paul II (1986). *The theology of marriage and celibacy*. Boston: St. Paul Editions.
Pope John Paul II (1984). *Apolostolic letter on the Christian meaning of suffering (Salvifici Doloris)*. Washington, D.C.: United States Catholic Conference.
Pope John Paul II (1992). *Catechism of the Catholic church*. Ottawa: Canadian Conference of Catholic Bishops.
Pope John Paul II (1993). *Veritatis Splendor*. Boston: Daughters of St. Paul.
Pope John Paul II (1995). *Evangelium Vitae*. Boston: Daughters of St. Paul.
Pope John Paul II (2000). Address to the International congress on transplants. *The National Catholic Bioethics Quarterly, 1(1)*, 89-92.
Pope Paul VI (1968). *Humanae Vitae*. In: J. Smith (Ed.) (1993), *Why* Humanae Vitae *was right: a reader* (pp. 537-567). San Francisco: Ignatius Press.
Pope Pius X (1930). *Casti Conubii*. Boston: Daughters of St. Paul.
Pope Pius XII (1957). Address to the First international congress of anesthesiologists. In: K.W. Wildes, F. Abel, & J. Harvey (Eds.) (1992), *Birth, suffering, and death* (pp. 209-215) Dordrecht: Kluwer Academic Publishers.
Porter, J. (1995). Individuality, personal identity, and the moral status of the pre-embryo: a response to Mark Johnson. *Theological Studies, 56*, 763-770.
Sacred Congregation for the Doctrine of the Faith (1974). *Declaration on procured abortion*. Boston: Daughters of St. Paul.
Sacred Congregation for the Doctrine of the Faith (1980). Declaration on euthanasia. In: K.W. Wildes, F. Abel, & J. Harvey (Eds.) (1992), *Birth, suffering, and death* (pp. 217-224). Dordrecht: Kluwer Academic Publishers.
Sacred Congregation for the Doctrine of the Faith (1987). *Donum Vitae*. Boston: Daughters of St. Paul.
Shannon, T. & Wolter, A. (1990). Reflections on the moral status of the pre-embryo. *Theological Studies, 51*, 743-763.
Smith, J. (1991). *Humane Vitae: A generation later*. Washington, D.C.: The Catholic University of America Press.
Smith, J. (1993). *Why* Humanae Vitae *was right: A reader*. San Francisco: Ignatius Press.
Texas Bishops (7 June 1990). On withdrawing artifical nutrition and hydration. *Origins 20*, 353-365.
Vatican Council II (1975). In: A. Flannery (Ed.), *The conciliar and post conciliar documents*. Collegeville, MN: The Liturgical Press.
Wildes, K.W. (1992). Life as a good and our obligation to persistently vegetative patients. In: K.W. Wildes, F. Abel, & J. Harvey (Eds.) (1992), *Birth, suffering, and death* (pp. 145-154). Dordrecht: Kluwer Academic Publishers.

Orthodox Christian Bioethics: Medical Morality in the Mind of the Fathers

H. Tristram Engelhardt, Jr.

I. Before and Beyond the Scholastic-Enlightenment Project

There is a continuity between the discursive, rational commitments of the Scholasticism that emerged in the 13th century and the Enlightenment project of providing a rational account of proper moral probity. Although the Enlightenment attempted to give an account of morality undirected by revelation and ecclesiastical authority, thus involving a substantive break with previous moral assumptions, the Enlightenment as well as Scholasticism share a substantive commitment to reason's abilities to provide outside of right worship and right belief a universal account of morality. Bioethics as it took shape in the 1970s reflected a late-Enlightenment attempt to provide a secular surrogate for the religious moral authorities that had once guided the West (Engelhardt, 2002). Secular and Western Christian bioethics have drawn on philosophical assumptions regarding the capacities of discursive reflection. They both have a penchant for attempting to identify moral truths with the deliverances of systematic moral reflections. In contrast, Orthodox Christianity lives in an understanding of morality uncompromised by Scholasticism, the Renaissance, the Protestant Reformation, and the Enlightenment.

Orthodox Christianity knows the moral life to be a whole, a way of life within which one can enter into union with God. Orthodox theology, morality, and bioethics serve to cure the soul of self-love. As a consequence, distinctions among dogmatic theology, moral theology, and liturgical theology threaten to distort and disorient the lived appreciation of theology as a practice transcending the confines of the academy and possessing a closer resemblance to a healing practice, albeit a special one aimed at bringing all into relationship with the Truth Whom the Orthodox recognize to be personal, namely, the Trinity (Vlachos, 1994). Morality is recognized as a kind of therapeutic regimen for purifying the person, inviting illumination by God's grace. As a consequence, the reader therefore must be warned: Orthodox Christianity does not offer a bioethics in the same way in which secular and Roman Catholic thought offers systematic reflections based on settled moral judgments elaborated philosophically towards the goal of developing ever clearer insights into the nature of morality. It contrasts as well with the bioethics of those Western mainline Christian bodies who have attempted in a progressive spirit to develop a moral theology adapted to the cultural concerns and demands of the contemporary age.

Orthodox Christian morality is a mode of reorienting persons away from themselves toward God and their fellow-man, thus giving Orthodox bioethics a homiletic rather than a scholarly character. Since theology *par excellence* is directed to purification of the heart and illumination by God's grace, all theological progress is personal, and the academic endeavors of Orthodox scholars at best clarify the use of terms and develop languages suitable for communicating reflections concerning the Church's unbroken experience of a timeless truth: the Triune God. The academic endeavors of scholars do afford commentaries on the experience and teachings of the Church Fathers over the centuries. However, such scholarly analysis and commentary are always secondary in authority and importance to theology as an experience of God. Because of the non-developmental character of the Orthodox Christian experience of God's presence, the age of the Fathers has not ended for Orthodoxy, as it did for the West around the 8th century. Strictly speaking, the age of the Fathers is coterminous with the unbroken presence in the Church of the Holy Spirit.

In summary, a number of points distinguish an Orthodox Christian bioethics. (1) First, Orthodox morality and bioethics form a seamless part of a way of life. Its various canons, directions, and prohibitions concerning medicine should be understood within a holistic approach to the goal of all Christian life: becoming a saint. (2) Orthodox moral reflection and bioethics have not produced an independent set of moral rules and principles that can be appreciated outside of an Orthodox Christian way of life. (3) Because Orthodox Christianity aims at a relationship with a fully transcendent God with Whom there is no analogy of being, general moral principles, casuistic analyses, and other discursive rational devices that might introduce a false Scholasticism are marginalized. Orthodox Christianity has not produced a moral philosophy independent of its theology because its morality and bioethics are spiritual-therapeutic rather than academic. They indicate how to pray rightly and live through discipline (i.e., asceticism) so as to come into relationship with God. (4) Because Orthodox morality is primarily therapeutic, it is not juridical. The goal is not to do justice but to bring God's mercy to the repentant. Although any falling short of the mark of saintly perfection is sinful, the response to sin is not punitive (e.g., penance is not punishment but treatment). Bioethics should be healing, aimed at restoring through repentance and purification the individual's focus on God. (5) Orthodox bioethics is not natural-law-oriented. Unlike Western Christianity, which came to look for traces of God in nature, Orthodox Christianity approaches nature as an icon, as a window through which to see God, with the result that Orthodox Christianity is innocent of the natural-law theory of the West (Foltz, 2001). (6) Orthodox Christianity is hierological: it relativizes the right and the good because of the overriding pursuit of the holy. Living rightly and justly is never sufficient, for the righteousness with which Christianity is concerned is holiness. In part, this is the case because the radical mercy of God transcends and sets aside the requirements of justice. More fundamentally, this is the case because the good, the right, and the just, apart from the holy, are always idols set over against God, the ultimate goal of all conduct. (7) Orthodox Christian epistemology is at root noetic or mystical; it acknowledges that the only way beyond a confining finite horizon of experience and texts is via a transforming relation with the transcendent God. For this reason, the theologians *par excellence* need not be academics or even literate. As Evagrios the Solitary (A.D. 345-399) stresses, "if you are a theologian, you will pray truly. And if you pray truly, you are a theologian" (Evagrios, 1988, p. 62).

The result is not just that Orthodox Christianity rejects the discursive rational commitments of Scholasticism and the Enlightenment; it also breaks through the fragmentation of the moral pluralism defining post-modernism. It reaches beyond the confines of particular narratives and texts, which are set within the horizon of the finite and the immanent. For example, the Scriptures are neither revelation nor a set of writings relevantly to be reassessed through historical, text-critical, and higher-critical methods. Instead, the Scriptures are records of a revelation whose significance can only be correctly experienced within the grace of the Church which is the body of Christ: their meaning is acquired on the model of Christ's unlocking the Scriptures on the way to Emmaus (Luke 24:13-35). Within the privileged ascetic and liturgically directed epistemological standpoint of the Church, the writings she has accepted, affirmed, and interpreted become, like an icon, a window so that one can look through the text to God.

II. The Past in the Present Tense

Neither medical ethics nor bioethics is a univocal term. Each has numerous meanings that depend on the background commitments and assumptions within which the terms are placed. Each context frames a particular understanding of appropriate action and moral probity. Guiding background assumptions are often unnoticed, insofar as they roughly comport with the presuppositions that structure the contemporary, dominant, secular culture. Against this background, it is difficult to imagine a radically different bioethics structured by fundamentally divergent moral commitments. Orthodox Christianity through its morality, bioethics, and theology provides a stark example of such differences. It is not just that Orthodox morality and bioethics possess a content different from that of the secular culture, as well as most religious communities; in addition, these perspectives diverge in terms of what a morality should be about. As a further introduction to the depth of these differences, one might consider the Orthodox Christian historiography of Christian morality and bioethics. Orthodox Christians hold that Christian bioethics is non-developmental in the sense of affirming the same moral commitments and insights that directed the Church of the first thousand years: it understands that all that has been essential for the appropriate moral life has been available since the time of the Apostles. This difference from Western secular and religious moral philosophical understandings is in part grounded in the Orthodox Christian recognition that truth is not merely a what (i.e., a set of discursive propositions referring to an objective truth), but a radically transcendent Who (i.e., the Trinity), with Whom since Pentecost right-worshipping Christians have had the possibility of a full relationship.

This non-developmental recognition of the full presence of truth in the Orthodox Church is expressed by the Fathers of the Seventh Ecumenical Council (Nicea II, A.D. 787):

> To make our confession short, we keep unchanged all the ecclesiastical traditions handed down to us, whether in writing or verbally ... Thus we follow Paul, who spake in Christ, and the whole divine Apostolic company and the holy Fathers, holding fast the traditions which we have received ... For we follow the most ancient legislation of the Catholic Church. We keep the laws of the Fathers. We anathematize those who add anything to or take anything away from the Catholic Church (Schaff & Wace, 1994, pp. 550-551).

Orthodox Christianity understands its morality to have been in its substance delivered to the Apostles once and for all. In particular, Orthodox Christianity does not regard moral theology as a cultural endeavor of the academy through which advances in moral insight and understanding are achieved.

Orthodox Christianity acknowledges its moral truth as nested within a liturgical Now, a moral experience that has existed and been sustained in its fullness since the age of the Apostles. For Orthodox Christianity, its moral theological past is in the present so that Orthodox Christians turn seemingly indiscriminately for guidance to any of the Fathers of any century. This epistemological standpoint within which the past is experienced as "now" is captured in the practice of its liturgical appropriation of the past as present. For example, the Vespers of the Sunday of the Holy Fathers of the First Six Ecumenical Councils declares: "Those God-mantled Fathers have proclaimed today in concert ..." (Nassar, 1979, p. 558). Despite the circumstance that these councils occurred from the 4th to the 7th centuries, liturgically they are encountered as present.

The Orthodox Church does not deny terminological development. The Church acknowledges that distinctions, terminologies, and analyses of theological experience take shape within a history. Yet, since Orthodox theology is not primarily an academic discipline but an immediate experience of God, these analytic, conceptual, and academic developments do not constitute theological developments *per se*. Rather, they are temporally and historically located responses to heresies and articulations of answers to particular questions and puzzles. The contributions of the Fathers from the 3rd to the 8th centuries can be understood as playing a role distantly analogous to the age of the Fathers for the West: they are a rich resource of theological reflection and Scriptural exposition that records the commitments and life of the Church of the first part of the first millennium so that one must think, believe, and act in one with their mind. However, because of the non-developmental character of Orthodox Christianity, the age of the Fathers has not ended, for the same Spirit Who inspired the Gospels inspires the holy Fathers of the 21st century. In this sense, one should understand the statement of Bartholomew I, the Ecumenical Patriarch of Constantinople:

> The manner in which we [the Orthodox and the West] exist has become ontologically different ... the Orthodox Christian does not live in a place of theoretical and conceptual conversations, but rather in a place of an essential and empirical lifestyle and reality as confirmed by grace in the heart [Heb 13:9]. This grace cannot be put in doubt either by logic or science or other type of argument ... However, the change of man's essence, theosis by grace, is a fact that is tangible for all the Orthodox faithful. Grace is not only obtained through the transformed relics of the saints, which is totally inexplicable without acceptance of the divine. Grace also radiates from living Saints who are truly in the likeness of the Lord [Luke 8:46] (Patriarch Bartholomew, 1997).

All the Fathers stand in the same privileged context of the Spirit, because all of theology is always fully available to all who, embedded within right worship and belief, experience God.

In approaching new technological developments, the present is set within the now of the past. In addressing issues such as cloning, the use of embryonic stem cells, and germ-line genetic engineering, Orthodox Christians will not seek new moral insights. There will not be a search for new medical-ethical or bioethical principles, but the recall of a permanent possibility for epistemic insight grounded in the consequences of the Incarnation. The goal will be to provide an expression of an abiding truth in part guided by the writings of the Fathers but always crucially sustained by the presence of the Holy Spirit, so as to express in a new context the enduring moral consciousness of the Church.

III. Bioethical Norms: Morality as Spiritual Therapy

Medical morality should be set within constraints integral to aiming one's life at holiness, at union with God. Because Orthodox Christianity has from the Apostles and Fathers had a concrete moral vision bearing on the fullness of human concerns from marriage, sexuality, and reproduction to suffering, dying, and death, contemporary moral issues ranging from abortion and cloning to the use of scarce medical resources and euthanasia are all approached within an already well-established framework. Given the recognition that all conduct should be aimed at the acquisition of holiness, concerns to avoid suffering and postpone death are radically relativized by a viewpoint that looks beyond the horizon of the immanent and finite to final judgment and beyond. Within this context, Orthodox Christianity affirms the importance of medicine and health care. As St. Basil the Great (A.D. 329-379) stresses, "Each of the arts is God's gift to us, remedying the deficiencies of nature ... the medical art was given to us to relieve the sick, in some degree at least" (Basil, 1962, pp. 330-331). One begins with the presumption that medicine should be used to restore health and preserve life, because good health aids in the discharge of one's duties to others. Yet, Orthodox Christianity recognizes the limits of life in a fallen world, acknowledging that this life ends in death and often involves considerable suffering. Nevertheless, suffering is not an end in itself. Suffering is recognized as having the possibility of leading not only to spiritual growth, but also despair. For this reason, Orthodox Christianity has endorsed the use of medicine to relieve pain and suffering. "...with mandrake doctors give us sleep; with opium they lull violent pain" (Basil, 1994, p. 78). So, too, one can understand the petition that is part of a litany in Vespers, Matins, and Liturgy: "A Christian ending to our life, painless, blameless, peaceful, and a good defense before the fearful judgment seat of Christ, let us ask" (Antiochian Orthodox Christian Archdiocese, 1989, p. 28). The Orthodox Church, which from the 4th century had established hospitals and supported the development of medicine, had by the fall of Constantinople (A.D. 1453) already reached a level comparable to the West of the early 19th century (Constantelos, 1991, p. 118).

The Orthodox Church affirms the proper use of analgesics, but she consistently rejects suicide, while recognizing that suicide can be the non-culpable result of mental illness (Peter, 1983, p. 746). Suicide is condemned not just because it involves a refusal to submit to suffering, even if this entails an excruciating death such as Christ's on the cross, but because, most importantly, suicide is self-killing. The taking of the life of anyone, but especially an innocent life, has always been viewed as sinful. Although humility in the face of suffering is required, the Orthodox Church, as already observed, endorses the use of analgesics. The Church also condemns the use of treatment to restore health, prolong life, or postpone death when such treatment becomes an all-consuming preoccupation setting the integrity of one's spiritual life in jeopardy. In this vein, St. Basil warns that one should avoid "whatever requires an undue amount of thought or trouble or involves a large expenditure of effort and causes our whole life to revolve, as it were, around solicitude for the flesh..." (Basil, 1962, p. 331). Unlike Roman Catholic moral theology, which has explored the question of the circumstances under which one's duty to preserve life can be defeated either by the costs or by the unlikelihood of success (e.g., as extraordinary treatment), the Orthodox Christian judgment regarding the appropriate limits to treatment is put in hierological terms: preserving the integrity of one's spiritual life. In part, the difference derives from the Roman Catholic attempt through natural reason to lay out understandings of moral duties outside of a Christian appreciation of the goal of life, suffering, and death, in contrast to the Orthodox Christian all-consuming focus on the pursuit of salvation. The result is a quite different sense of how one may appropriately withdraw and withhold medical interventions, including life-saving treatment.

Similarly, all sexual activity and reproduction are understood in terms of the marriage of a man and a woman pursuing salvation. The result is that any medical interventions aimed at supporting sexual activities of persons not in the marriage of a man and a woman are condemned. Although the ancient Church in its canons makes no reference to contraception, Orthodox Christianity regards both non-abortifacient contraception and natural family planning on a par. At stake is the condemnation of a contraceptive ethos that would tempt husbands and wives to fail in their obligation generously to bring children into the world. The focus is not on prohibitions grounded in a biological account of natural law, but on the nature of marriage and the requirement to trust unselfishly in God. Because the marriage of a man and a woman is the sole place for sexual activity and reproduction, cloning is appreciated as an attempt radically to set aside the interdependence of husband and wife in reproduction. As St. John Chrysostom (A.D. 354-407) notes in his commentary on Ephesians: "Nor did He enable woman to bear children without man; if this were the case she would be self-sufficient" (Chrysostom, 1986, p. 44). Because all sexual activity and reproduction should be within the union of husband and wife, the use of donor gametes as with artificial insemination or *in vitro* fertilization can be understood as a kind of adultery, although there may not be the full harm to the couple, as would occur with adulterous, carnal intercourse. In general, Orthodox Christian bioethics regards the intrusion of third parties in medically assisted reproduction as falling short of the mark when it breaks the intimacy of husband and wife. That is, there is moral concern regarding the use of *in vitro* fertilization, even when more embryos will not be created than implanted (the creation of surplus embryos would be seriously wrong in putting early human life at jeopardy).

Because of the Orthodox Christian recognition of the ontological significance of being male and female, there is a strong condemnation of any surgical intervention that obliterates sexual identity. In approaching the issue of castration, there are numerous and ancient canons rejecting castration when performed as a non-acceptance of one's sexual characteristics, thus giving grounds for understanding the evil of trans-sexual surgery. For example, the First-and-Second Council held in Constantinople (A.D. 861) reaffirmed a canon from Nicea I (A.D. 325)

> Wherefore the holy Council has been led to decree that if any bishop, or presbyter, or deacon, be proved guilty for castrating anyone, either with his own hand or by giving orders to anyone else to do so, he shall be subjected to the penalty of deposition from office; but if the offender is a layman, he shall be excommunicated; unless it should so happen that owing to the incidence of some affliction he should be forced to operate upon the sufferer by removing his testicles. For precisely as the first Canon of the Council held in

> Nicea does not punish those who have been operated upon for a disease, for having the disease, so neither do we condemn priests who order diseased men to be castrated, nor do we blame laymen either, when they perform the operation with their own hands. For we consider this to be a treatment of the disease, but not a malicious design against the creature or an insult to creation (First-and-Second Council, 1983, p. 465).

As this canon stresses, although castration is condemned when it involves a rejection of the sexuality God has given, it is accepted when undertaken for medical, that is, therapeutic purposes.

Orthodox Christianity categorically condemns abortion. In this, it sustains condemnations of abortion reaching back to Christianity's first century. For example, in the late 1st century or early 2nd century *Didache* (II.2), there are lists of proscriptions, including "thou shalt not commit adultery; thou shalt not commit sodomy; thou shalt not commit fornication; ... thou shalt not procure abortion, nor commit infanticide" (Lake 1965, 1:311, 313). This condemnation is joined with numerous canons prohibiting abortion, including one from a council held in Ankara (A.D. 315) (Council in Ancyra, 1983, p. 501), as well as canons from the Fathers (Basil, 1983, Canon 2, p. 789; John the Faster, 1983, Canon 21, p. 944) and the Quinisext Council or Council in Trullo (A.D. 691-692), which articulated the canons for the Fifth and Sixth Ecumenical Councils (Quinisext Council, 1983, Canon 91, p. 395). Unlike the Roman Catholic church, which has placed centrally the issue of ensoulment in its condemnation of abortion, Orthodox Christianity has prohibited abortion as an act having the spiritual impact of murder, whether or not the embryo is yet ensouled. As St. Basil notes, one is

> a murderer who kills an imperfect and unformed embryo, because this though not yet then a complete being was nevertheless destined to be perfected in the future, according to indispensable sequence of the laws of nature (Basil, 1983, p. 789).

It is important to note once again that the prohibition of murder and abortion must be appreciated in a therapeutic, not a juridical or punitive light, within which such offenses are often regarded in most Western moral, philosophical, and theological systems: the goal is not to subject the sinner to just punishment, but to bring the sinner through repentance and God's grace to holiness.

Because of this perspective, the Orthodox Church has never endorsed a doctrine of double effect, such as developed in the West, which allowed Roman Catholicism to approve of indirect abortions. The doctrine of double effect holds that when an action produces two effects, one good and one evil, one may nevertheless act, as long as the act is not evil in itself, the good effect is not produced by the bad effect, the evil effect is not intended, and there is a proportionate reason (more good will be produced than evil). According to the doctrine of double effect, when these conditions are fulfilled, one is held to be juridically innocent. In contrast, the Orthodox Church recognizes that close causal involvement in the death of another, whether a guilty or an innocent person, may harm one's spiritual life. Orthodox Christianity recognizes harms from both involuntary and "justifiable" homicide, including homicide in a just war, both of which incur excommunication not as punishment, but as spiritual therapy (Basil, 1983, Canon 13, pp. 801-802).

It is in this spiritually therapeutic context that one should understand the absolution of women who miscarry. The absolution expresses the Orthodox Christian healing approach to the involuntary loss of life.

> According to Your great mercy, be merciful to Your servant, N., who is in sin, having been involved in the loss of a life, whether voluntary or involuntary, for she has miscarried that which was conceived in her. Forgive her transgressions, both voluntary and involuntary, and protect her from every snare of the Devil. Cleanse her stain and heal her infirmities. And grant to her, O Lover of Mankind, health and strength of soul and body. ... Forgive this, Your servant, N., who is in sin, having been involved in the loss of a life, whether voluntary or involuntary, for she has miscarried that which was conceived in her. And, according to Your great mercy as the Good God Who loves mankind, be merciful and forgive all those who are here present and who have touched her (Monk, 1987, pp. 6-7).

The woman who has suffered a miscarriage is not held to be guilty in a juridical sense, but in need of God's loving grace. It is within this therapeutic perspective that the Orthodox Church approaches decisions made by women to engage in operations that will also incidentally lead to the abortion of a child (e.g., the removal of a cancerous uterus containing an unborn child), which in Roman Catholic terms would not count as an abortion. In such cases, the spiritual father must help the patient through repentance and love to repair the spiritual damage from the serious evil of involvement in the death of another person.

Orthodox Christianity departs also from Western understandings, both Protestant and Roman Catholic, which have been influenced by Augustine of Hippo's (A.D. 354-430) unequivocal condemnation of intentionally making false statements in order to deceive. Although Orthodox Christianity is committed to truth-telling, it recognizes that in a broken world one may be obliged to tell a falsehood to preserve life or serious moral-spiritual interests. Unlike Kant and Roman Catholics, Orthodox Christians are obliged if necessary to tell a falsehood to protect the innocent from being killed (e.g., lie to National Socialist officers searching for Jews). This view is rooted in the mind of the Fathers of the early Church. Clement of Alexandria (A.D. 155-220) stresses that one must at times "medicinally, as a physician for the sake of the sick ... deceive or tell an untruth" (Clement, 1994, p. 538). Although one may be justified, indeed obliged, to lie in some circumstances, one will usually also need spiritually to address the spiritual evil involved in lying, as Abba Dorotheos of Gaza (A.D. 506/508-580) stresses:

> But if a man did such a thing [as lying], in extreme necessity, let him not be without anxiety but let him repent and sorrow before God and consider it, as I said, a time of trial and not let it become a habit but done once and for all. ... Just as an antidote for snake poison or a powerful purge is beneficial when taken in time and in case of need, it does harm if taken habitually, without necessity (Dorotheos, 1977, p. 161).

The obligation to become involved in sin (i.e., to engage in an activity that by itself falls short of the mark) to pursue salvation requires confronting moral issues within a value framework that at times does not produce black-and-white choices (though idolatry, sexual impurity, and murder of the innocent are always forbidden).

Given this moral framework, the bioethics of Orthodox Christian physicians, nurses, families, and patients is often at odds with the reigning expectations of the surrounding secular society, as well as the moral views embraced by many Christians. This disparity of moral vision is expressed in competing understandings of proper professional conduct. For instance, Orthodox Christian physicians should not consider themselves obliged to be religiously and morally neutral in their care of their patients. Although they should avoid coercion of any sort (Canon CXIX of Carthage, A.D. 419), the ideal is to bring all who can be influenced into a life of right worship and right belief. For example, the Orthodox Church celebrates holy physicians such as St. Panteleimon (†304) who took advantage of their professional role to convert their patients. Rather than regarding the patients' vulnerability as a ground for not attempting to exert influence, Orthodox Christianity regards confrontations with pain, suffering, and death as opportunities to open the way to repentance and conversion. Traditional Orthodox Christianity does not affirm the abandonment by physicians of their Christian duties in favor of the norms of a secular medical ethics.

IV. Bioethics as Theology: Theology as Worship

At one with St. Paul in his first chapter of the letter to the Romans, Orthodox Christianity recognizes that moral knowledge is fully and rightly disclosed only within a life marked by right worship. "Therefore God gave them up in the lusts of their hearts to impurity, to the degrading of their bodies among themselves, because they exchanged the truth about God for a lie and worshiped and served the creature rather than the Creator, Who is blessed forever! Amen" (Rom 1:24-25). It should not be surprising to find contemporary Orthodox Christian studies of bioethics developing their analyses in the light of the prayers and liturgies of the Church (Guroian, 1996). Although content for reflection is drawn from liturgical texts, Scripture, the Fathers, and holy Tradition, it is placed within a confident appreciation that the ultimate guide for human conduct is fully revealed in the Church, the Body of Christ in the Holy Spirit, and that "Jesus Christ is the same yesterday and today and forever" (Heb 13:8). In the English language, a number of monographs have already been published embedded in this understanding of moral theology and bioethics (Breck, 1998; Engelhardt, 2000; Harakas, 1990). At one with the Fathers of the ancient Church and those of the 21st century, numerous contemporary authors are attempting to state for the contemporary world the enduring significance of the human struggle to God and its implications for the proper use of medicine and the biomedical sciences.

Bibliography

Antiochian Orthodox Christian Archdiocese (1989). *The liturgikon.* Englewood, NJ: Antiochian Orthodox Christian Archdiocese.

Bartholomew, Patriarch (1997). Joyful light. Address given at Georgetown University, Washington, D.C., October 21.

Basil, St. (1994). The hexaemeron. In: P. Schaff & H. Wace (Eds.), *Nicene and post-Nicene fathers* (Vol. 8, pp. 53-107). Peabody, MA: Hendrickson Publishers.

Basil, St. (1962). *The long rules.* Sister M. Wagner (trans.) Washington, DC: Catholic University of America Press.

Basil, St. (1983). The ninety-two canons of our father among saints Basil the Great. In: Sts. Nicodemus & Agapius (Eds.). D. Cummings (trans.), *The rudder of the Orthodox Catholic Church* (pp. 772-863). New York: Luna Printing.

Breck, J. (1998). *The sacred gift of life*. Crestwood, NY: St. Vladimir's Seminary Press.

Chrysostom, St. John. (1986). *On marriage and family life*. C. Roth & D. Anderson (trans.), Crestwood, NY: St. Vladimir's Seminary Press.

Clement of Alexandria (1994). The stromata. In: A. Roberts & J. Donaldson (Eds.), *Ante-Nicene fathers* (Vol. 2, pp. 523-567). Peabody, MA: Hendrickson Publishers.

Constantelos, D.J. (1991). *Byzantine philanthropy and social welfare* (2nd ed.). New Rochelle, NY: Aristide Caratzas.

Council in Ancyra (1983). The twenty-five canons of the holy regional council held in Ancyra. In: Sts. Nicodemus & Agapius (Eds.), D. Cummings (trans.), *The rudder of the Orthodox Catholic Church* (pp. 489-505). New York: Luna Printing.

Dorotheos of Gaza (1977). *Discourses and sayings*. E. Wheeler (trans.), Kalamazoo, MI: Cistercian Publications.

Engelhardt, H.T., Jr. (2002). The ordination of bioethicists as secular moral priests. *Social Philosophy & Policy, 19*, 59-82.

Engelhardt, H.T., Jr. (2000). *The foundations of Christian bioethics*. Lisse: Swets & Zeitlinger.

Evagrios the Solitary (1988). On prayer. In: G.E.H. Palmer, P. Sherrard & K. Ware (eds. and trans.), *The Philokalia* (pp. 55-71). Boston: Faber and Faber.

First-and-Second Council (1983). The seventeen canons of the so-called first-and-second council. In: Sts. Nicodemus & Agapius (Eds.), D. Cummings (trans.), *The rudder of the Orthodox Catholic Church* (pp. 455-474). New York: Luna Printing.

Foltz, B.V. (2001). Hidden patency: On the iconic character of human life. *Christian Bioethics, 7(3)*, 317-331.

Guroian, V. (1996). *Life's living toward dying*. Grand Rapids, MI: Wm. Eerdmans.

Harakas, S. (1990). *Health and medicine in the Eastern Orthodox tradition*. New York: Crossroad.

John the Faster, St. (1983). The 35 canons of John the Faster. In: Sts. Nicodemus & Agapius (Eds.), D. Cummings (trans.), *The Rudder of the Orthodox Catholic Church* (pp. 931-952). New York: Luna Printing.

Lake, K. (trans.) (1965). The didache. In: *The apostolic fathers* (pp. 303-333). Cambridge, MA: Harvard University Press.

Monk of St. Tikhon's Monastery (trans.) (1987). *Book of needs*. South Canaan, PA: St. Tikhon's Seminary Press.

Nassar, S. (Ed.) (1979). *Divine prayers and services of the Catholic Orthodox Church of Christ*. Englewood, NJ: Antiochian Orthodox Christian Archdiocese.

Peter, St. (1983). The 15 canons of our father among saints Peter, archbishop [Pope, fl. 304] of Alexandria and a martyr. In: Sts. Nicodemus & Agapius (Eds.), D. Cummings (trans.), *The Rudder of the Orthodox Catholic Church* (pp. 740-756). New York: Luna Printing.

Quinisext Council (1983). The 102 canons of the holy and ecumenical sixth council. In: Sts. Nicodemus & Agapius (Eds.), D. Cummings (trans.), *The rudder of the Orthodox Catholic Church* (pp. 290-412). New York: Luna Printing.

Schaff, P. & Wace, H. (Eds.) (1994). *Nicene and post-Nicene fathers*, Second Series. Peabody, MA: Hendrickson Publishers.

Vlachos, H. (1994). *Orthodox psychotherapy*. E. Williams (trans.), Levadia, Greece: Birth of the Theotokos Monastery.

Bioethics in the Episcopal Tradition

Cynthia B. Cohen and David H. Smith

I. Introduction

A. History and Governance

The Episcopal Church is an historic descendant of the Church of England. In the wake of English colonial expansion, the reach of the mother church gradually spread to North America, Europe, Africa, Asia, Latin America, the Caribbean, and the Pacific. Despite political changes (including revolutions), these roots provided the basis for the formation of the Anglican Communion in the mid-nineteenth century (Butler, 1999; Wright, 1999). This world-wide communion consists of approximately 100 million Christian churches in 167 countries each of whose members stand in loose affiliation with one another. The Protestant Episcopal Church is the branch of the Anglican Communion in the United States of America. A grasp of the history of the Church of England, therefore, is important for an understanding of the development of the Episcopal tradition.

Christianity was brought to England by the Romans early in the second century. The Angles and Saxons soon took over Christian Roman Britain, however, and it was not until the seventh century that a distinctively English church emerged due to the work of Christian missionaries. Reforms introduced in the Church of England in the sixteenth century distinguished it as a separate ecclesiastical body from the Church of Rome. These changes were catalyzed by King Henry VIII's efforts to father a male heir, in particular by his attempt to have his first and childless marriage annulled by Pope Clement VII. The Pope had been taken prisoner after his failed war against the nephew of Henry's wife and was unable to grant this fairly ordinary request due to his dire situation.

The ensuing ecclesiastical reforms were set in motion by Thomas Cranmer, appointed by Henry as Archbishop of Canterbury, the chief clergyperson of England. Cranmer worked to make the Bible accessible in English and wrote the first Book of Common Prayer in 1549 with set services in English. The Anglican reformers aimed to return to the Christianity of the church councils of the first five centuries and carved out an Anglican identity that comprised a unique blend of Roman, Lutheran, Reformed, and Orthodox elements (Haugaard, 1999). Their reforms were consolidated by Queen Elizabeth I, who took pains to see that bishops maintained a continuous line of succession from the earliest times (Avis, 1999).

English colonists brought this form of Christianity to the New World colonies of Roanoke and Jamestown, Virginia and later to the middle colonies (Pritchard, 1999).

Its association with the crown made it controversial before, during, and after the Revolution. In the decade following the American Revolution, therefore, Anglican settlers sent clergy back to Scotland and England to be consecrated as bishops, and upon their return in 1789 established the Protestant Episcopal Church in the United States of America. Even as this church retained ties with the mother church, it broke significant new ground in that it was independent of a state connection and included not only bishops and clergy, but also laypersons in its governance (Pritchard, 1999). Today the Episcopal Church includes about 2.3 million members.

The governance of the Episcopal Church is carried out by a bicameral legislature comprised of the House of Deputies (including both laypersons and clergy) and the House of Bishops. They meet and deliberate at the General Convention, the major gathering of the church, held every three years. Between sessions of the General Convention, the work of the church is carried out by an elective Executive Council of 40 members and the Presiding Bishop, who is elected for a nine-year term by the House of Bishops with the concurrence of the House of Deputies.

B. *Distinctive Features of Anglican Ethics and Bioethics*

Anglican moral theologians and ethicists have included among their number casuists, natural law theorists, principlists, communitarians, liberal individualists, and situation ethicists who have differed widely in their approaches and emphases. They have tended to agree that the community, with its past wisdom and experience, shapes the individual conscience and provides the framework of moral values from which reason operates (Chadwick, 1999).

A distinctively Anglican form of casuistry sprang up in the sixteenth century that continues to provide a leading form of moral thinking within the communion. Its originators viewed this "casuistical divinity" as a comprehensive moral science that included not only the resolution of specific conflicts of conscience but also a systematic body of teaching (Wood, 1986). They rejected a Roman Catholic approach focused on the application of canon law to cases and instead developed broader accounts of Christian faith and life that often combined the moral and the ascetical (i.e., the practices of religion or what is often spoken of today as "spirituality") (Sedgwick, 1999). In particular, the casuists rejected the "probabilism" of the Jesuits, which held that any one of several probably correct opinions could justify a moral choice. Instead they held that the opinion that "in the whole conjunction of circumstances and relative considerations" is most reasonable should prevail (Taylor, 1996).

This reformed casuistry was succeeded in the seventeenth century by an approach grounded more firmly in general moral principles, although it also revealed an empirical strain that took account of the complexity of moral life (Butler, 1970). Anglican evangelicals and social reformers of the eighteenth and nineteenth century used this approach to campaign relentlessly for social reforms; they sought industrial legislation designed to ameliorate hardship and injustices suffered by the poor (Wood, 1986).

The quest for a distinctively Anglican moral theology was continued in the twentieth century by Kenneth Kirk, who revived the casuistical style while rejecting what seemed to be the rigorism of some of his Anglican predecessors (Kirk, 1999). "Situation ethics," introduced by Joseph Fletcher in the middle of the twentieth century (Fletcher, 1966), utilized a form of casuistry based on the commandment to love understood in utilitarian terms.

Fletcher held that love is the only moral norm, the end justifies the means, and decisions ought to be made in view of the uniqueness of each situation. Although this provoked a storm of protest from Anglican and other Christian moral thinkers, it provided yet another moral approach attractive to some Episcopalians.

Spiritual liberty has been important to Anglicans; they have exhibited considerable variation in belief without censure. Consequently, no single document expresses the final teachings of the Episcopal Church concerning bioethics and healthcare. Only canon law passed by the General Convention is binding; canon law, however, generally addresses matters of governance and does not specifically address matters of health and morals. The Holy Bible assumes great importance as a source of fundamental Anglican convictions concerning ethical questions related to healthcare, exerting much of its influence through the *Book of Common Prayer* with its largely biblical content (Booty, 1986). Writings of the Church Fathers and classical Christian theologians also figure significantly in Anglican thought about bioethics.

Episcopalian understandings of questions of medical ethics and healthcare have also been enhanced by a variety of other writings, including the following:

- Resolutions of the General Convention
- Reports from the House of Bishops
- Reports and special studies from standing commissions, committees, and task forces of the General Convention
- Reports and special studies from Executive Council committees
- Pastoral letters from the Presiding Bishop and diocesan bishops
- Articles and books by Episcopal scholars

Episcopalians also take heed of the reports and pastoral letters of the Lambeth Conference of the Anglican Communion (Lambeth Conference, 1998), resolutions of the General Synod of the Church of England, and reports of its Board for Social Responsibility (Board for Social Responsibility 2000, 1996, 1961), as well as resolutions and reports from other branches of the Anglican communion. These wide-ranging resources reveal the mind of the church, but none is considered juridically binding upon Episcopalians.

II. Issues in Bioethics

A. The Patient-Professional Caregiver Relationship

The value of the human body is stressed, rather than denied, in Anglican thought. The doctrine of creation, always important in Anglican ethics, is reinforced and underlined by the identification of God with humankind in the Christ. The fact that God became human, experiencing human life not only in mind and spirit, but also in body, indicates that human embodiment is important to what it is to be human. The Anglican focus on creation and incarnation suggests that we are to care for our bodies as temples of God, promoting physical health by seeking medical treatment, engaging in preventive care, following healthy diets, performing regular exercise, and avoiding substance abuse (Resolution A098, *Journal of the General Convention*, 1991; hereafter *JGC*.).

Healthcare professionals play an important role in assisting individuals to achieve these ends. Given the importance of the values of fidelity and community in Anglicanism, the relationship between patient and healthcare professional, at its best, is collaborative and collegial (Cohen et al., 2000, pp. 61-65; Smith, 1986, pp. 54-63). Patients and health care professionals are not isolated atoms, but, as human beings, are essentially social. They are, as sixteenth century Anglican divine Richard Hooker observed, "sociable parts united into one body ... bound each to serve unto other's good ..." (Hooker, 1977, Section I.3.5). Thus, service to others, including care for those with impaired health, and consideration of the common good are important Anglican values.

The Anglican tradition recognizes that adults with the capacity to make decisions have the right and responsibility to choose among treatment options and to refuse available treatments (Cohen et al., 2000, pp. 61-62). The social autonomy of individuals is, however, set within the context of the relationship of the individual to God and others. This means that patients are not only free to choose their form of treatment, but bound to do so in ways rooted in their lives in community and in God's purposes. This Anglican emphasis on individual choice with regard to care of the body is grounded in the recognition of human dignity, which derives from the special relationship in which each human being stands to God, rather than any particular qualities that an individual might possess. The dignity of each person, the noted twentieth century theologian William Temple stated, means that "[t]he Church must make respect for freedom its most fundamental principle of action." (Temple, 1949, p. 219). Indeed it is entirely consistent with the spirit of the tradition to regard work in the helping professions as a form of ministry (Mohrmann, 1995).

Healthcare professionals are also individuals whose choices should be respected. If the healthcare requests of patients would violate the moral or religious principles of healthcare providers, the latter should explain this to patients and, if possible, refer them to other caregivers willing to honor those requests. Carrying out such transfers exhibits respect for the freedom and responsibility of patients to make important decisions about their own healthcare (A093a, *JGC*, 1991).

Healing is not only of the body. Healing is of the whole person – spirit, mind, and body, as the General Convention of 1991 observed (A062, *JGC*, 1991). Therefore, others in addition to health care professionals, can offer an efficacious ministry of spirit and mind. A church commission has recognized that clergy and spiritual healers also serve as agents through whom God works to achieve human health (*JGC*, 1964, p. 654).

A.1. Informed Consent

Anglicans share the conviction that healthcare professionals should speak openly with patients about their condition and the therapeutic alternatives available to them. Physicians should inform patients of the probable benefits and risks of treatment options and offer them the opportunity to give or to withhold their consent to a course of therapy (Cohen et al., 2000, p. 63). Moreover, disclosure of information and statements made by health care professionals should be made in light of the individual patient's world-view, cultural background, and moral framework. "The need to be sensitive to our relational, as well as our informational needs may be particularly important outside a generalized Anglo and middle-class culture" (Cohen et al., 2000, p. 64).

Parents should serve as custodians for children for whom health care decisions must be made and should be committed to their physical, emotional, and spiritual well-being. "[T]he love that binds them together ... because they have a history of a life together in which they have shared values, joys, and sorrows" grounds the right and responsibility of parents to make decisions about medical care for their children (Cohen et al., 2000, p. 70). Episcopalians presuppose that parental decisions represent considered judgments about the good of the child, although in rare cases, this may be called into question (Smith, 1986, p. 54). Although children who are very young cannot be considered capable of participating in decisions on their behalf, as children mature, they should join in decisions about their care to the degree possible to (and desired by) one their age and individual level of maturity. Most physicians and medical ethicists recognize the importance of seeking the assent to treatment of a child who is sufficiently mature to participate in decisions directly affecting his or her health and physical integrity (Cohen et al., 2000, p. 70).

A.2. Truth-telling and Confidentiality

The Anglican tradition stresses both honesty – accurately speaking what one believes to be the truth – and candor – volunteering information of relevance when not specifically asked for – in healthcare (Cohen et al., 2000, pp. 62-65). Honest communication among persons is fundamental to Christian life, for unless we acknowledge the dignity, personhood, and status of others as neighbors to be treated openly and honestly, we fail in our duty to promote right relationships with others.

However, there are important issues of timing and wording that arise when caregivers communicate troubling news. To speak the truth in love (Ephesians 4:15) requires professionals to avoid providing poor prognoses in ways that can terrify or estrange vulnerable persons (Cohen et al., 2000, pp. 64-65). Furthermore, the failure to retain confidences and to be trustworthy erodes any relationship. Therefore, confidentiality is also demanded as a component of the relationship between healthcare professionals and patients (Smith, 1986, p. 15).

B. Sex, Procreation, and the Family

The importance of the body and sexual intercourse in marriage is emphasized within the Anglican tradition. Hooker commented in the sixteenth century that:

> parties married have not anie longer intire power over them selves but ech hath interest in others person, it cannot be thought an absurd construction to saie that worshipping with the bodie is the imparting of that interest in the bodie unto another which none before had save onlie our selves (Hooker, 1977, Section V:73:7).

Similarly, John Donne, in his seventeenth century sermons, reiterated the Anglican view that the joining of two persons, body and soul, in matrimony is not inferior, unworthy or unclean (Donne, 1955, Section II, p. 340). Human sexuality is tied to the embrace and care of the other in a loving marital relationship within the Anglican tradition.

In the twentieth century, the Anglican tradition tempered an earlier emphasis on procreation as the major end of sexual intercourse in marriage and adopted a more explicit recognition that mutual affection, support, and care are at the core of marriage. It thereby set aside Augustine's views that sexual intercourse is illicit when it is grounded in sexual desire and that such intercourse can be excused only by the intent to procreate (Smith & Cohen, 2003, pp. 78-85). Thus, the "The Celebration and Blessing of a Marriage" in the 1979 *Book of Common Prayer* frames sex within a generous love for the other, recognizing the need of married persons to complement and fulfill each other and to establish a durable partnership. The purposes of marriage are described as follows:

> The union of husband and wife in heart, body, and mind is intended by God for their mutual joy; for the help and comfort given one another in prosperity and adversity; and, when it is God's will, for the procreation of children and their nurture in the knowledge and love of the Lord. Therefore marriage is not to be entered into unadvisedly or lightly, but reverently, deliberately, and in accordance with the purposes for which it was instituted by God (*Book of Common Prayer*, 1979, p. 423).

This suggests that, in some situations, which are not necessarily confined to infertility, it may not be God's will that a married couple have children.

Yet the Anglican tradition also recognizes that children are a blessing and a joy. They are cherished not only as symbols of the mutual commitment of couples, but also as beings with their own integrity and uniqueness. Parents serve as their procreators, rather than their creators, meaning that their children are not parents' possessions, products, or projects, but their trusts (O'Donovan, 1984). Children are beings with a fundamental human dignity who are not to be viewed as extensions of the parental self or as a means of securing parental identity (Smith & Cohen, 2003, pp. 85-92).

B.1. Contraception

The use of contraception was generally frowned upon within the Anglican tradition until the last century. At the Lambeth Conference of 1930, however, the Anglican Communion introduced a new openness to the use of contraception, indicating that it was morally appropriate for couples to pursue responsible family planning to control the number and spacing of children. This view was subsequently reaffirmed by several General Conventions of the Episcopal Church. Responsible parenthood, they observed in various resolutions, requires wise stewardship of the resources and abilities of the family, as well as consideration of the varying population needs of society and the claims of future generations (D-016, *JGC*, 1982; D009 *JGC*, 1994).

B.2. Sterilization

A decision to employ sterilization, according to a Church of England working party, can be justified when there is a need for lower population growth within a community and when a family seeks to limit its growth so that it can provide adequately for its members (Board for Social Responsibility, 1961). Sterilization can also appropriately be considered by those who wish to avoid conceiving children because they might pass on to them serious genetic disease (Committee on Medical Ethics, 1998, pp. 67-73). Sterilization however is not just a decision for oneself and one's own body. It is a choice with implications for present or future spouse, existing children, potential grandparents, and indeed the larger human community. Therefore, the following are among the questions those considering sterilization should ask: Is sterilization the least drastic means available to attain a necessary end? Has the person involved considered the effects of sterilization on his or her identity and self-image? Is the decision a collaborative one? (Smith, 1986, pp. 79-80).

Compulsory sterilization, however, is morally unjustifiable. The forced sterilization of families of the People's Republic of China was deplored in a 1994 resolution of General Convention (D091, JGC, 1994). Sterilization of those who are developmentally disabled, an English working party observed, should be rejected; instead we should integrate such persons "into the life of the community, providing such support and protection as they need in the conduct of their lives," (Board for Social Responsibility, 1961, pp. 40-41). Moreover, our history of eugenic sterilization does not provide reason to believe that we would necessarily use this technique wisely in the future. Smith concludes that "[c]ompulsory sterilization is wrong, then, because it involves serious risks to the person of the patient, because of its dubious effect and necessity, and because it is unclear that we can formulate criteria for its fair use" (Smith, 1986, p. 81).

B.3. Abortion

Theologians in the early Christian tradition generally opposed abortion. However, a greater openness to abortion for the sake of the life and health of the woman has become evident within the Anglican and several other Christian traditions in recent times. The question turns on at least three issues: the importance of procreation as an outcome of sexual activity, the moral status of the embryo and fetus, and the welfare and self-determination of the pregnant woman. Episcopalians maintain that each of these values is to be respected, but they differ about the relative priority to be accorded to them in cases where they conflict.

The Christian tradition has generally maintained that there is no defining scriptural text detailing when individual human life begins. The Church Fathers, by and large, agreed with Aristotle that there is a biological and moral difference between "unformed" embryos (those at 40 days gestation or below for males and 80-90 days for females) and "formed" fetuses (those past the 40 or 80-90 day point respectively). "Formed" embryos, they maintained, no longer have a vegetative or an animal soul but have been "formed" with a human soul. They therefore considered it seriously wrong to end the lives of "formed" embryos. However, to end the life of an "unformed" embryo was viewed as a lesser wrong, not because it destroyed an individual human entity but because it, like contraception, frustrated the primary end of sexual intercourse – procreation.

The distinction between the "formed" fetus and the "unformed" embryo was maintained in the thirteenth century by Aquinas and continued to be influential until the eighteenth century. The discovery of the oocyte at that time led some within and without the Anglican tradition to declare that the fetus should be protected from the moment of conception, since they now concluded that the merger of sperm and oocyte at fertilization created an actual or potential human being.

Currently, there is no unanimous view within the Anglican tradition about the moral status of the human embryo. Some maintain that the same protection should be accorded to the newly fertilized egg as to a born human being because the unique genetic component of the individual is largely established at conception. They hold that the same individual subject is present throughout the process of prenatal development, for they can find no obvious threshold beyond conception at which the embryo seems to become distinctively different and an individual human being (O'Donovan, 1984; Banner, 1999).

Others have taken cognizance of scientific findings that the early embryo can divide during its first two weeks into two or more separate fragments, each of which can develop into a distinct human being. They have also noted that if a cell is removed from an early embryo and put into a hospitable environment it can be grown into a separate embryo distinct from the original. They have concluded from this and other evidence that the physical basis for human individuality is not settled until the primitive streak, the precursor of the central nervous system, has formed at about two weeks after fertilization and the path that the embryonic cells will take as they grow into various bodily organs is settled (Dyson, 1992; Dunstan, 1988, 1984; Habgood, 1998, pp. 249-252, 277-281; Smith & Cohen, 2003, pp. 113-125). Some in this latter group reinforce their conclusion by pointing to the fact that a large proportion of embryos (in the range of 75-80%) is aborted spontaneously early in pregnancy. They find it difficult to accept that God allows three-quarters of individual human beings to die after having brought them into life (Smith & Cohen, 2003, pp. 113, 123).

Furthermore, understandings of the values at issue in abortion have shifted over the years. Procreation is no longer considered the primary purpose of sexual intercourse; marital love and union are taken to be equally, if not more, important. In addition, women have been granted greater social and moral autonomy and there has been an increased openness to the right of women to decide whether or not to bear children. The defining question concerning abortion has now become whether there is a certain point at which fetal life is owed the same protection due an infant such that it cannot be set aside in favor of the welfare and autonomy of the pregnant woman. The doctrines of Creation and Redemption weigh toward preserving fetal life, but also direct the concern of Christians to the preservation of the life and health of the woman.

The Episcopal Church generally views the decision about abortion as a matter of individual conscience. Any proposed legislation regarding abortion, the General Convention of 1988 resolved, must support respect for individual moral deliberations (C047a, *JGC*, 1988). However, the Episcopal Church opposes both abortion on demand and an absolute ban on abortion, tending to accept it mainly in those cases in which the life or health of the woman is at risk. The General Convention of 1994 reaffirmed earlier statements according to which abortion has a tragic dimension and should be carried out only in extreme situations, not as a means of birth control, family planning, sex selection, or convenience (A054, *JGC*, 1994; C047a, *JGC*, 1988; A065, *JGC*, 1982). The resolution goes on to urge those considering abortion to seek the counsel of members of the Christian community and the sacramental life of the Church as they explore the alternatives available to them. The church's approach to abortion, however, has not been without its internal critics, who maintain, among other objections, that this approach is self-contradictory in that it affirms the sacredness of human life and yet allows the destruction of human fetal life (Scott, 1992).

In 1991, the General Convention opposed legislation requiring that parents be notified or required to consent when a minor seeks an abortion, unless such laws allow for a non-judicial bypass in cases when a minor is unable to notify parents or where family dysfunction may put the minor "at serious physical, psychological or emotional risk." In the latter circumstances, minors should be allowed to make an informed decision, but should notify a responsible adult, such as a clergy person, teacher, guidance counselor, mental health professional, or other family member (C037s, *JCG*, 1991).

B.4. New Reproductive Technologies
Interest in new reproductive technologies skyrocketed at the end of the last century as infertile persons sought assistance in bringing children into the world. A stunning repertoire of new methods of medically-assisted reproduction was developed in response to these couples and to those who wished to avoid having children with inherited serious genetic disease. Questions have been raised within the Episcopal Church about where to draw limits around human control over procreation. Some of these questions have been addressed in General Convention resolutions and by various Episcopalian scholars. The latter have been especially concerned about what it would mean to procreate children in a world in which we might be able to bring forth offspring according to our own design.

a. IVF. The Episcopal Church has taken a cautious but generally accepting position about the use of *in vitro* fertilization (IVF), or fertilization of an egg with sperm in a laboratory dish and subsequent transfer of the resulting embryo to a woman's uterus (Cohen, 2002). Use of this technology was approved by the General Convention of 1982 for married couples who are experiencing infertility (A067, *JGC*, 1982). A couple's attempt to use IVF to bypass physical obstacles to procreation can be a responsible and loving choice, an Episcopal Church task force has maintained (Smith & Cohen, 2003, pp. 91-92). Couples considering the use of this reproductive technology were advised by the 1991 General Convention to seek the advice and assistance of a qualified professional counselor (A101, *JGC*, 1991). They should consider not only this new technology, but also adoption as one of the options open to them, the General Convention declared. Thinkers within the Episcopal Church have not endorsed the use of IVF and other new reproductive technologies unreservedly but have maintained that more needs to be done to protect those involved from their physical and psychological risks and to develop appropriate ethical and social limitations on their use (Smith & Cohen, 2003, pp. 91-92; Cohen, 2002).

b. Artificial insemination by husband. The use of artificial insemination, or the impregnation of a woman with sperm by medical or other artificial means, by married couples using the sperm of the husband was approved by the Standing Commission on Human Affairs and Health in 1988 (*Blue Book*, 1988, p. 159). No resolution has been passed by the General Convention, however, in support of the use of this reproductive technique.

c. Sperm and egg donation. The introduction of third party donors into the creation of children has not been endorsed as an option by the General Convention the Episcopal Church. Artificial insemination by donor was considered problematic by the Standing Commission on Human Affairs and Health of 1988 because it viewed it as morally questionable to hide knowledge about one of their biological parents from the resulting children. A donor should not be allowed "to refuse moral and legal responsibility for a future child that his or her choice helped procreate" (*Blue Book*, 1988). Yet revealing the identity of the donor, the commission also opined, raises "difficult issues of parenting, family identification for the child, and, potentially, legal issues of parental responsibility..." In addition, the use of a third party donor can create difficult issues of parenting and can complicate the marital relationship for the spouse who did not contribute gametes to the creation of the child, the commission observed.

A Church of England working party has maintained that the use of third party donation to overcome infertility is acceptable, for "[t]here is no offence against the married partner, there is no breaking of the relationship of physical fidelity and there is no relationship with a person outside of marriage" (Board for Social Responsibility, 1996). Anthony Dyson, an English commentator, has observed that the principal question raised by third party donation is whether the rearing parents will provide a stable environment in which the welfare of the child is a central focus of concern (Dyson, 1995, pp. 108-120). In this context, an American task force has stated that "... it is difficult to judge third-party donation wrong" without qualification (Smith & Cohen, 2003, p. 93).

d. Surrogate motherhood. Another reproductive practice, surrogate motherhood, or contracting with a woman to be impregnated with a male's sperm, bear the resulting child, and deliver that child to the contracting man and his wife, was rejected by the General Convention of the Episcopal Church in 1982 (*Blue Book*, 1982) and in 1988 (*Blue Book*, 1988). In 1988, the Standing Commission on Human Affairs and Health pointed out that this practice poses physical risks to the surrogate and raises the possibility that she will be exploited economically (*Blue Book*, 1988). The commission called for more complete study of this and other new forms of reproductive technology by the church, keeping in mind the distinctive Christian vision of sexuality, marriage, and parenting.

e. Reproductive cloning. The possibility of using reproductive cloning in order to have biologically related children is morally abhorrent to many Episcopalian thinkers, although some others consider this merely another way of bringing wanted children into the world. Reproductive cloning involves using the gamete of one person, the female egg, inserting a single cell from another person into the nucleus of that egg, and then giving it an electrical or chemical shock to initiate its growth as an embryo.

Those who oppose reproductive cloning view human beings as unique and precious creatures who should not be reproduced by a process that they believe stands the very meaning of procreation on its head. They are concerned that reproductive cloning might destroy the core Christian view of procreation as a biological and relational partnership between two people in a loving, committed union. Moreover, it would introduce confusion into our understanding of parenthood. Who would be the parent of the cloned child? The cell donor? The egg donor? The cloned child's grandparents? The lines between family members, which seem integral to human identity and well-being, would be blurred in a way that they are not by coital procreation were reproductive cloning introduced, these critics maintain (Smith & Cohen, 2003, pp. 97-99). Those who would welcome reproductive cloning maintain that it is an appropriate way to enable otherwise infertile parents or those who might pass genetic disease to their children to have healthy children (Smith & Cohen, 2003, pp. 97-99).

An Episcopal Church task force has maintained that sufficient questions have been raised about the risks of reproductive cloning for the health of the resulting children, for our understanding of procreation and for our view of the parent-child relationship to lead it challenge the use of this technology (Smith & Cohen, 2003, pp. 98-99). Moreover, the General Convention of 2003 resolved that it is not morally acceptable to use reproductive cloning at this time.

B.5. Embryo Research

The Standing Commission on Human Affairs and Health of the Episcopal Church stated in 1988 that Christian thought widely judges the use of human embryos for experimentation to be immoral and went on to say that it could not affirm such experimentation for members of the Church (*Blue Book*, 1988). The commission also rejected freezing fertilized human ova "for later thawing, experimentation, possible implantation, or discard" on grounds that the safety and efficacy of this procedure were still in doubt.

The question of whether it is morally acceptable to carry out embryonic stem cell research has not been addressed broadly within the Episcopal Church. However, the narrow question of whether stem cells derived from embryos remaining after completion of IVF treatment should be used in such research was addressed by an Episcopal Church task force in 2003. The task force maintained that it is morally acceptable to use these embryos, which would otherwise be discarded, provided that those donating the embryos have given their informed consent, the embryos were not deliberately overproduced for research, and they were not obtained through sale or purchase (*Blue Book*, 2003). This view was endorsed by the General Convention of the Episcopal Church in 2003.

C. Genetics

A long tradition of thought within Anglicanism encourages humans to pursue scientific knowledge and to develop more accurate ways of understanding the natural world. The conviction that humans are called to shape and renew the natural order in accord with God's purposes is a prominent feature of Anglican moral thinking (Committee on Medical Ethics, 1998, pp. 15-18; Board for Social Responsibility, 1996, pp. 24-26). In particular, Anglicans maintain that we are to use our God-given abilities to gain scientific knowledge to alter the progression of disease (Committee on Medical Ethics, 1998, pp. 15-18). Yet our obligations as stewards of God's creation also constrain our interventions into nature, requiring us to respect its integrity and order (O'Donovan, 1984, p. 29). There are limits to what we may do with and for our bodies, according to the Christian tradition. They are not to be treated as mere instruments but are to be honored in their own right (Board for Social Responsibility, 1996, pp. 29-30). Therefore, human beings are to proceed cautiously in efforts to understand and rework the human genome and thus affect the human body; we are to respond to disease and disability in ways that fulfill God's intentions.

C.1. Genetic Interventions

The importance of research into the human genome was cited by the General Convention of 1985, which acknowledged its potential benefits even as it noted that such research raises ethical concerns. A resolution adopted in that year encouraged "genetic engineering research to increase human understanding of vital processes, recognizing that human DNA is a gift of God, at the center of life and directing our development, growth and functioning" (A090, *JGC*, 1985). A 1988 report of the Standing Commission on Human Affairs and Health endorsed gene therapy studies that are approved by peer review boards and that are intended for publication in recognized scientific journals (*Blue Book*, 1988). In accord with these resolutions, the 1991 General Convention stated that there is no theological or ethical objection to gene modification aimed at preventing or alleviating serious suffering when it poses no undue risk to the patient (A095, *JGC*, 1991). It also indicated that the Episcopal Church has "no theological or ethical objection against the production and use of medicinal materials by means of genetic manipulation for therapeutic or diagnostic purposes aimed at the prevention or alleviation of serious suffering" (A095, *JGC*, 1991).

Gene transfer research (sometimes termed "gene therapy") was viewed as morally acceptable by the General Convention of 2003 to treat disease, but only if it is rendered safe and effective. Intervening in the human germline by altering the genes of sperm, egg, or embryo, and thereby modifying the genetic make-up not only of the child to be born but also that of his or her descendants, was deemed morally acceptable in principle by the General Convention of 2003. It accepted the view of a leading Episcopal thinker that if such interventions can be used to eliminate terrible disease within a family that would be a gift of God that we should celebrate (Smith, 1999). However, the General Convention also made a strong statement to the effect that there would have to be compelling scientific evidence that germline interventions were safe and effective in humans before it would be appropriate to proceed with them. Moreover, it maintained that using this and other forms of genetic interventions to enhance or improve children beyond a point necessary to sustain health should not be done without prior review by a national body authorized to oversee this and other forms of genetic research. The possibility of enhancing tomorrow's children, is troubling, according to the Ethics and New Genetics Task Force, not least because of the possibility of the abuse of power and the impossibility of changing the results (Smith & Cohen, 2003, pp. 55-68).

New genetic techniques may be used in conjunction with *in vitro* fertilization, the General Convention of 2003 held, to avoid procreation of human beings with serious genetic or chromosomal disorders.

C.2. Genetic Testing and Counseling

As stewards of creation, we have an obligation to use our developing capacities for genetic testing in ways that serve God's purposes, a report from the Committee on Medical Ethics of the Diocese of Washington stated (Committee on Medical Ethics, 1998, p. 17). We need to become aware not only of the benefits of such testing, but also of its drawbacks for individuals and for society.

Genetic testing may reduce anxiety and uncertainty for those whose family history suggests that they might inherit gene-based disease. It may indicate that they are free of the gene at issue and do not need treatment or, for those who test positive, may lead them to investigate possible treatment. It may also assist the latter in making decisions about the future, inform their decisions about having children, and draw them closer together as families. Yet such testing also has its drawbacks. It can heighten anxiety, yield results that are difficult to interpret, create uncertainty, impair planning for the future, expose individuals to discrimination in insurance and employment, and strain family relationships (Smith & Cohen, 2003, pp. 29-34). The General Convention of 1991 maintained that "the use of results of genetic screening of adults, newborns and the unborn for the purpose of discrimination in employment and insurance is unacceptable" (A095, *JGC*, 1991).

Such drawbacks can make it difficult to decide whether to undergo genetic testing. It is advisable for those considering such testing to call upon genetic and pastoral counselors for assistance in deciding whether to proceed (Smith & Cohen, 2003, pp. 29-30; Committee on Medical Ethics, 1998, pp. 36-40). It is also wise for individuals to discuss the possibility of testing beforehand with their family and to reach an understanding about how other family members would respond to the test results (Smith & Cohen, 2003, pp. 33-34, 47-48; Committee on Medical Ethics, 1998, pp. 26-30). The decision by one person in a family can have implications for other family members as well. When a family has a history of a serious genetic disorder and a member tests positive for the relevant gene, others in the family will have to decide whether they, too, wish to learn whether they have the gene. Thus, consultation with a family in advance can prepare members for the possibility that they, too, may have to confront the decision whether to be tested.

Genetic testing also creates certain social risks, for it opens the door to the reintroduction of a eugenic ethos into the community. For instance, decisions by individuals to use prenatal testing to abort fetuses with disabilities or unwanted characteristics might, when taken together, have a disastrous cumulative effect. They might create a culture in which those who are "defective" are weeded out and only those deemed of excellent quality – according to sometimes arbitrary and perverted standards – are considered worthy of coming into the world. While it is tempting to want to bring a "perfect" child into the world, such a desire is unrealistic and uncharitable. Christians should embrace diversity within the human family and the equal value of all of God's children as they work to overcome social stereotyping (Smith & Cohen, 2003, pp. 39-42; Committee on Medical Ethics, 1998, pp. 102-104).

D. Organ and Tissue Transplantation

The Episcopal Church has supported the use of organ transplantation and has encouraged members to consider seriously the opportunity to donate organs, blood, and tissue after death (A097, *JGC*, 1991; C024, *JGC*, 1982). The church has not discussed the possibility of serving as living organ donors.

The Standing Commission on Human Affairs and Health raised important questions in 1988 about ways in which organ transplantation should and should not be used. Often use of this procedure is morally sound. Accepting tissues such as cornea or skin can enhance the quality of life of a person without imposing serious burdens. However, the situation is more complicated in the case of the transplantation of organs such as kidneys, pancreas, or heart. The standing commission recommended careful reflection about such issues as: What is the risk to living donors? Is one obliged to undergo severe burdens to avoid death or, to the contrary, should one forgo transplantation when it would be disproportionately burdensome? Because these questions are complex, the commission urged their further study (*Blue Book*, 1988, p. 161).

In 1991, the General Convention urged members of the church to consider seriously the opportunity to donate organs after death so that others might live. A decision about donating bodily materials to others should be made well ahead of time so that any tissues or organs needed for donation may be removed as soon after death as possible. That decision should be clearly stated to family, friends, church, and attorney (A097, *JGC*, 1991). Although it is morally appropriate to decide to donate an organ to another in need, special care must be taken by those making inquiries to avoid coercing living donors (*Blue Book*, 1988).

The conception and deliberate abortion of fetuses to obtain fetal tissue for medical research was rejected by the 1991 General Convention, as was the use of fetal tissue aborted for profit (A096, *JGC*, 1991). The Convention recommended further study of the use of tissue from fetuses that have been aborted to save the life of a woman.

E. HIV/AIDS

As the terrible scope of the AIDS epidemic became apparent, the Episcopal Church responded with measures designed to bring care and comfort to those afflicted with this disease. In 1985, the General Convention recognized "with love and compassion the tragic human suffering and loss of life involved in the AIDS epidemic" and repudiated "indiscriminate statements which condemn or reject the victims of AIDS." It went on to urge the development and funding of programs of awareness, education, and prevention concerning AIDS and of ministry to those affected by this illness (D062, *JGC*, 1985). Resolutions adopted by succeeding General Conventions repudiated discrimination against those with AIDS; approved of anonymous testing and counseling for HIV; urged the creation of accessible drug treatment, needle access, and safe sex programs, as well as monogamy in sexual relationships; and authorized funds for AIDS education programs in dioceses and congregations (D062, *JGC*, 1985; A086, B007, D101, D104, D109, *JGC*, 1988; A002-A006, A008, A009, B025, D096, *JGC*, 1991; A002, A003, A006, A007, B028, *JGC*, 1994; A047, A048, D099, *JGC*, 1997; A050-A052, D049, *JGC*, 2000).

An Episcopal Commission on AIDS and a National Episcopal AIDS Coalition were established to focus on the theological, ethical, and pastoral concerns raised by this illness, develop strategies to increase awareness of the AIDS crisis throughout the church, and advocate concern for those affected with HIV/AIDS to the world (A128, *JGC*, 1994). In 1997, these bodies were authorized to convene consultations to examine the impact of HIV/AIDS in communities of color, clarify the role of racism in responding to AIDS, and identify actions that Episcopalians must take in response to such racism (A046, *JGC*, 1997).

In 1991, the General Convention set out "Ten Principles for the Workplace" to govern the way in which Episcopalians relate to people with HIV/AIDS at places of employment. These support the equal rights and opportunities of those with this illness, nondiscriminatory employment policies, educational programs about HIV/AIDS, protection of the confidentiality of employees' medical records, appropriate infection control procedures, and no pre-employment or workplace HIV screening (A007, *JGC*, 1991). The Washington Office of the Episcopal Church was instructed to work for increased funding, research, preventive education, and comprehensive service delivery related to those with HIV/AIDS at all levels of government (A005, JGC, 1994). Aware that a global AIDS epidemic was developing, the General Convention urged various international agencies to respond to the emerging AIDS crisis (D110, *JGC* 1988; A004 *JGC*, 1994).

F. Mental Health

The needs of those suffering from mental illness have been of particular concern to the Episcopal Church. The General Convention of 1985 called for the development of a means of assisting homeless persons who are mentally ill and without an adequate support system through various agencies of the church, other social agencies, and the healthcare delivery system (D127, *JGC*, 1985). The 1991 General Convention reiterated this concern and encouraged the development of programs to equip clergy and laity to minister to the mentally ill and their families. More specifically, it called for the development of "support groups, drop-in centers, housing and employment opportunities" for those with mental illness, particularly the homeless (D088, *JGC*, 1991). Dioceses, congregations and individual parishioners were encouraged to become advocates for funding that would provide comprehensive community-based services, hospital care, and research into the causes and treatments of mental illness. The National Alliance for the Mentally Ill was recommended as a resource for congregations and families of the mentally ill in a 2000 resolution (C032, *JGC*, 2000).

G. *Alcohol and Drug Abuse*

Alcoholism and other forms of substance abuse, the 1985 General Convention declared, are treatable disorders that can affect any individual, "regardless of financial situation, education, employment, race or creed" (A083, *JGC*, 1985). These conditions affect not only their victims, but also family and friends. Furthermore, they represent a major health concern of our society (A083, *JGC*, 1985). The General Convention encouraged each diocese to appoint a committee to educate members about the nature, prevention, treatment, and pastoral care of alcoholics and drug abusers and their families. Spiritual care should be provided to those addicted to substances, it specifically stated in 1991 (A100, *JGC*, 1991). In 2003, the Standing Commission on National Concerns provided more detailed guidelines for forming a Diocesan Alcoholism and Drug Dependency Committee and suggested steps to follow in carrying out an intervention and obtaining treatment for an affected person (*Blue Book*, 2003).

Employees of the Episcopal Church who are alcohol or drug dependent have been of special concern to the church. The General Convention of 1985 maintained that they should be offered treatment and counseling during recovery and that every effort should be made to offer them job protection and re-employment, as well as salaried sick leave should they require hospitalization (A083, *JGC*, 1985). The Standing Commission on National Concerns in 2003 also recommended that certain specific barriers to treatment that clergy and church staff face should be addressed. These include the existence of few clergy and employee assistance programs, inadequate use of resources for assistance and education within dioceses, and inadequate health insurance coverage for clergy and church staff (*Blue Book*, 2003). The General Convention of 2003 approved a resolution to this effect.

H. *Death and Dying*

Sixteenth century Anglicans, who lived in a society in which plague swept away vast numbers of people and childbirth often ended in death, drew a close connection between sickness, death, and sin. Thus, the "Great Litany," published in 1544, ended with the prayer: "Have pity upon us miserable sinners, that now are visited with great sickness and mortality, that like as thou didst command thy angel to cease from punishing, so it may now please thee to withdraw from us this plague and grievous sickness ..." (*Book of Common Prayer*, 1559, p. 76). A steady flow of books taught those who were sick to repent, meditate upon "last things," and to go on to die well (*ars moriendi*). Chief among these tracts was Jeremy Taylor's guide to holy dying, which emphasized the need to prepare for death over a lifetime, but especially when visited by sickness (Taylor, 1989).

The 1979 *Book of Common Prayer* tends to view illness as result of a disordered universe, rather than as retribution directed against evil doers. Thus, it offers the prayer to God that the sick, "accepting your healing gifts through the skill of surgeons and nurses, ... may be restored to usefulness in your world with a thankful heart" (*Book of Common Prayer*, 1979, p. 459). Death, in the service for burial of the dead, is viewed as comforting rather than condemning, triumph rather than defeat (Booty, 1986, p. 259). An Episcopal Church task force asserted that "Christian faith enables us to look upon our own dying, and that of people we love, as a journey with Christ through death into the life of God" (Cohen et al., 2000, p. 16).

H.1. Forgoing Life-sustaining Treatment

Human beings are precious, cherished creations of God, yet their lives need not be extended at all costs. When individuals are near the end of life and medical powers can no longer stave off death, there is no moral obligation to prolong their dying. In such circumstances, it is morally appropriate to withhold or withdraw life-sustaining treatment and to allow their lives to come to their end (A093, *JGC*, 1991). Although it can be enormously difficult to acknowledge that someone who is deeply loved cannot be kept alive, recognizing when this is the case and removing burdensome medical measures to allow the natural course of events to proceed is an act of care and compassion (Cohen et al., 2000, pp. 39-42; Committee on Medical Ethics, 1999, pp. 31-40).

Decisions to withhold or withdraw life-sustaining treatment should be made by the individuals whose lives are involved. However, as an End-of-Life Task Force reaffirmed, when such individuals no longer have decisionmaking capacity, a surrogate or family members (when no surrogate has been named) should make decisions about the use of such treatment for the sick person on the basis of the values and preferences they expressed earlier (Cohen et al., 2000, p. 65; Committee on Medical Ethics, 1999, pp. 18-19). Caregivers should allow those who are near the end of life to die peacefully in a setting that enables them to maintain dignity free from unwanted and inappropriate technology.

When persons are in a comatose state from which there is no reasonable hope of recovery, it is appropriate to contemplate withholding or removing life-support, including artificial nutrition and hydration (Cohen et al., 2000, p. 44; Committee on Medical Ethics, 1999, pp. 42, 49-50, 115-117; Lambeth Conference, 1999; A093a, *JGC*, 1991).

Not only adults, but also newborns and children for whom cure is not possible and who face a life that amounts to a form of dying should not be subjected to useless life-sustaining treatment. Instead, they should be provided with all available comfort measures as their lives come to an end (Smith, 1986, pp. 48-54). Children who are developmentally disabled or mentally challenged should not be considered to be dying solely on account of their disabilities and should receive care that is appropriate to their needs.

A service for a time when life-sustaining treatment is withdrawn developed by the Committee on Medical Ethics of the Diocese of Washington offers pastoral support to those who are dying and those who care of for them in those circumstances when burdensome life-sustaining treatment is removed (Cohen et al., 2000, pp. 156-161; Committee on Medical Ethics, 1995, pp. 31-39).

H.2. Proxy Decision Making and Advance Directives

Several reports from church working groups and General Conventions have encouraged the use of advance directives by individuals to inform relatives, friends, and future caregivers about the sort of treatment they wish to receive near the end of life should they become unable to speak for themselves (Cohen et al., 2000, pp. 65-69; Committee on Medical Ethics, 1999, pp. 21-23; C008, *JGC*, 1991; C002a, *JGC*, 1982). Ethical questions related to preparing such documents are specifically addressed in a book from the Committee on Medical Ethics of the Diocese of Washington (Committee on Medical Ethics, 1995). It points out that it is important to prepare these documents *before* a serious illness so that those caring for persons near the end of life will know whether or not they wish to have life-sustaining treatment, what sorts of supportive care they want, and whether or not they plan to donate organs and tissue to others. It urges Episcopalians to discuss their advance directives with family members and friends as they develop them, so that those close to them will be aware of their values and concerns and will be able to make medical care decisions for them should they later become incapable of deciding for themselves.

H.3. Pain Control and Palliative Care

It is widely accepted within the Anglican Communion that caregivers have an obligation to provide palliative care and pain-relieving medication to those nearing the end of life, even if this should inadvertently shorten their lives (Cohen et al., 2000, pp. 45-51; Board for Social Responsibility, 2000; Lambeth Conference, 1999; Committee on Medical Ethics, 1999, pp. 61-72; A056, *JGC*, 1994; C008, *JGC*, 1991; C002a, *JGC*, 1982). The General Convention of 1994 emphasized that "[p]alliative treatment to relieve the pain of persons with progressive incurable illnesses, even if done with knowledge that a hastened death may result, is consistent with theological tenets regarding the sanctity of life" (A056, *JGC*, 1994). The report of the End-of-Life Task Force points out that recent research indicates that providing medication to patients to alleviate pain in doses that are gradually increased to meet their individual needs rarely shortens their lives (Cohen et al., 2000, pp. 49-50). Instead, giving such drugs in carefully titrated doses prolongs the lives of many who are near death because they become more comfortable and more apt to take greater amounts of nourishment.

However, there is a pressing need to provide more adequate and extensive palliative care for those approaching death. Several General Conventions have urged healthcare professionals, families, patients, and legislative bodies to prevent intolerable suffering among the dying caused by the under use of pain medication, including narcotic drugs (A078, *JGC*, 2000; A056, *JGC*, 1994; C008, *JGC*, 1991; C002a, *JGC*, 1982). The General Convention of 2000 urged the healthcare professions to improve the quality of palliative care by offering physicians and nurses more extensive education about the most recent research. It specifically declared that healthcare professionals should provide sufficient levels of pain-relieving drugs to those near the end of life to relieve their pain and discomfort and should make timely referrals to hospice for them (A078, *JGC*, 2000).

H.4. Hospice Care

The great renewal of care for the dying, the hospice movement, originated with the work of Dame Cicely Saunders, a physician and nurse whose outlook has been deeply formed by Anglican practical piety. The basic goal of the hospice movement, to provide comprehensive end-of-life care that will achieve a good quality of life for each person by meeting his or her physical, emotional, and spiritual needs, has been widely approved within the Anglican Communion. The concept of hospice was introduced in 1976 in the first edition of *On Dying Well*, a Church of England report to which Dame Cicely contributed (Board for Social Responsibility, 2000). It has since been embraced in subsequent reports from within the Anglican Communion, including those from the Episcopal Church (Cohen et al., 2000, pp. 45-48; Committee on Medical Ethics, 1999, pp. 86-91). The General Conventions of 2000 strongly supported the hospice goals of providing interdisciplinary hospice care and communal support for the patient and family during the dying process, as well as care for families during bereavement (A078, *JGC*, 2000).

H.5. Suicide, Assisted Suicide, and Euthanasia

Reports from within the Anglican Communion express the almost universal Christian belief that suicide is wrong and that assisting persons to kill themselves or killing them outright is also wrong (Cohen et al., 2000, pp. 51-58; Lambeth Conference, 1999, pp. 101-106; Committee on Medical Ethics, 1999, pp. 73-84; Board for Social Responsibility, 2000, pp. 20-25; A056, *JGC*, 1994; A093a, *JGC*, 1991). Our lives are not our own, to dispose of at will, but are a gift from God, to whom they ultimately belong. Suicide is the expression of a refusal to trust in God, an embracing of death for its own sake, a form of self-justification. The great moral danger of suicide and assisted suicide is that they will be egotistical and manipulative, symbolic of an unwillingness to play the role of dependent when it falls to our turn. Moreover, the end of a person's life is not simply a private matter, but has import for those who surround him or her.

The question whether it is more compassionate to kill those who are in excruciating pain and suffering near the end of life, rather than allow them to die in misery can arise in unusual, extreme cases. Any honest person will acknowledge that he or she would wish for a hastened death in such circumstances (Board for Social Responsibility, 2000, p. 23). However, there should be no need for anyone to undergo such radical suffering today. The End-of-Life Task Force declared: "Where there are drugs available to hand to a despairing person near death so that he or she can commit suicide, there are also drugs available to provide to that person that will afford relief from pain and allow a peaceful death" (Cohen et al., 2000, p. 57). A*gape* or neighbor love may be "better expressed and more deeply nourished by the careful accompanying of a person in his dying than by any established practice of voluntary euthanasia" (Board for Social Responsibility, 2000, p. 22).

The Anglican Communion has consistently held that euthanasia should not be legalized, for if this practice were to become socially accepted, those who are vulnerable, such as the elderly and chronically ill, might well have to cope with the question, "Why aren't you dead yet?" (Committee on Medical Ethics, 1999, p. 81). That is, some might be pressured into ending their lives in order to relieve others of the burden of their care rather than because of pain and suffering that they experience. Others could elect assisted suicide to save their families the costs of maintaining them in a health care system that may drain them of their life savings. Rather than allow such persons to end their lives prematurely for the sake of others, we should reemphasize that we value all who are living and wish to provide them with care and support as their lives draw to a close.

I. Justice and Access to Healthcare

The Anglican Communion has been actively involved in providing healthcare. Indeed, many of those who practiced medicine and surgery in England and America before the nineteenth century were clergy. As the subject matter of medicine became more complex, however, fewer Anglican clergy found themselves able to devote time to the study of both theology and medicine, and the medical and clerical professions gradually separated. Even so, the close historical connection between pastoral caregivers and medical practitioners, as well as the theology of healing of the Anglican tradition (see above, The Patient-Professional Caregiver Relationship) has lead to a deep commitment within the communion to ensuring that all persons receive healthcare of good quality in a just manner.

As hospitals and other healthcare facilities were developed in England and the United States, it was not uncommon for some to be established under Anglican auspices. Moreover, as the Anglican Communion spread, various branches of the communion sent medical missionaries to found hospitals on various parts of the globe. Hence, by the twentieth century, the provision of healthcare formed a major element of Anglican church life (Booty, 1986, p. 255).

The General Convention has expressed concern about the provision of adequate degrees of healthcare for those in need many times over the years. For instance, in 1985 it called for the creation of a national commission on healthcare reform and urged congregations to increase their support for such health services as food kitchens, shelters for the homeless, legal aid centers, and neighborhood health clinics (A088, *JGC*, 1985). In 1988 it urged the church's Office of Government Relations in Washington D.C. to advocate for "all persons suffering from illness by creating appropriate levels of cost-effective healthcare, for example, hospices and alternative healthcare facilities" (B009, *JGC*, 1988). In 1991, it decried the inequitable healthcare delivery system of the United States and called for universal access to healthcare (A099, *JGC*, 1991). It also enunciated four principles regarding healthcare that included care of the whole person – physiological, spiritual, psychological, and social – and attention to preventive care (A057, *JGC*, 1991). Moreover, it encouraged the creation of legislation offering comprehensive medical benefits at all levels, including "diagnostic tests, primary and tertiary care for acute and chronic conditions, rehabilitation care, long-term care, mental health services, dental care and prescription drugs" (A010, *JGC*, 1991). Increased attention to matters affecting the healthcare of women, including "domestic violence, AIDS, heart disease, breast, ovarian and endometrial cancer, safe and effective contraceptives, and other methods of pregnancy prevention, maternity care, menopause and chronic illnesses unique to or prevalent among women" was called for by the 1994 General Convention (A055, *JGC*, 1994).

In 2000, the Office of the Bishop for Armed Services, Healthcare and Prison Ministries was directed to advocate for a healthcare system in which all may be guaranteed decent and appropriate primary healthcare, keep abreast of the changing healthcare market, and collect resources related to access to healthcare for the use of the church at all levels (A079, *JGC*, 2000). Two major conferences were held during the following three years on healthcare. The Standing Commission on National Concerns recommended to General Convention in 2003 that such efforts be continued through a church commission (*Blue Book*, 2003).

Bibliography

Anglicanism (1996). In: H.J. Hillerbrand (Ed.), *Oxford encyclopedia of the Reformation, vol. 1*: (pp. 38-44). New York: Oxford.

Avis, P. (1999). What is Anglicanism? In: S. Sykes, J. Booty, & J. Knight (Eds.), *The study of Anglicanism* (pp. 459-476). Minneapolis, MN: Fortress.

Board for Social Responsibility, Church of England (1961). *Sterilization: An ethical inquiry.* London: Church Information Office.

Board for Social Responsibility, Church of England (1996). *Personal origins, 2nd revised edition.* London: Church Publishing House.

The book of common prayer and administration of the sacraments and other rites and ceremonies of the Church together with the psalter or psalms of David according to the use of the Episcopal Church. (1979). New York: Church Hymnal Corporation.

Booty, J.E. (1986). The Anglican tradition. In: R.L. Numbers & D.W. Amundsen (Eds.), *Caring and curing: Health and medicine in the western religious traditions* (pp. 240-270).

Butler, J. (1970). *Fifteen sermons preached at the Rolls Chapel.* T.A. Roberts (Ed.). London: SPCK.

Butler, P. (1999). From the early eighteenth century to the present day. In: S. Sykes, J. Booty, & J. Knight (Eds.), *The study of Anglicanism* (pp. 30-51). Minneapolis, MN: Fortress.

Chadwick, H. (1999). Tradition, fathers and councils. In: S. Sykes, J. Booty, & J. Knight (Eds.), *The study of Anglicanism* (pp. 100-114). Minneapolis, MN: Fortress.

Cohen, C.B. November (2002). Protestant perspectives on the uses of the new reproductive technologies. *Fordham Urban Law Journal 30*, 135-145.

Cohen, C.B., Heller, J.C., Jennings, B., Morgan, E.F.M., Scott, D.A., Sedgwick, T.F., & Smith, D.H. (2000). *Faithful living, faithful dying: Anglican reflection on end of life care.* Harrisburg, PA: Morehouse.

Committee on Medical Ethics, Episcopal Diocese of Washington (1995). *Before you need them: Advance directives for health care, living wills and durable powers of attorney.* Cincinnati, OH: Forward Movement.

Committee on Medical Ethics, Episcopal Diocese of Washington (1997). *Assisted suicide and euthanasia: Christian moral perspectives.* Harrisburg, PA: Morehouse.

Committee on Medical Ethics, Episcopal Diocese of Washington (1998). *Wrestling with the future: Our genes and our choices.* Harrisburg, PA: Morehouse.

Committee on Medical Ethics, Episcopal Diocese of Washington (1999). *Toward a good Christian death: Crucial treatment choices.* Harrisburg, PA: Morehouse.

Donne, J. (1955). *The sermons of John Donne*, G.R. Potter & E.M. Simpson (Eds.), 10 vols., Berkeley and Los Angeles.

Dunstan, G.R. (1984). The moral status of the human embryo. *Journal of Medical Ethics, 1*, 38-44.

Dunstan, G.R. (1988). The embryo, from Aristotle to Alton. *Cross Currents, 38(47)*, 6-8.

Dyson, A. (1992). At heaven's command?: The Churches, Theology, and Experiments on Embryos. In: A. Dyson & J. Harris (Eds.), *Experiments on embryos* (pp. 82-105). London: Routledge.

Dyson, A. (1995). *The ethics of IVF.* London and New York: Mowbray.

Fletcher, J. (1966). *Situation Ethics.* Philadelphia, PA: Westminster.

Habgood, J. (1998). *Being a Person. Where Faith and Science Meet.* London: Hodder & Stoughton.

Haugaard, W.P. (1999). From the reformation to the eighteenth century. In: S. Sykes, J. Booty, & J. Knight (Eds.), *The study of Anglicanism* (pp. 3-29). Minneapolis, MN: Fortress.

Hooker, R. (1977-1981). *Of the lawes of ecclesiastical politie, Folger Library Edition.* W.S. Hill (Ed.). Cambridge, MA: Harvard University.

Horner, S. (Ed.) (2000). *On dying well: An updated contribution to the euthanasia debate* (2nd ed.). London: Church House Publishing.

Journal of the General Convention of the Episcopal Church. New York: General Convention. (multiple years).

Kirk, K. (1999). *Conscience and its problem: An introduction to casuistry*. Introduction by David H. Smith. Louisville, KY: Westminster John Knox.

Lambeth Conference (1999). *The official report of the Lambeth conference 1998*. Harrisburg, PA: Morehouse.

Michael, B. (1999). *Christian ethics and contemporary moral problems* (pp. 86-135). London: Cambridge University.

Mohrmann, M. (1995). *Medicine as ministry: Reflections on suffering, ethics, and hope*. Cleveland, OH: Pilgrim Press.

O'Donovan, O. (1984). *Begotten or made? Human procreation and medical technique* (pp. 49-66). London: Oxford University.

Pritchard, R. (1999). *A history of the Episcopal church, Revised Edition*. Harrisburg, PA: Morehouse.

Reports of the committees, commissions, boards, and agencies of the General convention of the Episcopal church (multiple years). In: *The blue book*: New York: Episcopal Church Center.

Scott, D.A. (1992). Changing teachings on abortion. In: T. Sedgwick & P. Turner (Eds.), *The crisis in moral teaching in the Episcopal church* (pp. 56-73). Harrisburg, PA: Morehouse Publishing.

Sedgwick, T.F. (1999). *The Christian Moral Life*. Grand Rapids, MI: Eerdmans.

Smith, D.H. (1986). *Health and medicine in the Anglican tradition: Conscience, community, and compromise*. New York: Crossroad.

Smith, D.H. (Fall 1999). Creation, preservation, and all the blessings ... *Anglican Theological Review 81*, 567-588.

Smith, D.H. & Cohen, C.B. (2003). *A Christian response to the new genetics: Religious, ethical and social issues*. Lanham, MD: Rowman and Littlefield.

Taylor, J. (1989). *Holy living and holy dying*. (2 vols.), P.G. Stanwood (Ed.). Oxford: Clarendon.

Taylor, J. (1996). *Doctor dubitantium*. London: J.O. Luke Meredith.

Temple. W. (1949). *Christus veritas: An essay*. London: Clarendon.

Wood, T. (1986). Anglican moral theology/ethics. In: J.F. Childress & J. Macquarrie (Eds.), *Westminster dictionary of Christian ethics* (pp. 22-28). Philadelphia, PA: Westminster.

Wright, J.R. (1999). Anglicanism, *Ecclesia Anglicana*, and Anglican: An Essay on Terminology. In: S. Sykes, J. Booty, & J. Knight (Eds.), *The study of Anglicanism* (pp. 477-482). Minneapolis, MN: Fortress.

Gospel Truth and Societal Consensus: Recent Bioethics Statements by the Protestant Church in Germany (EKD)

Corinna Delkeskamp-Hayes and Matthias Zierenberg

This essay will investigate the voice of German Protestantism[1] in the public debate on bioethical issues. The most important "Protestant voice" belongs to the "Protestant Church in Germany" (EKD, the Evangelische Kirche in Deutschland).[2] What are German Protestantism's contribution to contemporary debates concerning the biomedical and medical ethics problems of our time, and what does that contribution tells us about how that church perceives her role within society?

Our investigation will focus on the two most important recent EKD documents. The first, *Gott ist ein Freund des Lebens*,[3] (which occupies Section II) is the result of an ecumenical work group that was jointly installed by the council of the EKD and the German conference of Roman Catholic bishops in 1987, to secure a seemingly deepened cooperation between the two major German churches in their effort to strengthen Christianity's voice in societal discussions of biomedical issues.[4] The second, *Im Geist der Liebe mit dem Leben umgehen* (which occupies Section II), was issued by the EKD's Chamber for Public Responsibility (exclusively)[5] in 2002. This document bears particularly illuminating witness to the more specifically Protestant emphasis on freedom of conscience[6] in portraying two different, but equally "Protestant", ethical positions concerning pre-birth human life.

Both documents are distinguished by their quest for comprehensiveness. Large portions of the texts are devoted either to endorsing – wholeheartedly or with different shades of reservation and concern – positions which are also accepted in Germany's secular society or incorporated in German law. To isolate any particular position or claim, or to get at any possible bones of contention, one must traverse vast spaces of introductory, context-securing, horizon-delineating, relativizing, concessionary, precautionary material, that is devoted to the posing of questions, to the pointing out of "ethical dimensions", the issuing of warnings and the offering of dialogue and cooperation concerning those generally accepted positions. Since the EKD is recognizably reluctant to overtly infringe on any believer's or unbeliever's right to individual conscientiousness, the task of delineating what that church specifically stands for is not easy. To secure some general bearing for our interpretation, the EKD's recently stated understanding of her task of publicly pronouncing will be summarized in a short introduction.

I. Introduction: How Does the EKD Understand Her Public Role?

From the more important recent statements which the Protestant Church in Germany has issued concerning her public role, two major church projects emerge. Both projects follow from her responsibility for the future life of the faith (EKD, 2001a ed., EKD Text 68, Section I.1). On the one hand, that responsibility imposes the task of representing her theological position. The church takes seriously her missionary task as devoted to an ascertainment of faith in Jesus Christ, an enlivening of the Christian life, and an attractive giving forth of the Gospel (EKD, 2001a, Preface; Section III.1). She enhances awareness of her own message and wishes to help people in coming to their own experience of faith (EKD, 1999, Section III.1). She takes seriously the questions from those outside the church concerning the significance of the Gospel for our future (EKD, 2001a, Section I.1). Accordingly, she assumes the task of critically accompanying cultural developments (EKD, 1999, Preface) in her contemporary societal context by reference to the Christian faith (EKD, 1999, Section III.3). She wishes to encourage a "distinction between the spirits" according to the criteria of (among others) respect for God's honor, and denial of violence (EKD, 1999, Section III.2), as an encouragement to fight evil,[7] and with a view to identifying heresies (EKD, 2001a, Section III.4). She takes a stand in the question of truth in religion and advocates the triune God (EKD, 2001a, Section II.3). She musters her powers of composure and profile sharpening for opposing the secularizing tendencies in her environment (EKD, 2001a, Preface). With regard to biomedical problems, a previous document, *Zur Achtung* (1987), declared the church's obligation to participate in the public discussion by invoking the foundations which her faith provides for ethical decisionmaking, even among non-Christians (I, §4).

On the other hand, Protestant responsibility for the future life of the faith is seen to impose a certain openness with regard to the secular environment, into which that faith is to be introduced. "Enhancing awareness of the church's message" must, therefore, avoid endorsing a mere niche-existence for that church (EKD, 1999, Preface). She is to encourage change in her own cultural manifestations in response to changing cultural givens in her societal environment. She must learn from the critical arguments (concerning toleration, social service and ethical failure) of those outside the church and devise an invitingly evangelizing language (EKD, 2001a, Section I.1), which "reaches" the people. The commitment to not imposing on Christians one schematic form of life is also understood as the commitment to respecting different degrees of belonging to and working within the religious community (EKD, 2001b). The task of critical "distinction between the spirits" is also to encourage a culture of enlightenment and of a critique of (even Christian) religious superstition and ideology (EKD, 2001b).

In keeping with this twofold project, the church, especially in each local community, is conceived of as a place where people can find a home. The difficulty, that different groups of people conceive of their respective "homes" quite differently, is to be solved by reference to the fact they are to find "more" in church than their own selves, and more than what they expected. Traditions must be preserved but not idolized. Responsiveness must not be confused with appeasement (EKD, 2001a, Section I.3). The cultivation of communication with those outside the church must be accompanied by taking a precise and distinct stand vis-à-vis other institutions and worldviews (EKD, 2001a, Section III.3).

How does this subtle equilibrium between a commitment to faithfulness towards her theological roots and a commitment to societal relevance manifest itself in the pronouncements of that church concerning recent developments in biomedicine?

II. Gott Ist ein Freund des Lebens

The church's[8] bioethical position, as endorsed in this declaration, is placed in the context of a forceful call towards "common efforts for the protection of life" (EKD, 1991, Preface, Introductory survey). This call is motivated by a scenario of acute endangeredness of human life (§1) in view of its foundations and dignity. The project of the declaration can thus be subsumed under the "critical accompanying cultural developments" category featured under the faithfulness-aspect of the Protestant church's public mission. However, since that call is to elicit a cross-societal common effort (§2), its critical impact does not seem to concern that church's particular position. Accordingly, her biblical backing is designed to be acceptable to non-Christians as well (§3). In what sense, then, could one hope to extract from the declaration a particular Protestant stand in bioethics?

On closer scrutiny, the call is not quite as general as the initial survey suggests. While threats to the conditions of biological life on earth (§5) touch a value that is recognized as indispensable by adherents of any worldview, the threat to human dignity (§6) is later specified in view of a right to life even among the unborn, the severely, and even mentally, handicapped, and the permanently unconscious. Understood in such a radical sense, the value of dignity is not acknowledged by secular society. "Concern for life" has insensibly moved from the "basic level" universal to the "higher level" religious value domain.[9] The project of mustering universal agreement and cooperation thus indeed involves some (even if minimal-content-) missionary undertaking, the (anti-niche-aspect imposed) secular acceptability of which will have to be separately ascertained.

To what, then, does the Protestant church's pro-life position in bioethics specifically amount? And, how does it realize that church's twofold public commitment? Our concern with Christian specifics makes it advisable to leave aside whatever was generally acknowledged by secular society in Germany either at the time of the publication or today,[10] and was added to the declaration because of the churches' commitment to "truth" as "the whole". We will restrict ourselves to those ethical positions which the churches endorse on their own, and in the face of a non-universal and non-majority secular consent. These can be divided into prohibitions and enjoinders.

The most important prohibition concerns the killing of innocent human life (IV 2, §1). This prohibition encompasses human beings from the moment of conception (IV 4, a) through all phases of ever so handicapped, reduced, suffering and care-intensive, *in vitro*, *in utero*, and *extra utero* existence up to the completion of the dying process (IV 5, §2). Abortions, whether for eugenic or medical reasons, are illegitimate (VI 2, c, §1#1, and b, §2).[11]

Another firm prohibition concerns the integrity of the human genetic heritage. Genetherapy, gene-transfer and other interventions in the human germ-line are classified as ethically unacceptable (III 3, b). Somewhat in contrast to that overall opposition, in a later chapter the declaration permits germ line interventions, even if these do affect future generations, as long as they are designed to treat the particular fetus in question (VI 3, i, §5). Here the German churches were even more permissive than the *European Bioethics Convention* (Council, 1997).[12]

Enjoinders addressed to individuals, (church-) communities, and society at large (both with respect to its normative culture and to its political institutions and legal structure) permeate the document as a whole. They all are centered around, on the one hand, efforts at protecting life and opposing abortions (see I 3 §1, IV 4 f, V 3, §5, with suggestions concerning supportive measures occupying the very extensive section 2 of chapter VI) and the instrumentalization of pre-birth human beings (VI 1, §5). On the other hand, these enjoinders supporting families in general, and respecting, caring for and socially integrating the handicapped in particular (VI 3, c, §2, F §§1, 3, 5, g) as well as respecting and caring for the old and the dying (VI 5, a, §§2, 3, f). Both educational efforts at raising society's value consciousness with regard to human life in all its forms, and practical solidarity for preventing situations of suffering and helplessness are demanded. Thus, the two major causes of threats to human life, ignorance and need, are to be removed.

The two following sections (A and B) will explore how this determined pro-life stand is both supported by Protestantism's biblical foundations and rendered secularly acceptable. As a result, the Protestant view of the relationship between those two commitments can be specified in greater detail (C) and interpreted in view of what it means for Christianity to be thus publicly presented. In a final section, the implications of this interpretation for the Protestant church's role vis-à-vis her surrounding, largely secularized society will be drawn out (D).

A. *The Underlying Biblical Truths*

God is the source of life, which encompasses both created (natural) and promised life in Christ, through Whom created life was made (II 1, §1). Thus, natural life is permeated with God's own life. And thus, if we may supplement the text, life on earth, as a gift of its Creator, has not thereby been "given away", but remains in God's hand, subject to His exclusive disposition. In particular, no infringement on innocent human life can, therefore, be licit (II 4, §2).

Restricting our consideration to human life, the fact that its natural aspect is "permeated" by God's own life is taken to explain that humans' natural life does not constitute an ultimate value. Accordingly, dying is not the ultimate evil but can be accepted. Even more so: "whoever wants to secure his <natural> life will lose it", and "whoever loses it for my <Christ's> sake, will save it <the promised life>" (Mt. 16:25 ff., cf. II 1, see also III 3, c, §1#4). Accordingly, human judgments about a life's value (which could motivate infringing on it) are illicit. Even more, devoting one's life to the service of one's neighbor, as in the care for a handicapped child or a sick or dying relative, is not an ultimate evil but instead realizes humans' highest calling and permits them to find their own life (IV 3, c, §1#3).

The world in which we live is fallen (II 3): it is characterized by sin, which ultimately rests on the hubris of not acknowledging the limits imposed by one's createdness and wanting to determine what is "good" independently of God, and by the wrong attitude toward death. The commandment "thou shalt not kill" (II 4, §2, IV 2, §1) does not exhaust what is required of humans: they are enjoined to invest the works of the life-giving spirit (love, peace, goodness, faithfulness, gentleness, justice) in their dealings with every living being (II 4, §3).

It is not death itself, but only the sinful desire to altogether abolish death, which is evil (II 5). Thus, not only is the prospect of one's own dying not in itself an evil (as developed already above), but the non-accepting of one's eventual death is sinful and must be overcome by reference to a life in God that overcomes death. The experience of painful or early death generates the desire to escape death. This is why the Bible enjoins us to remember our own mortality.

The fallen world longs for deliverance; its suffering is placed in a perspective of hope (II 6, §1). Humans are unable to work out that deliverance on their own, they must be patient (§2). Yet, just as in present human life there are signs of the coming salvation of eternal life (II 7), so too the promised new life can be realized "as through signs" with the help of human action (VII, §3). That promised eternal life, thus, is not restricted to humans' afterlife (VII, §1). Through Christ's victory over death it is already present for faith (§3). It rests on confidence in God's faithfulness and on a hope that defies whatever encumbers and endangers the present life: none of it will be permanent, therefore, none of it is ultimately decisive (VII, §2).

Creation is entrusted to man's cultivation and preservation (III 3, §1). But this position of dominance is limited by accountability to God (III 3, §§1, 2): it must be exercised in the service of life (§4), preserving the multiplicity of species and preserving what is "natural" about nature and "human" in humans (III 3, b).

In what concerns man's dealing with his fellow men, the fact of his having been created in the image of God (IV 1 §1) constitutes his unique dignity, which – along with his life (IV 2, §3) – must be unconditionally respected and valued in each individual (IV 1, b). This value of human life rests not on any function or achievement (IV 2, c, §1#1), but on his having been accepted by God in Christ (§1). Such value also encompasses unborn humans (IV 4, d, VI 2, c, §1#1). This image-relationship implies a Divine call into community with God (IV 1, d). Humans are thus enjoined to serve life (VII, § 4) and to protect it with all their might.

Whatever God gives, especially in the form of human life, is a blessing for the bearers of that life and all fellow humans (IV 6, §2). This includes the sick, the handicapped, the elderly (IV 6, a) and young children (b). These blessings may take the form of difficult challenges, but God's help is near (IV 7, §2). Unexpected events, even if they present hardships, will be transformed for the good among those who love God (IV 8, §3). Moral education is oriented toward the forming of conscience, and rests on the conviction that humans' conscience is oriented towards God's creative will and His promise (V 1, §3).

Looking back at the biblical truths thus invoked and at the manner of their invocation in the text, at the bioethical problems addressed, and at the bioethical positions taken, a number of critical observations present themselves.

A.1. The Testimony of the Biblical Authors is Relativized as Insufficient for Answering the Bioethical Challenges of Today (II, §2)

The authors claim that technological progress has rendered questionable much that was taken for granted in biblical times (II, §2). Yet, insofar as the church's encompassing pro-life stand could be adequately backed by reference to God's creation and the acceptance and salvation of all forms of human life, the enhanced technical possibilities for even well-meaningly jeopardizing such life do not seem to make much difference. Moreover, the causes for such jeopardizing were said to lie in human inconsiderateness, sloth and conscious passivity (IV 8, §2), value-ignorance and situations of suffering and need. Accordingly, contemporary Christians do not seem to be in a position much different from that of biblical times (at least, when one thinks of regional devastation and depopulation through war, infectious diseases (II, §2), and abortion).

A.2. *Categories that Traditionally Belong to a Biblical Account of Ethical Prohibitions and Obligations, and that are Pertinent to the Biomedical Issues at Stake, are Either Treated with Considerable Discretion or Avoided Altogether*

This holds for – at the very least – sin, chastity and the command to multiply.

a. Sin. In its first occurrence that term is bracketed as a "way of speaking" that occurs in the Bible.[13] A little later, the authors endorse that way of speaking, but only by calling the biblical insight into man's evilness "valid" (II 4). In III 2, §5, "the power of sin" is said to "show itself in man" through "denial of life, obliviousness, hatred..." and so forth, suggesting the occurrence of sin in man to be something like a natural phenomenon (see, for example, §1). Moreover, even though killing an innocent human being violates God's command, the act of destroying embryos in medical research (VI 1, §4), or in abortion (at the scale of 200,000 per year, VI 2, §1) is never explicitly classified as "sinful".[14] The only unconditional affirmation of the term occurs in the context of atomic weapons and gene technology (III 3, §5).

b. Chastity. The fact that unwanted pregnancies occur as an unforeseeable event (IV 8) is noted as one of the difficulties that confront women who are not ready for a child. The authors rightly distinguish between principally unforeseeable disasters and the results of carelessness, inattention or voluntary passiveness (IV 8, §2). But when they draw the pertinent conclusion that such attitudes are irresponsible, they address exclusively technological and scientific developments, not, for example, pre-(extra-) marital sex. Accordingly, the term "renunciation" is used in the context of ecology exclusively (as in III 2, §6). To be sure, the authors set the goal of strengthening responsibility in partnering and sexual relationships (VI 2, b, §2#1), but neither abstinence nor chastity are mentioned.[15]

c. The enjoinder to multiply. This Divine command (1. Mos. 1, 28) is entirely absent from the church's discussion of abortion. In a document portraying God as "a friend of life", and in a societal context (Germany) that is not particularly harassed by problems of overpopulation, this absence is surprising.[16]

A.3. *The Church's Position with Regard to These Three Categories is Presented in much Weaker Terms than the Biblical Foundations Warrant*

a. With regard to abortion. Both in the introductory survey (§9) and in the main text (IV 4, b), the goal of protecting life *in utero* is relativized by reference to the specific dependence of the fetus from its mother (the fetus cannot be protected against her will) and the fact that it is psychologically difficult to perceive an early embryo as a human being (IV 4, c and e, §1##2, 3). The text here becomes ambiguous (IV 4, e §1#1): children may be a burden (IV 6, b, §2), sufficient time for considerate decisionmaking is often lacking (IV 2, a, §1), pregnancies may disrupt someone's life plan (VI 2, a, §2) or a couples relationship (VI 2, a, §2), families may exert pressure (VI 2, a, §2),[17] and special emphasis is given to the fact that the limits of what someone can bear cannot be generalized (IV 7, §3), even if such limits never justify denying another's right to life (§4, see also VI 2, c, §1#3). The final part of the statement is immediately trivialized by reference to cases in which the life of the fetus endangers the life of the mother. The preceding part is weakened by a turn to the mother's environment: to her need of help and, when she opted to have an abortion, to the necessity of a charitable response.

While such self-critical (VI 2, c, §1##4, 7) charity is repeatedly endorsed, the traditional task of the church to proclaim clearly against trespasses (in order that the sin – which must be judged – can even effectively be distinguished from the sinner – who should not be judged) is neglected.[18] Moreover, the trespass of God's commandment is disassociated from a self-centered infringement on another's life (VI 2, c, §1#6). Since self-centered (rather than God-centered) ways of defining what is "good" and "evil" for oneself had once constituted the essence of sin (II 3), that disassociation separates sin from trespassing God's commandment. The conclusion seems to be that we sometimes simply have to trespass, and that what ultimately counts is whether we do so in an inconsiderately self-centered way or out of desperation. Here as well, the authors de-emphasize clarity in exposing sin in favor of charity in not exposing sinners.[19]

b. With regard to chastity. In the rather extensive section that enters more deeply into responsibility in partnering and sexuality (VI 2, e, 2), marriage is acknowledged as the divinely indicated institution (§2).[20] Yet in the following sub-sections, premature sexual relationships among young adolescents are considered only in view of their lacking psychological independence (#1), of their (claimed) earlier biological maturity (#2) that is not matched by emotional maturity, of general egoism (##2-5), and of fears that stand in the way of commitment to marriage. The wide-spread disregard for the latter's divine institution is thus represented in terms of psychological and sociological impediments, rather than in terms of simple disapproval. On the contrary, the realization of one's own sexual feelings and openness for the partner's needs are claimed to "require, especially among adolescents, possibilities for development" (§3).

c. With regard to multiplying. The declaration mentions family planning. That concept, of course, in secular contexts is usually associated with reducing, rather than increasing the blessing children are affirmed to constitute. The issues recommended for consideration in this regard – including the well-being of the potential child, the well-being of the parents, their soul- and spirit-capacities and material means, the well-being of the siblings, of the family as a whole, as well as of society in general, and the need to protect women from too short an interval between pregnancies – each seem rather more relevant for reducing than augmenting the number of one's potential children.

A.4. Some of the Positions Go Beyond What the Biblical Foundations Warrant

Human dominance over creation must be exercised "in the service of all life" (III 3, §4). It must preserve the right to existence of other living beings – except for the sake of satisfying man's survival and averting danger (III 3, §4). Gene-therapy on humans (III 3, b, §1) is considered ethically illegitimate not because of presupposed research involving the instrumentalization of fetuses (since that latter argument is introduced by "furthermore"). The main reason offered concerns a regard for "the human" in humans (b, §1). Yet, disease had been classified under life threatening powers, the opposition to which was legitimate. Man's victory over infectious diseases was even hailed (III 3, §3). Thus, if diseases are not linked with human-ness in a way that would warrant objecting to their extinction, and to the annihilation of viruses causing such disease, why should genetic disease (apart from the risk presently involved in its therapy) be treated differently?

The exploitation of nature's genetic material for the development of medicines is objected to not only in view of risks to the environment, but also in view of the preservation of species multiplicity. The theological principle according to which natural entities' right to existence may be overruled to avert danger is thereby violated.

The peculiar manner in which the document's biblical foundations are treated can be explained when we turn to the second commitment of its author-churches.

B. Secular Acceptability

In invoking their biblical sources, the authors were guided by the conviction that what these sources suggest should be acceptable to non-Christians as well (Introductory survey, §4, again verbatim II, §1). The document's overall goal is the awakening of a will in all members of society to actively protect life in all its phases and against all dangers. While for Christians this goal represents a divinely imposed obligation as well as a demand of neighbor love, for politicians it corresponds to the demands of justice and solidarity, and for all non-Christians it is an issue of self interest (Survey, §16). Accordingly, the protection of life is a task not only for Christians. When practically implementing this task, the ability to identify one's actions (as "Christian", so we must add) is less important than cooperating with others of different world views (I 3, §1). Moreover, "even though the concept of person is construed differently today in theology, the law, and philosophy", what the document establishes as a "matter of fact" concerning persons is held to be "independent of such conceptual construals" (IV 3, final §).

On the basis of such confessions, it becomes understandable why the value of the Bible for providing ethical orientation for modern biomedicine should have been a little downplayed, why unfashionable biblical categories and claims were treated somewhat obliquely, and why general ecological concerns were presented strongly, whereas the illegitimacy of abortion was presented rather more muffledly. While biblically not supported, these differences in outspokenness were obviously designed to meet the expectations of a secular audience.

Let us disregard the question of whether the bioethical pro-life position endorsed by the churches could in fact be hoped to win secular support. Let us attend exclusively to what the author churches intended. If what Christianity has to offer is thought not to add anything ethically substantial to what is secularly assessable, why were biblical foundations invoked in the first place?

But it may perhaps be altogether inappropriate to reduce the declaration's purpose to the defending of ethical positions. The unique contribution of Christianity, which could render issuing a church position paper still worthwhile, if it does not exist on the content level, may still lie in its evocative power, or in its empowering function for rendering those ethical positions operative in humans' lives. The introductory survey, after all, does not promise ethical analysis but rather places a call towards common pro-life efforts, which the Christian perspective encourages (III 2, §6). Let us pursue this hypothesis by asking why there should have been any need for encouragement in this regard.

With regard to the protection of life in general, as addressed above, the text implicitly addresses a series of dilemmas concerning the finitude of man's life, the forces of destruction threatening the environment, the place of human life within that environment, and the problem of misfortune in individuals' lives.

First dilemma: If the principle that each human life must be treated with awe is no longer sustained by a society, that society will gradually degenerate into accepting more and more encompassing murderous practices. On the other hand, if each human life is held to be infinitely precious, a society may develop more and more senseless medical activism for the sake of keeping humans alive. How should pro-life activity be thought to steer between such equally undesirable alternatives?

Second dilemma: Faced with the ever more overwhelming impact of natural as well as man made forces of destruction, we have noted a contrast between, on the one hand, reckless unconcern, exaggerated demands, blind realization of self interest, the illusion that everything can be managed, unethical dispositions and, on the other hand (and in part even as underlying these life denying tendencies), a widely experienced sense of fear, of disorientation, lack of meaning, loneliness, and resignation (I 2, §2).

Third dilemma: Still, wherever such extremes have been avoided, concern for the environment has often given rise to exaggerated conceptions of man as "partner" of the animal and plant population, with a resulting overall hostility to scientific and technological infringements on nature. These hinder a fruitful cooperation between different segments of society for the protection of life on earth. How should the line between "awe-" and "utility-" motivations be drawn?

Fourth dilemma: Dramatic negative occurrences in individuals' lives acutely disrupt their confidence in life's benevolent design, and render them unable to see any sense in ethical striving.

Quite clearly, the biblical backing the churches have offered for their bioethical as well as their more general pro-life positions provides a resource for resolving those dilemmas, and thus for removing their efforts-discouraging impact.

First: Once humans' life (and health, see V 5, §1) is acknowledged as a gift of God, its inviolability can be asserted. At the same time, its finitude (as well as the uncertainty of health, V 5, §3#2) can be accepted in view of the divinely promised afterlife (and of the hidden blessing Christians recognize in illness and suffering, V 5, §3#2).

Second: Once God's promise that He will not desert this world is taken seriously, no threats of catastrophe can be experienced as ultimately disturbing. On the other hand, once God's enjoinder to life serving work is accepted in the context of that promise, a strong motivation for cooperating with God's creative will can be derived. That is, once God's loving gift of our life-world is gratefully acknowledged, both abstaining from life-destroying actions and the call for active resistance against such actions becomes universally compelling.

Third: Once humans' call to responsible tutorship is adequately understood, both the evil-averting and the utility-enhancing ways of exercising that human dominion can be rendered compatible.[21]

Fourth: Once God's closeness to every form of human life, and His particular closeness to human weakness, suffering and handicap, is taken as an expression of His life sustaining love, even personal hardships can be "actively" accepted (IV 5, §3#2) and sustained.

In all four cases, the specific contribution of the invoked biblical sources – a contribution which indeed is utterly unavailable in secular (philosophical) terms – consists in rendering conceivable a subtle balance between accepting and pursuing the good, while yet not idolizing it, and between sustaining courage and composure in fighting or accepting an evil, the removal of which lies not in humans' power, while not losing hope. Throughout the text, the authors place strong emphasis on precisely that illusion-expelling, depression-defeating (VII, §4), meaning-asserting, exaggerated ambition-averting, yet also relaxing, confidence-instilling impact, through which their Christian perspective can be seen to encourage an active commitment to the respecting and protecting of human (and all earthly) life. The purpose of the document thus seems to lie not so much in providing a (bio-) ethical orientation, but rather in providing a (bio-) ethical motivation.

Yet, if the secular world has thus been diagnosed as beset by fear, uncertainty, lack of meaning, resignation and psychic illness (I §1, I 2, §2), how do the authors account for the fact that all have not long since flocked under the wings of so empowering a faith? Can the reason really lie in the churches' previous failure to present their message in a properly inviting, palatable, threats-avoiding form?

The problem with the suggested secular acceptability of biblically founded encouragements lies in the author churches' obliviousness with regard to the details of their implicit reasoning. Even if we disregard any difficulties which secular minds may have concerning a benevolent creator God and assume that any well disposed mind must embrace some sort of deism, still some important Christian inferences from such a deism are hard to render consistent. Let us sketch the most important clusters of problems.

1. Why, if God is a friend of life (II 1, §1), did He create life on earth as finite and reserve His ultimate pro-life stand for a promised afterlife? This is bioethically important, because accepting the finitude of one's life in this world, and achieving a balanced regard for life-sustaining medical technology, was argued to depend on there being such "another" life.[22]

2. That humans' this-worldly life has an ethical value even if they discontinue enjoying it (and that they may, therefore, not throw it away) is derived from the fact that God accepts even un-enjoyable this-worldly life (II 2, §2, to cite just one of the many places). The importance for this-worldly humans of such Divine acceptance is explained by reference to the anthropological fact that all human life has a social dimension. Yet, why that dimension, as referring to inter-human acceptance (and, in addition, often withheld from "useless" or "burdensome" human life), should be relevant for the normative fact of God's acceptance (even where humans refuse to), is secularly incomprehensible.

3. Why, even if God created earthly life as finite, is not His acceptance of that finite life sufficient? Why should there be an "ought" concerning humans' keeping God's orders (II 1, §1), and even giving up that earthly life in Christ's service (with the bioethical relevance of shouldering the burden of caring for someone else), in order to attain the promised better life? And why, if that other life is promised anyway, should we be bothered with keeping God's commands and devoting this life to the service of Christ, rather than to more immediate satisfaction, by sacrificing some others' lives if necessary?

4. How, if wishing to escape death was defined as the origin of sin (II 5), and thus the origin of the world's fall from perfection, can the wish to overcome death "arise" from that very premature and painful death that belongs to the world only "after the fall"? And how, if wishing to escape death is the origin of sin, can killing non-human fellow creatures be justified if undertaken in order to avert the danger of starving to death? And why does death, as "shaped" (II 5) by sin (i.e., by humans not wanting to die), still also need to be "overcome"? And why, if death in the fallen world is an evil that separates man from God, can it be overcome, not by (and here the bioethical problem recurs) postponing it for ever longer stretches of time, but by a life "out of God", which is (and in what sense, since we are going to die anyway) "victorious" over death (II 5, §1)?

In sum: How can an encouragement to pro-life ethical acting be derived from an account that is so deeply wrought with incomprehensibilities and incoherence? This question is especially important if that encouragement is to sustain individuals in situations which entirely disrupt their professional and private life plan, their psychological and economic means, their capacity to shoulder substantial losses in opportunity, and even to lose the basic freedom of creatively structuring their lives to "prove themselves" (IV 2, §3), and possibly for many years, or even for the whole of their earthly existence, all the while sustaining prolonged hardship and suffering, public contempt, loss of social standing. Such challenges must be addressed if that encouragement is to sustain the difficulties of mothers faced with an unwelcome pregnancy, parents faced with the prospect of a handicapped child, or children and spouses faced with the illness or permanent handicap or prolonged periods of utter helplessness of their spouses or parents. How could such a feeble base be hoped to strengthen those who also have easy access to "medical solutions" which merely sacrifice some (defenseless) one's life?[23]

Perhaps the Christian perspective provided by the declaration could still serve one important function: of recommending hope in God's help and the consolation of God's acceptance in cases where all other hope and consolation fails. Thus, as long as there is no therapy for certain kinds of handicaps or diseases, those afflicted by such a fate as well as those who devote their lives to taking care of them can console themselves with the idea that God is especially close to the weak. And once a therapy has been developed (VI 3, §3), they can gratefully abandon that last resort position. Yet, how could, secularly speaking, such a reference to God as a final *pièce de résistance* be even conceived to constitute anything but a merely cheap escape (for both the consoler and the one letting himself be consoled)?

But perhaps there is still another way of understanding the document's claimed secular acceptability. On reading the document, one is struck by the human kindness and caring that inspires its discussions. The authors go to great length in expressing their sympathetic regard for the difficulties and irresolvable conflicts in which the individual addressees of their bioethical positions may find themselves, and which stand in the way of their ability to obey God's commands. As noticed above, they even demand respect for those who are incapable of that obedience (VI 2, d, §7), and take great care to protect such unfortunate ones from others' disparagement. Quite clearly, the Gospel of God's encompassing love is being communicated in a humanly loving manner. Thus, in the final analysis, the claimed harmony between biblical backing and secular acceptability may be cashed in in terms of this persuasively witnessed sympathetic charity, or in this truly humane extension of "love, peace, goodness, …, gentleness and justice" which surely will be acceptable to non-Christian readers as well.

C. *The Price of the Church's Double Commitment*

The previous section has shown how the Christian message of the bioethical declaration, in order to secure its secular acceptability, had to be reduced to the humaneness of its messengers. The document's heavy emphasis on education and the media, however, bears witness to the fact that the text was not meant (as with a sermon) to stand for itself. Its purpose lies in inspiring further society-wide activities designed for the formation of consciences. It is difficult to conceive how a message that had been transformed into the medium could be helpful in this regard.[24] Would any other manner of presentation have been conceivable that could have served the Protestant church's double commitment in some more substantial sense?

What would it have taken both to remain more encompassingly true to the biblical sources and to offer a more clearly orienting guidance to even non-Christians' conscience formation? At the very least, such a strategy would have to remove the embarrassing questions compromising the rational conceivability of the churches' biblical account.

Quite obviously, the critical questions posed in the preceding section could have been answered, and the document's account of God's relationship to human, and all created, life rendered consistent, if that very Divine plan of salvation had been more thoroughly discussed, which surfaces once in a remark on God's calling humans into community with Him (IV 1, d), and another time only vaguely (and in a not salvation-oriented, but merely early-death oriented sense) in the context of "human life's ever failing to reach its design" (II 5).[25] The central question concerning the finitude of a life created by a life-loving God would have required a more faithful account of the relationship between sin and death: that death is not a natural property of created life, as the authors would have it (II 5)[26] but came into the world as a result of man's sin which consisted, as the authors aptly recognize, in his hubris.[27]

Bioethically speaking, a more candid emphasis on humans' God-given task, as placed in the horizon of their fallen nature, might have permitted the churches to take a more explicit stand on a problem which their end-of-life discussions conspicuously shun: the problem of artificial nutrition of PVS patients. The declaration's determined pro- (biological) life stand (VI 5, b, §2) disregards the question of what it means for medicine technologically to force a human being to keep living, once that human being, while clearly not dying, equally clearly has completed his task of repentance and cooperation with the Divine will.[28]

Why have the author churches introduced such substantial changes into their biblical backing? Perhaps they subsumed the causal connection between human sin and human mortality, as well as the more unsettling aspects of a final judgment, under the "religious superstition and ideology" (see p. 4) which the EKD had committed herself to criticizing. But from where would she derive her criteria for thus critically distinguishing (within her *sola scriptura* heritage) "between the spirits"? We can only guess. The consoling, reassuring, encouraging impact of their document would have been jeopardized, had they came right out with those truths. Their conspicuous silence regarding any afterlife-related details of God's plan of salvation thus becomes understandable as well. If there is a Divine plan every human is required to cooperate with, the chance of failing becomes conceivable. Trespasses on God's commandments (as in the kinds of killing the innocent or wishing to kill oneself, which are addressed in the declaration's bioethical discussion) might be recognized as likely paths towards such failing. Since the idea of a final judgment, and of salvation as requiring loving efforts at repentance and conversion, is hard to reconcile with the goal of proclaiming the Gospel to those not prepared for such a turning of heart in a non-threatening, merely inviting manner, it is conceivable that the authors considered it preferable to present human death as an integral part of life (similar to the ancient Greek philosophical idea of "becoming and perishing"), and to reduce the promised blissful afterlife to something that awaits just naturally every human being.

Quite in contrast to what the authors seem to have supposed, however, it has turned out that only by including the proper biblical understanding of sin and man's Divine calling can the vexing incoherence of the manner in which God is presented as "a friend of life" be overcome. Only on the basis of such an understanding is there at least a chance of offering something substantial, into which a secular reader could be non-trivially invited.[29] Such "inviting", of course, would be understood not as a predominantly worldly and humane *diakonia*, but as missionary in the traditional sense.

Why have the churches abandoned that traditional task? The answer for Protestantism must be sought by attending to that church's more general institutional self-understanding, to its view of its place in the world.

D. *The EKD's Understanding of the Protestant Church's Place in the World*

The most important addressee of the document, or at least the addressee to whom the most space is devoted, is society as a whole and its individual members, insofar as they take part in, shape and influence the life of that civil, legal, and political society (V 4, §6).[30] The particular manner in which the authors address society reveals that they understand their churches as societal forces. They acknowledge the secular, liberal democratic framework not in the sense of merely obeying its laws and policies, but of "basing themselves on" those laws and policies (V 1, 3, §2). They pervasively endeavor to challenge society in view of that framework's own normative commitments. The proclamation of the church's own bioethical position is explicitly designed for seeking a general societal consensus (V I, 3, §2).[31]

That this is no trivial undertaking is recognized by the authors. They point to the contradictory tendencies characterizing public opinion in view of the ethical status of unborn life (IV 4, §1) and of abortion (VI 2, b, §1). Still they consider it both "necessary and promising to define a common goal for the whole of society" (VI 2, b, §1, see also survey §9).[32] Obviously, such a difficult goal demands that the threshold for the articles of faith to be invoked must be kept low. Rallying for political influence is incompatible with confessing any truths that go beyond what is – at least in theory – widely acknowledged (or what, if not acknowledged, at least hurts no moral majority's feelings). This appeal to a common foundation underlies the whole (Albert-Schweitzer-preciousness-of-life and Hans-Jonas-responsibility-dyed) of part I. The churches' own contribution reduces to demanding consistency[33] and embellishing the secularly professed values with a halo of biblical stories. Quite clearly, those stories must be clipped a little (especially with regard to sin and death), so as not to awaken secular concern.[34] One must also abide by the rules of political correctness: one may chime in with popular concern about technological hubris, castigate eugenic tendencies as a heritage of Nazism (IV 5, §1), sympathetically respond to fears concerning natural disaster, demand more public funds for humanitarian purposes, but avoid touching on a socially unwelcome notion such as chastity, and tread altogether lightly on the issue of abortion. That is, the churches certainly castigate the practice of abortions in general as a deplorable social phenomenon (this is even expected of them), but they must carefully avoid appearing judgmental on a personal level, since this would violate the liberal taboo against intolerance.[35]

A church that understands her mission of cooperation with God's kingdom on earth as contributing (somewhat at odds with Christ's apocalyptic warnings) to a life-friendly society, and that pursues this mission by influencing the public's value awareness and by pressing for public solidarity funds and policy support, does not ultimately rely on the individual's grace-supported change of heart. Such a church sees the origin of life destroying acts not as lying in individuals' free (and wrong) decisions, but in normatively environmental and economic factors (VI 2, e, 5, §5, VI 2, c, §1#2). She consequently invests her energies in supporting secularly acceptable ethical positions, and in preventing those situations of need and hardship, in which the conflict between individuals' worldly cares and their – still desirable – obedience to God's commands must appear irresolvable, and where disobedience for that reason is excusable.[36]

To secure the societal consensus needed to retain that political influence indispensable for realizing her societal goals, the Protestant Church in Germany, as far as her declaration *Gott ist ein Freund des Lebens* goes, has adjusted her theological commitments to such an extent that her Christian position appears blurred.[37] Those whom the Protestant church wished to invite into her faith perspective on bioethics can follow that invitation only if they vigorously avoid thinking clearly, and instead faithfully abide by the vagueness of the concepts that are made available.

III. Im Geist der Liebe mit dem Leben umgehen

The document *Im Geist der Liebe mit dem Leben umgehen* is noticeably not the work of an inter-church-committee (as was the previous declaration), but of a more homogeneously Protestant working group. Perhaps due to the greater portion of lay members among its authors, this document places greater emphasis on argumentative stringency.[38] Surely the fundamental and irresolvable disagreement among the members of the chamber developing the document, which concerned the crucial question of pre-birth humans' entitlement to full protection, rendered some presentational discipline in portraying the consequences of and exposing the grounds for that disagreement imperative.

We shall assess the resulting changes in the Protestant church's bioethical positions and in what she conceives to be her role within secular society under four perspectives regarding the relationship of Christianity to the secular world (A), the specific nature of Christian ethics (B), constraints for Protestant position taking (C), and the public role of the Protestant church (D).

A. *"Heil" Versus "Heilung": Christianity as an Added Option*

Greater stylistic cogency has its price. Whereas the combination of thematic treatment and the "bits and pieces" of theological reasoning that were strewn throughout the former document left a certain space for interpretations that might emphasize a more comprehensive regard for the truths of the Christian faith, the more streamlined argument of the latter document fixes its meaning to a more clearly circumscribed account. The tendency to posit a homogeneity between Christian and secular experiences of and attitudes towards death, disease, and the endangered-ness of life in general, or to conceive of Christianity as something that can be superadded to an otherwise integral secular life, which was observable already in the former document, is thereby strengthened. The declaration still wavers between, on the one hand, both the *memento mori* principle as a moral and spiritual component of the Christian life (II 5) and the interpretation of human suffering in the context of "God's transforming a burden into a blessing" (IV 7, §2) and, on the other hand, the acknowledgement of the blessings of modern medicine in postponing death and curing disease (III 3, §3). In contrast, the latter document not only acknowledges the fact of disease and death as givens of human life, but also endorses avoiding or postponing them (respectively) as worthy pursuits (p. 9). It thus establishes a common ground for both secular and Christian understandings. The specific contribution of Christianity reduces to granting greater immunity against exaggerations concerning those latter pursuits: Christians know that apart from cure and life in this world (concern for which they share with their secular environment) there exists a salvation in another world (p. 10). The idea that this additional hope may have something to do with a non-worldly manner of shaping one's life in one's worldly environment has effectively vanished.

B. "Love" Before "Law": Christian Ethics as Accommodating Secular Constraints

Greater argumentative stringency encourages explicit acknowledgement. Such acknowledgement integrates into the church's ethical self-understanding what could only be hypothetically imputed in the earlier document: the side-by-side proclamation of general norms (the law) and of the need for charitable leniency in cases of extreme conflict (*Einzelfallgerechtigkeit*, p. 15). In the former document that two-tier account had been interpreted as indicative of a weakness in biblical orientation, or of a compromised biblical faithfulness in view of secular acceptability that could not be understood but as motivated by a quest for political influence and a betrayal of the Gospel's truth to societal consensus. Here, in contrast, that two-tieredness is advertised as a consequence of the fact that life can present very real normative impasses (p. 14) and as a realization of the principle that love should rule supreme (p. 15). As Christianity imposes a loving regard for "individuals' particular needs" and limited possibilities, as well as for the constraints of their situation, acknowledging that tragic exceptions to the imposed rule-obedience are possible is presented as bearing witness to that humane sensitivity in the context of which "the law" must be understood. Thus, some cases of eugenic abortion are classified as "action in a dilemma" (p. 26).[39]

"Christian love", defined as "protecting and furthering the other even with regard to his perceived needs and vulnerability" (p. 15) is here conceived in exclusively human terms. It leaves no room for questioning individuals' perceived needs and vulnerability by reference to a Divine love for humans that expresses itself in the saving gift (not only, but clearly also – see Mt. 5:17-19, 7:21) of the law. Neediness and vulnerability are thus taken as absolute, and are separated from underlying, perhaps mistaken or misguided, value choices and life decisions. Even though there is still a sense for the Christian inappropriateness of, for example, excessive obsession with planning and self determination (p. 26), the perception of the Christian life as imposing very specific (and secularly inaccessible) value choices and life decisions is lost. Or while the (Judaeo-) Christian interpretation of neighbor love traditionally gave priority to the context of "loving God with all one's heart and with all one's might and all one's powers" (Mt. 22:37, thus making obedience supreme), here a resolutely human understanding of neighbor love is given priority over love of God, and is engaged as a criterion concerning when obedience to His commandments is "livable" and, therefore, imperative.

C. *The Protestant Culture of Ethical Disagreement*

The "dialectic" (p. 15) of rule and exception thus endorsed as an integral part of Christian ethics is claimed to be responsible for differences in the ethical evaluation of individual cases (p. 15) and thus for ethical dissension within the church. This conclusion once again illustrates the purely human character of the authors' conception of Christian love: at least traditionally that latter principle had been thought to unify, rather than to divide the church (Eph. 4:2 ff).

But this conclusion also does not even support the ethical dissension subsequently discussed. That dissension concerns not problems in the application of generally acknowledged rules, but a problem in the formulation of such a rule: under what conditions is a "becoming human" entitled to full legal protection? According to one view (which will be called "strict"), that entitlement unconditionally holds from the moment of conception, because this moment establishes the beginning of a human being whom God has accepted. According to the other ("lenient") view, a fertilized egg is a "becoming human" in the full sense only within a properly supportive environment, but does enjoy some limited protection even independently of such an environment. Only the latter, not the former position, therefore, accepts IVF (and also limits the fertilization of ova to those which will be implanted, p. 45) and PID, irrespective of the destructive implications of both techniques for the early fetus. Only that latter position also accepts research on embryos that were discarded in the course of these techniques.

There is a strange duplicity in the council's attitude to that dissension. On the one hand, it is presented as harmless: ethical judgments belong to the sphere of each individual's personal responsibility before God.[40] The Protestant church's obligation to provide unequivocal guidance (and shun dissension) is restricted to fundamental questions of faith (p. 4). On the other hand, the invocation of the love-inspired virtues of honestly facing conflicts (p. 3), listening to one another, correcting and accepting corrections, as well as the cultivation of mutual recognition among the opponents (p. 42) is situated in a context of hope for an eventual agreement (pp. 16, 29, 43).[41] This hope cannot entirely be restricted to concern for the social consequences of the lenient position (p. 28). It reflects an uneasy feeling vis-à-vis the claimed harmlessness of intra-church ethical disagreement, which might even reveal a sense of the difficulties involved in thus separating dogma from ethos, with only individuals' respectively different consciences as a buffer in between. And indeed, when it comes to asserting dogmatic unity in the face of ethical dividedness (p. 15), that dogmatic unity is not specified. It is replaced by "some view toward man and human life"

(p. 15) that is claimed to be derivable from the supposedly common dogmas. As the bioethical dissension however reveals, it is precisely that supposedly common view of man (in view of the normative significance of factors influencing his becoming), which is split between an "absolutist" and an "environmentalist" approach. The Protestant church's anthropological commonality is thus merely verbal.

Moreover, as further discussion shows, the "lenient" position restricts ethical legitimacy not only in view of the biological environment of the embryo, but also in view of the human-life-producing agent's intention towards realized humanity. Accordingly, the fertilization of human eggs for research purposes is illegitimate (pp. 33, 45), whereas the use of clones from a developing human for therapeutic purposes is legitimate (p. 33). Or more specifically: manufacturing human beings for the purpose of instrumentalizing them is not permitted by the original egg-plus-sperm method (which would be an illegitimate trespass onto God's creative design), but is permitted when achieved by extracting totipotent cells from a developing human being (who will not thereby be damaged). The difference then between the ethically strict and lenient positions cannot be restricted to the ethical realm after all. Contrary to what the document claims concerning the common theological assumption of acceptance through God as the root of the human being as a person and of his dignity (p. 23), the ethical difference does imply a difference in the theological perception of that to-be-believed Divine will, which unconditionally obliges humans' cooperation and which determines, how the law "thou shalt not kill" must be understood. According to one account, God accepts humans unconditionally from the moment of fertilization as His beloved creatures. According to the other account, (for which no specific biblical support is offered) God is much more complicated: He withholds His loving acceptance until a proper biological environment has been secured (with the question left undecided of how He would respond to artificial uteri that might be designed to save some human life within a dying mother), but retains enough loving acceptance even for those outside of such an environment to oppose having them simply fabricated. Still, however, He must limit His opposition to having them fabricated "from scratch", while not worrying at all about those developing human beings who are cloned into existence, but only for therapeutic purposes, and as long as they are efficiently kept from ever becoming full humans (as in reproductive cloning). In short, on the one hand, we are enjoined to believe in an entirely inflexible, conceptually satisfying but human-freedom-limiting God, on the other hand in a rather research-friendly and humanitarian-intention-accommodating one. Which is to say: the doctrinal integrity of a Protestant church that responds to the bioethical challenges of our time can be maintained only at the price of strategic vagueness.

D. The Church as a Societal Risk Factor

Given these rather more fundamental disagreements, it is understandable that the council responsible for publicizing the document restricted its project to "Argumentative support concerning burning medical and bioethical questions". The project of providing ethical orientation had to be abandoned in favor of an endeavor of mapping out what it means to be a Protestant Christian of the one or other variety. Acceptable Protestantism in ethics is not limited to the two positions portrayed: it encompasses whatever can be packed into the notion of theology- and church-related considerations (p. 16). Moreover, the two positions presented are merely ideal types, so that numerous combinations between elements of the one with elements of the other present a bioethical *Markt der Möglichkeiten* (to take up a famous motto that is included in any Protestant church festival in Germany).

With regard to the church's public role in secular society, facing such internal disagreement has led to a greater affinity with the German law's pro-human-life implications. Whereas *Gott ist ein Freund des Lebens* simply assumed the strict position and simply claimed that this is also what the German constitution endorses, this later document acknowledges the indecisiveness of what the German constitutional court has been ruling during the last 30 years (p. 11). The church's already very modestly relativized claim for providing ethical orientation within secular society has been abandoned in favor of merely "posing ethical questions" and "opening ethical horizons", which the ever more liberal (official) German Protestantism of the last decades has been practicing all along (as a kind of fallback position).

Yet underneath disagreement concerning (different varieties of) strict and lenient positions in bioethics, there lurks a more fundamental disagreement concerning the significance of such ethical dissension for society. Some members of the chamber work group believe that ethical dissension, while tolerable within theology, can reach a level of seriousness that hurts[42] secular social cohesion. Others believe that what theology can accommodate in terms of value pluralism can also be accommodated by a secular society (p. 42). Whereas in the olden days society had been believed to need the cohesive glue of a common religion, at least modern Protestantism is thus acknowledged as having lost its glue-factor. It is even discussed whether its disunity might threaten social life. But then it is also no longer clear, whether the mapping service the document wishes to offer is helpful or harmful for secular society. The very project of the church's entering the public arena has become problematic.

The authors are confident that the church still has something important to contribute to her secular environment. Irrespective of internal dissent, there are common enemies out there worth defeating: the exaggerated and irresponsible speed with which new technological developments are implemented (p. 43), the undifferentiated presentation of bioethical problems in the media (pp. 43 f, see also p. 26 note 16), the reduction of humanness to the biological (pp. 17 f), and utilitarianism (pp. 46 f). And there are, of course, all those bioethical positions concerning which – as a kind of residual consensus – all Protestants can still agree (pp. 44 ff).

If we look at these contributions in more detail, they are not impressive. With regard to tutiorism, secularly grounded warnings are also available. One does not need a Creator-God (and in particular a triune personal one) to take an (already merely) utilitarian interest in natural resources and conceptual clarity. With regard to utilitarianism and biologism, there exist secular philosophical resources to oppose them. Perhaps these resources are not as audible in public as when supported by the church. But that support in turn is problematic already in view of utilitarianism itself. After all, like Christian ethics (p. 15), utilitarianism opposes exclusive attention to principles. Like Christian ethics (p. 15), at least rule utilitarianism also respects rules. And just like the Christian ethics the Protestant church endorsed, certain types of utilitarianism endorse a humanly loving concern for the particular individual with his needs and vulnerabilities, and for the kinds of consequences rule obedience would have for any such individual cases. Such utilitarians, just like the Protestants of this document, will therefore accept exception-making even to the rules they endorse.

Moreover, if we consider that residual consensus which still links the different ethical positions acknowledged by the Protestant church as represented by this document, it does not stand much closer scrutiny. Just consider the supposedly common ban on abortion. Why should (for the lenient position) God's withholding His loving acceptance from those becoming humans who lack their needed environment not extend beyond the biological? Why should this not include the mother's psychological ability "to accept" what she might otherwise keep providing the biological environment for? Why should that withholding not also extend even further, to parents' post-birth psychological or economic ability "to accept" what they might otherwise keep providing the social environment for. Once environmental considerations are permitted to enter into one's conception of what God lovingly accepts (and only subsequently imposes definite no-kill obligations), it becomes hard (given that in this analysis there are no biblical bearings to guide one concerning how to distinguish normatively among different kinds of environment) to draw a conceptually compelling line. The authors of the document rightly observe this with regard to IVF connected to PIDs (p. 27): that becoming humans will be subjected to life-worth-living-judgments, can be extended to very general, murder-friendly ethical conclusions against which the lenient position provides no conceptual or theological safeguards.

Accordingly, it seems that it may be dangerous to give the church a public voice in a secular society which still sustains a broad bioethical consensus against killing infants before they have the ability of surviving outside of their maternal (or even parental) environment.

IV. Conclusion

Our examination of those characteristic positions, in which the bioethical statements issued by the Protestant church in Germany (EKD) during the last 27 years differ from what is generally acknowledged in secular society (and has framed its laws and policies), has revealed that the biblical backing offered for those positions has become somewhat diffuse. Most significantly, the evaluation of human mortality and morbidity has changed in such a way as to remove the difference Protestant Christianity once made with regard to the meaning of life, of suffering and human finitude. Christianity's specific orientation towards a promised after-life is in the great majority of documents either explicitly or implicitly disassociated from sin as the origin of that mortality and morbidity (and thus from a final judgment concerning the character of one's personal afterlife). Accordingly, the validity of Christianity's moral norms is either disregarded (as with chastity and the enjoinder to multiply), or limited by a regard for "what is livable" among humans (as with the "do not kill"-commandment, as directed against biomedical practices such as abortion, IVF, PID, research on human embryos, physician-assisted suicide, and euthanasia). Concern for that latter commandment has been transferred to the securing of societal conditions which support such "livability".

With the weakening of the biblical (and liturgical) anchoring of the Protestant church's public pronouncements, the endorsement of ethical dissension (in the last document *Im Geist der Liebe mit dem Leben umgehen*) comes as no surprise. The more the German

Protestantism embodied in those pronouncements is intended to secure their secular acceptability at the price of theological substance, and the more the Protestant church publicly embraces some faintly Christian shade of generic religiosity (as in the idolization of biological survival at the expense of regard for their spiritual journey to God, which the unlimited endorsement of life-sustaining technology among patients who are not yet in the process of dying suggests), the more German Protestantism weakens its normative resources. It is incorporating that normative pluralism in secular society, which it had traditionally been intended to restrain. The more concern for the truth of the Gospel is limited by concern for societal consensus, the more that very consensus will be jeopardized.

Acknowledgement

We wish to thank Kurt Schmitt for his kind help in finding the relevant literature.

Notes

1. The predicate "Protestant" does not quite do justice to how that church understands itself. Yet the commonly used term "evangelisch" in German is distinguished from "evangelikal", and thus from a group of (rather more Bible oriented) Protestant communities and churches which sometimes (as for example with regard to negotiations with Roman Catholics on common doctrine) take a critical position vis-à-vis the EKD. This (rather crucial) distinction is lost in the English "Evangelical". The term "Lutheran" is also occupied by a somewhat less mainstream German church association.
2. To be sure, the EKD does not exhaust "German Protestantism". She is "the" organizational federation of local German churches and understands herself, and is acknowledged by society as well as by politicians and by the Roman Catholic church, as representative for German Protestantism (and in this sense as "the" Protestant Church of Germany), to be sure. Yet, a sizeable number of local churches and their associations do not take that representation to extend to doctrine. Since most of those other organizations have in the past been less concerned about partaking in predominantly secular debates (they restrict themselves mostly to traditional missionary undertakings and work within the communities), it makes sense to concentrate on the statements issued by the EKD, and to refer to the other prominent public voice (that of the Evangelicals) in the notes.
3. "God is a friend of life". That document also addresses gene-technological and ecological issues which will be considered only in view of their either bioethical or theological relevance.
4. This declaration, as the authors term it, has served as point of reference for most subsequent bioethical statements which were co-authored by both churches (or by the EKD alone), as well as for the Evangelical Alliance (*idea* 3/93, p. 3). Wherever the positions of these further statements significantly differ or provide substantial additions, this will be indicated in the notes.
5. "Dealing with life in the spirit of love". Previous hopes for progress in ecumenical "growing together" had been disappointed by the failure to win the necessary universal cooperation among the German Protestant churches as well as by Cardinal Josef Ratzinger's "Dominus Jesus" pronouncement.
6. This principle is also emphasised in other EKD pronouncements, see for example the EKD president Kock's opening of the EKD bioethics conference (Pressestelle der EKD, 28 Jan. 2002, §2).
7. EKD: Kundgebung der Synode der EKD auf ihrer 4. Tagung in EKD 2001b.

8. In referring to both author churches collectively, we still shall focus on Protestantism exclusively.
9. The survey, just as the declaration as a whole, takes great pains to blur over that difference: "No one can maintain credibility", so the survey argues, if he restricts his attention to only one side of the threat (Survey §3, Section I 3, §2 f.). (The appropriateness of such blurring will be discussed further on.) The comprehensive pro-life efforts called for are claimed to be derivable from the political requirements of justice and solidarity, and from individual self interest, just as from Christian premises (§16). Yet there exists no secularly compelling argument for repudiating the possibility of separating the ban on abortion either from ecological catastrophe (the opposite seems more likely in some parts of this world), or from the legal principle of respect for autonomy, or finally from individuals' fears that their eventual chances of securing their own or their burdensome loved ones' voluntary euthanasia might be jeopardized.
10. This acknowledgement covers, apart from the general principles of respect for autonomy, limitations restricting biomedical research on human subjects (V 4, §§1-3), the appeal to individuals' personal responsibility with regard to their health (V 5, §3), objection to IVF (VI 1, §§2, 4) and to instrumentalization of embryos for research (§3), the insolvability of the conflict where a fetus threatens the life of the mother (VI 2, c, §3), the advisability of genetic counselling before marriage (VI 3, h, §2), opposition to forced sterilization for eugenic purposes (VI 3 §2) and to eugenic population programs (§3), conditions for organ donation after death (VI 4, §§2, 6 ff), the opposition to either voluntary or involuntary euthanasia (VI 5, b, c, e) and the acceptance of pain relief even under the risk of accelerating the death of a dying person (d). Other secularly not endorsed reproductive practices, such as heterological insemination, donation of ova or sperm, surrogate motherhood, and cloning were already excluded by the 1987 proclamation *Zur Achtung* (III c, d, j). In that document, the right to "genetic privacy" is also endorsed (III f). The 1990 declaration *Organspende* also endorses the secular ban on organ sale (1.2 §3). The issue of research on human stem cells will be discussed in Part II.
11. Already parents' firm decision to permit only a healthy baby to come to term is illegitimate (VI 3, h, §3). Reproductive techniques, such as IVF (in vitro fertilization), PND (pre natal diagnosis), and PID (pre implantation diagnosis), are illicit, insofar as they either from the very start involve the destruction of fertilized eggs or encourage eugenically (not even to speak of sex preference-) motivated embryo destructions or abortions. The latter two techniques might become legitimate once they permit an early therapy (VI 3, h, §3). The "Common Word" *Wieviel Wissen* specifies that even in that latter case, PID would not be legitimate if conducted on toti-potent cells (App. §1 f.).
12. This well-balanced regard for genetic integrity is present already in 1985, 1.8. A more restrictive view which forbids already somatic gene therapy (because in practice not separable from germ line interventions) is taken by the Evangelical Alliance (*idea* 3/92, p. 12).
13. "The Bible ... is characterized by the perspective that natural life ... is deeply disrupted. It denotes the powers of life disrupting and destruction with the concept of sin." (II 3).
14. There is one sentence stating that "God does not want abortions to be" (VI 2, c, §1#1). But even that is bracketed as a "sentence" that is cited "to remind the reader of the unconditional claim contained in God's commandment which wants to exclude any killing of humans" – an oddly roundabout way of proclaiming, as a church in charge of the truth of the Gospel might, "do not abort!". The Evangelical Alliance, on the other hand, does invoke the idea of guilt (*idea* 10/98, p. 7).
15. Given this quotational abstinence, it becomes significant that among the works of the Spirit of life (which were enumerated in the quote of II, §4), chastity was the only one omitted from the series. This oversight matches poorly with the fact that two of the three quotes adduced for indicating signs of the coming life in this life (II 6, §§2) pointedly proclaim against fornication: Gal. 5:16 ff, Eph. 4:17 ff).

16. We might add that the 1990 declaration *Organtransplantation* extensively discusses the subject of human dying without ever invoking the concept of God's final judgement. The 1996 *Common Word on Dying* does discuss "Paul's notion" of such a judgement, but immediately trivialises it by reference to Christ's accomplished atonement, which assures each dying Christian of a happy issue (*idea* 10/98, p. 38 f.). What is entirely lacking in the Protestant treatment of the dying process is any reference to repentance and to the need of even asking for forgiveness. Especially in that latter document, the emphasis is on "not indoctrinating" dying patients (p. 39), on respect for their closeness or distance to God, and on the sacraments, with the conspicuous exclusion of confession.
17. In IV 4, a, §2 we find the statement that "Pre-birth human life must be protected and may not be arbitrarily manipulated". Yet as neither medical researchers nor abortion seeking mothers would consider their undertakings "arbitrary", but would each adduce strong justifying reasons (either of beneficence or of irresolvable conflict), this statement does not address the relevant issue (of manipulation, merely as such, and irrespective of justifying reasons).
18. There is merely a warning concerning the physical and psychological damage such a woman might incur (VI 2, a, §3).
19. Similarly, in the treatment of PND, there is no clear demand that it should be offered exclusively to parents who expressed their willingness to accept even a handicapped child. Instead, the authors restrict themselves to demanding that the technique should not become routine (§7#1), may only be administered with consent (#2), and only if the mothers' worries cannot otherwise be alleviated (#3). These weak demands are amplified again by reference to the hardships which a handicapped child involves (§5). (A more consistently restrictive position is taken by the Evangelical Alliance, *idea* 3/93, pp. 4, 6 ff., 10).

    To be sure, the authors emphasise the ethical illegitimacy of eugenic abortions. But since they restrict God's position in the matter to be one of "inviting" into life, they implicitly leave open that what cannot be ethically justified occupies an ethically merely problematic space. This relativizing tendency is strengthened by the generalizing perspective of the following paragraphs: The consequence of habitually aborting imperfect foetuses for "changes in ethical guidelines" which "one" endorses, the ensuing changes in how "one" relates to the sick, the old, and the handicapped in general, and the corresponding changes in society's normative culture (§8) and their likely legal consequences (§9) all contribute to removing the problem from the individual to society at large (see also VI 3, I, §§2, 3).
20. Similarly, in the 1987 document on criteria for gene technology and procreative medicine, the discussion of heterologous insemination and sperm or ova donation disregards issues of chastity or of that spiritual integrity of marriage which (at least according to the 1997 *Wieviel Wissen*, §10) also encompasses a regard for the body.
21. The assumption of man's "partnership" with non-human creation also can be repudiated. This position designates an important modification of the 1987 *Zur Achtung* pronouncement, which still speaks of a "right to life" in non-human creation (II 1, II 2).
22. In the text, the fact that this-worldly life is "permeated" by God, and therefore more than merely "natural" gets "explained" in view of humans' concern for the quality of life. Surely that concern will keep a secular person from regarding the mere fact of his life as not the "only and highest value". But why that should lead one to give up continually working towards improved quality of "this" life's ever prolonged duration (and instead pursue a "better" afterlife) is secularly incomprehensible.
23. The authors seem to have sensed something of this incongruence. Rather than relying entirely on their theological conclusions, they supplement them with secular sounding appeals, which however regularly fail to be secularly compelling. Just one of the many examples: VI 2, c, §1#5 argues against abortion on the ground that a woman's right to self determination has a limit where the right to life of another human begins. Of course it is precisely the classification of a

foetus as "a human entitled to human rights" which is secularly contested. (As the authors also admit, IV 4, §1.)

24. For the two most pressing bioethical problems addressed: termination of unwanted pregnancies, merely as such, and abortion for eugenic reasons, the authors themselves admit the ineffectiveness of their value-consciousness-raising undertaking: In spite of a generally developed awareness of the problematic nature of the former, "this tendency has ... so far not yet found its expression in changed behaviour" (VI 2, e, 1, §2), and in spite of a grown acceptance of handicapped persons and a wide voluntary financial support of the "Aktion Sorgenkind" which finances services to them, still eugenic indications (which at the time of publication were still legal) continue to be widely demanded. (The corresponding law was changed in 1995, but only to permit eugenic indications to resurge under the heading of medical indications concerning danger for the mother's physical and psychological health. [see EKD 1997 *Wieviel Wissen*, 1. §7.])
25. Taking more thorough issue with that design could have made it clear that
    - "this life" is a preparation for the promised after-life, and that this is why the former's finitude is a threat wherever that preparation has not been adequately realized, but acceptable for dedicated Christians who devote their lives to that preparation, because what it leads to may be a reason for joy;
    - that that very design concerns God's ultimate goal of unifying His creature humans, through their freely offered love with His own Tri-une life of love, which is why humans' this-worldly life presents their (after the fall only) chance to freely offer that love;
    - that offering that love (rather than throwing one's life away or not caring about one's Divine design) consists in giving up "this life", and thus is indispensable for attaining the promised joyful "after-life";
    - that the this-life-defying aspect of such giving up results from efforts at placing this life not under this-worldly, but under other-worldly priorities, as prefigured in Christ's option for the weak and the suffering;
    - that that option results from efforts at rendering humans aware of God's power (and realizing the nothingness of their own) to transform even already this life into an anticipated afterlife-bliss; and
    - that therefore Christ's promise of an "other life" does not defeat the relative but crucial significance of this life.
26. The authors' reference to Moses 2,9 does not support their thesis. Only the tree of knowledge was forbidden. The fact that God expelled humans from paradise in order that they not eat of the tree of life does not prove that humans were mortal beforehand, but only that He did not want them to continue to be immortal after sin. The authors' claim that mortality does not belong to the consequences of God's after-the-fall curse (II 5, see also III 2, §2) conflicts with the content of the curse. Whereas before the fall, humans' having been created from earth was made up for by God's breathing His life into them, after the fall that original "material" is transformed into humans' (earthly) final destiny: "you are made from earth, you will again become earth." Keeping them from eating from the tree of life (Gen. 3:9) makes sense, since that would defeat His curse. In associating sin with the obsession with the desire to avoid mortality, the authors confuse cause and effect. (The 1990 declaration on *Organ Transplantation* does recognize death as the "wage of sin", 4. §3, but immediately weakens that statement by describing death as the "sign" of man's alienation from God.)
27. In the authors' account, the salvation which all creation awaits with sighing (II 6) is not related to Christ's victory over death but left in a haze of pining and longing. In place of a proper explanation of death as the result of human sin, some odd (Manichean) references to "the dark powers" as opposed to the "good creation" are offered (II 3, III 2, §§1,3), along with references to "corresponding ancient oriental texts" (i.e., heathen sources) which speak of the destructive powers of chaos (§6).

28. Where representatives of the EKD have addressed the issue of PVS patients, they invoked the principle of (putative) human self determination exclusively (*idea* 10/98, pp. 10,12). The same difficulty in justifying (not, of course, conservative basic care, but) medical infringements on bodily integrity that serve no medically assessable purpose (of – at the very least – supporting some residua of self-conscious life) concerns severely brain damaged new-borns. Separating God's creative "friendship" for life in general from God's spiritually demanding friendship for humans introduces the danger of a specifically tutiorist Christian biologism. (The Evangelical Alliance, always given to more determined position taking, seems to fall for that temptation when questioning "brain death" as medical criterion (*idea*, 10/98, pp. 7,10).
29. Such an account would have to acknowledge the scandal which a personally loving God, Who became incarnate, Who overcame death and promises a blessed afterlife, the effects of which already permeate life on this world, presents even for a deism-trained secular mind. Only such an account, on the other hand, could encourage humans to turn to a properly spiritual life in Christ by fundamentally re-orienting their priorities in loving obedience to God's commandments, so as to keep, what to a worldly mind appears an "irresolvable conflict", from becoming quite as irresolvable. By attending to the fullness of their teaching, the author churches' bioethical account might have both preserved the Gospel's pristine consistency and fulfilled its empowering function – even for non-Christians, provided they have "ears to hear". Such an alternative way of realizing the Protestant church's double commitment would pursue its "inviting" goal not by leaving the secular world where it is, and endeavouring, with all the human capacities at her disposal, to work out the encouraging, or at least the reassuring and consoling purpose of her mission within the secular environment. Instead, it would call that secular world away from itself, and into the faith.
30. This becomes especially obvious from the way in which discussions of conflicts in the lives of individuals – as with regard to abortion, the acceptance of handicapped children, of helpless patients and parents, to the problem of voluntary and involuntary euthanasia – are unfailingly supplemented by references to what it would mean for society, would such a practise be generally adopted. Since it is hard to imagine that such Kantian generalizing could exert any influence on – say – pregnant mothers or persons confronted with unhelpful relatives, such references move the discussion from the individual to a societal level. Accordingly, the most forceful ethical enjoinder of the whole document (I 3, §1), which categorically demands that one should not comply with actions that disrespect life, only refers to life-destructing tendencies generally, and the need to awaken a sense of awe vis-à-vis life generally, not however to each person's struggle against his health, comfort, or career-idolizing tendencies.
31. This also explains why the churches have not restricted themselves to "the religious" but have tried to cover the secular ground of bioethical arguments as well. Thus they implicitly recommend their position as both Christian and "universal". That their message is designed to cover "the whole" gives it not so much a spiritual but a pragmatic impact.
32. By contrast, the Evangelical Alliance quite boldly defines its societal context as "post-Christian" (*idea* 3, 92, p. 14).
33. Ecological pro-life-ness should not shun the issue of abortions (survey §3), the constitutions' commitment to human life (and health) protection (IV 2, §2, IV 5, §§2-4) should be extended to all forms of that life (VI 2, 4, IV 4 f, VI 1, §5), and the state's commitment to the principle of protection of human life and to solidarity should be cashed in (VI 2, 3).
34. They may be supplemented by popular folk beliefs concerning destructive powers and original chaos (which are not quite as heresy-proof as the Protestant church's declared self-understanding promised). And understandably, one must never mention the fact that the secular world, in resting on the claim of humans' right to know "god and evil" on their own, without reference to God, altogether falls under what the document rightly describes as "original sin".

35. In the same spirit, the German legislative's decision to render abortions (under certain conditions) non-punishable is accepted (even though not found entirely satisfactory, VI 2, e, §5) by the Protestant church, and the introduction of IVF (against which she had protested on theological grounds in the 1985 document *Von der Würde* (1.1, 1.2, 2.6, 2.7) is reluctantly accepted. The issue of legal punishment in the case of abortion is not considered in the perspective of Romans 13 (as a divinely authorized obligation), but as a question of efficiency for hindering abortions (survey §9, IV 2, a, §3), even though the church admits the extensive abuse of the legal permissiveness (VI 2, e 4, §§6-8). Even though that church assumes the task of "critically accompanying cultural developments ... by reference to the Christian faith" (p. 3), she altogether abstains from clearly protesting and condemning both legal decisions. (That she should be so cooperative concerning laws and policies she recognizes to be incompatible with Christianity strikes one as odd, if one considers what an important role the recognition of her failing during the time of National Socialism plays for her current self-understanding, V 3, §4, VI 3, a, VI 3, I, §3).
36. Or, to state the contrast still more pointedly, such a church (except in her own, very substantial engagement with supporting the handicapped, and in her call for people who are willing to sacrifice a more attractive career for the sake of such support, VI 3, e, §1) trusts not in encouraging and personally witnessing to the lived cooperation of individual humans with their supporting and redeeming Creator, but in what is achievable on a large scale, and with a human help exclusively that is theologically anchored in a predominantly theoretical (and thinned out) way. (Quite in harmony with this interpretation, the 1997 Common word *Wieviel Wissen* sees the goal of the Christian life no longer in community with God, but in enhanced humaneness (final section), understood in the sense of increased human maturity. For a contrast, see the Evangelical Alliance which emphasises that "humanitarianism without reference to God leads to bestiality", *idea* 10/98, p. 8.) Very oddly, such a church thus ultimately endorses that very hubris (II 3, III 2, §5) of trying to know what is "good and evil" by herself, which she herself had classified as constituting man's original sin.
37. Most German Protestants would not accept such an interpretation. The authors of the declaration might claim that doing what is humanly possible, even if on a societal level (and with her extensive material and human resources contributions to boot), as long as it was done in a neighbourly loving fashion and with God in mind, is "tantamount enough" to cooperating with God's creative will. And to the question of why their biblical presentation of that will had been so selective, weak, and distortive, they would probably invoke the change of times, and that some manners of speaking and thinking bioethically (just as ethically in general) are right for some times, but not for others. They would thus suppose that either the Divine creative will itself keeps adjusting to changing times (up to one moment opposing IVFs, and, once a law permitting IVF was passed, accepting it under certain conditions, and so for all issues), or, perhaps even, that the changing times have altogether left that old creative will behind.
38. In spite of the large lay involvement in the work of the chamber, the council of the EKD published the document. We may, therefore, take the position endorsed there as the one endorsed by "the" Protestant church in Germany (with the reservations stated in the Introduction).
39. By paraphrasing such action in a dilemma as something that "stays behind what ought to have been accomplished", the authors show that their notion of sin can no longer differentiate between *anomia* (trespass of a prohibition) and *hamartia* (missing the mark). Christ's placing law-obedience in the context of love (Mt.22:37 ff.) in order to forestall loveless legalism (and adherence to human traditions at the cost of violating the loving spirit of the law) is taken to suggest an opposition between love and the law.
40. It seems that the Evangelical Alliance, in contrasting ethical responsibility before God with both responsibility in view of the interest of society and with one's own conscience, has

expressed some reserve with respect to the EKD's rather individualist understanding of the Protestant ethos (*idea* 3/92, p. 14).

41. The council confesses that it endorses only one of the two positions, but does not claim to determine what is "right" for Protestantism (p. 4). This is understandable, because even the proponents of the strict position seem unwilling to "take the consequences" of regarding even spontaneously aborted foetuses as human beings and discouraging nidation blockers with the same force as they discourage IVF (p. 23).
42. While the document speaks only of the foundation of societal life being "touched" by such pluralism, it is obvious that the touch is not friendly, but hurtful.

Bibliography

Council of Europe. 1997. *Convention for the protection of human rights and dignity of the human being with regard to the application of biology and medicine: Convention on human rights and biomedicine.* Adopted by the Committee of Ministers on 19 November 1996. Directorate of Legal Affairs, Strasbourg.

EKD. 1985 ed. *Von der Würde werdenden Lebens, Extrakorporale Befruchtung, Fremdschwangerschaft und genetische Beratung. Eine Handreichung der Evangelischen Kirche in Deutschland zur ethischen Urteilsbildung,* EKD Texte 11, Hannover

EKD. 1999 ed. *Gestaltung und Kritik zum Verhältnis von Protestantismus und Kultur im neuen Jahrhundert,* EKD Text 64. [On-line.] Available:, http://www.ekd.de/EKD-Texte/2139

EKD. 1987 ed. *Zur Achtung vor dem Leben – Maßstäbe für Gentechnik und Fortpflanzungsmedizin, Kundgebung der Synode der EKD, Berlin.* [On-line.] Available: http://www.ekd.de/ EKD-Texte/2078

EKD. 1990 ed. *Organtransplantationen, Erklärung der Deutschen Bischofskonferenz und des Rates der EKD, Bonn/Hannover.* [On-line.] Available: http://www.ekd.de/EKD-Texte/2086

EKD. 1991 ed. *Gott ist ein Freund des Lebens, Herausforderungen und Aufgaben beim Schutz des Lebens.* [On-line.] Available: http://www.ekd.de/EKD-Texte/2086.html

EKD. 1996 ed. "Im Sterben: Umfangen vom Leben, Gemeinsames Wort zur Woche für das Leben", *idea Dokumentation* 10, 1998, p. 36.

EKD. 1997 ed. *Wieviel Wissen tut uns gut? Gemeinsames Wort der Deutschen Bischofskonferenz und des Rates der Evangelischen Kirche in Deutschland zur Woche für das Leben.* [On-line.] Available: http://www.ekd.de/EKD-Texte/2086

EKD. 2001a ed. *Das Evangelium unter die Leute bringen, Zum missionarischen Dienst der Kirche in unserem Land.* [On-line.] Available: EKD Text 68, http:/www.ekd.de/EKD-Texte/2059

EKD. 2001b ed. *Kundgebung der Synode der Evangelischen Kirche in Deutschland auf ihrer 4. Tagung.* [On-line.] Available: http://www.ekd.de/EKD-Texte/2059_evangelium_Kundgebung_2001.html

Idea-Pressedienst. 1998 ed. "Das Recht des Menschen auf Leben – Stellungnahme der Deutschen Evangelischen Allianz zu Lebensrechtsfragen", *idea Dokumentation* 10, p. 5 ff.

Informationsdienst der Evangelischen Allianz. 1992 ed. "Darf nur noch der gesunde Mensch überleben? Sieben Empfehlungen des Hauptvorstandes der Deutschen Evangelischen Allianz zur gesetzlichen Regelung der Anwendung der Genanalyse", *Dokumentation* 3.

Kirchenamt der EKD. 2002 ed. Kammer für Öffentliche Verantwortung der EKD: *Im Geist der Liebe mit dem Leben umgehen,* EKD Texte 71, Hannover.

Kongregation für die Glaubenslehre (Josef Ratzinger), *Erklärung "Dominus Jesus".* [On-line.] Available:www.vatican.va/roma_curia/congregations/cfaith/documents/rc_con_cfaith_doc_20000806_dominus-iesus_gl.html

Pressestelle der EKD. 2002: Kock rät Abgeodneten: Stammzellenimport nicht zustimmen, Auftakt des Bioethik-Kongresses der EKD in Berlin, 28.Jan. [On-line.] Available: http://www.ekd.de/presse/397_6803.html

Reformed Perspectives in Bioethics

Ruth Groenhout

I. Introduction

The Reformed tradition traces its legacy to the Protestant Reformation in 15th and 16th Century Europe. Having made this fairly straightforward claim, however, one finds that it immediately must be modified, suggesting to the alert reader, perhaps, that defining the Reformed tradition is no easy matter. Although Martin Luther's historical status as the instigator of the Reformation might suggest that the Lutheran tradition is one of the members of the Reformed tradition, most Lutheran thinkers would define themselves as a separate tradition, and with good justification. Likewise it is difficult to know whether contemporary Anglican thought can or should be included in the Reformed tradition – there are clear historical connections, and yet historical separation as well. Finally, and complicating matters even more, many thinkers choose to write as representatives of Protestant thought. Clearly the Reformed tradition is one variety of Protestant thought, and its theological resources have been crucial to the development of contemporary Protestantism, but it is just as clearly true that much of contemporary Evangelical thought arises out of the Anabaptist tradition rather than the Reformed.

For the purposes of this essay, the Reformed tradition will be defined broadly, using two separate sets of criteria. First, the Reformed tradition will be used to refer to those churches and denominations which define themselves as belonging to the Reformed tradition, particularly in terms of membership in contemporary councils and alliances defined by a Reformed theological perspective. The World Alliance of Reformed Churches, for example, which represents 215 member churches in 106 countries, totaling more than 74 million Christians worldwide, clearly identifies itself as one major component of the Reformed tradition. Many members of the WARC are Congregational, Presbyterian, Reformed, or United Churches. In addition, the Reformed Ecumenical Council includes a number of other denominations world wide.

In addition to this very broad definition of the Reformed tradition, I will also be relying heavily on certain central thematic concepts, which are typical of thinkers in the Reformed tradition and frequently invoked by thinkers who identify themselves as Protestant, as aspects of contemporary Reformed bioethics. The concepts which I will be using as typical are certainly not found in every thinker one might identify as Reformed, nor are all of them unique to the Reformed tradition. Analogues to several can be found in the Catholic tradition, as well as branches of the Jewish tradition, as one should expect given the shared heritage of all of them. But they nonetheless offer a framework that is recognizably Reformed and are an important part of contemporary Reformed bioethics. The specific concepts I will note (and develop in more detail below) are: Calling, or vocation; Covenant; a Creation/Fall/Redemption historical and social perspective; Worldview or *Weltanschauung*; and an Augustinian notion of sin.

One final note should be added to this introduction. In what follows I will be discussing many aspects of the Reformed tradition which have counterparts in other religious traditions, both other Christian groups and Jewish and Islamic traditions. Nothing that follows is necessarily unique to the Reformed tradition; what I discuss are the ways in which these concepts, principles and practices play out in this particular tradition. Concern to provide support and care for the dying, for example, is expressed in all of the traditions I have mentioned, and the theological justification for such care is very similar. This essay will discuss how topics of this sort have been understood in the Reformed tradition, but nothing in this discussion should be taken to imply that any particular theological concept is the exclusive property of the Reformed tradition.

II. History

Questions we would today identify as bioethical are not strange to ethical reflection in the Reformed tradition. Theodore Beza, a follower of John Calvin, addressed the issue of the physician's duty to risk fatal illness to care for patients. Unlike Martin Luther, who argued that remaining with one's patients was an obligation of Christian charity, Beza held that the physician could leave such patients if the preservation of the physician's life was in the interests of the commonwealth (Jonsen, 2000, p. 46). The Reformed, Calvinist teachings on the doctrine of providence were influential in the development of English medicine in the 15th and 16th centuries, particularly in the development of "experimental religion", which provided a congenial context for the development of empirical medical knowledge (Harley, 1993, p. 102). And the treatises on the duties of a physician written by both Dr. John Gregory and Dr. Thomas Percival likewise show some evidence of the generalized influence of the Reformed tradition on Scottish and English thought of the 18th and 19th centuries.

But the notion of a consciously Reformed perspective offered as one voice in what is assumed to be a pluralistic discussion is a more contemporary phenomena. In the Reformed tradition two separate strands of philosophical thought have contributed to the phenomena. The first, which can be traced back to Abraham Kuyper, involves the philosophical development of the notion of a worldview, or *weltanschauung* (Kuyper, 1981, p. 20). For Kuyper, this conceptual notion was connected to an understanding of social structures in terms of separate spheres of authority (that is, family, business, science, and the like as relatively autonomous social structures) (Kuyper, 1981, p. 90). In the political sphere, as Kuyper understood it, it was necessary to develop state structures which support alternative faith commitments, and these provide important components of contemporary Reformed conceptions of ethics in a pluralistic society (Kuyper, 1981, p. 106). (One cannot laud Kuyper for this without also noting and condemning the role of his thought in providing the theoretical underpinnings for the deep evil of Apartheid, another historical offshoot of Kuyperian thinking.)

The second development, which provided the context for a Reformed theological assessment of bioethical issues, was the development of moral reflection that accompanied the flourishing of modern medical science in the mid-1900s. As the medical sciences increased in power and effectiveness, reflection on the proper use of those sciences also began to gain a new urgency, and theologians from a number of traditions provided the theoretically sophisticated concepts in which that reflection was carried out (Jonsen, 1998, pp. 34-42). Several of the major figures from this time, including Paul Ramsey and James M. Gustafson, drew explicitly on the thought of Reformed and neo-Calvinist thinkers such as Karl Barth, Reinhold Neihbur, and H. Richard Neihbur, making the Reformed influence central in the early days of the development of bioethics.

Reformed bioethics in the contemporary world is carried out in a number of spheres. There are theologians and philosophers who bring explicitly Reformed perspectives to bioethics as their academic specialization, such as Allan Verhey and Kenneth Vaux. Others understand themselves to be developing a Protestant bioethics, but one that is profoundly shaped by Reformed theological concepts, as in the case of Paul Ramsey. But bioethical thought is not carried out only in the academic context. Various churches in the Reformed tradition have spoken out on a variety of bioethical issues, and church councils and synods frequently debate bioethical issues and produce careful, reflective discussions of the dimensions of a Reformed moral response. Individual members of various Reformed churches debate these issues and frequently must make decisions in their professional and personal lives that reflect and are faithful to their Reformed commitments. So bioethical thought occurs on many levels, and this essay can only hope to give some flavor of the many and complicated aspects of that thought.

Before moving to specific aspects of bioethics, however, a few words about the general framing concepts, mentioned above as characteristic of Reformed thought, are in order. Earlier I listed Calling, Covenant, Creation/Fall/Redemption, Worldview, and Sin as characteristic of a Reformed perspective, and I would now like to develop in a bit more detail what they are and how they have shaped Reformed thought.

The notion of calling or vocation is grounded in the Christian doctrine that humans are created in the image of God and developed further by Luther's and Calvin's articulations of the value of ordinary life. These two theological concepts, brought together, yield a recognition that all humans have an inherent value, and part of that value is the role they are created to play in bringing the peace of God's kingdom to a broken world. This role need not be in church ministry. Almost all occupations have a redemptive aspect, an aspect which is clearly present in the health care professions, and Christians are called to such professions in precisely the same way they may be called to be pastors or deacons. In both cases, the call is to become an agent of God's will in the world, bringing peace, justice, and relief to the oppressed. This conception of vocation radically reconfigures any division between sacred and secular and has provided the framework for discussions of, for example, the physician's moral obligations.

The notion of calling has also contributed to the strong emphasis many Reformed thinkers have put on individual liberty. If each person is called by God to play an important role in Kingdom building, then there is reason to respect and protect individual autonomy. This autonomy is not absolute, of course, and Reformed thinkers have always understood it as freedom for obedience to God, not simple license, but it has nonetheless been an important component in most Reformed discussions of bioethical issues.

Second, Reformed theology is marked by the notion of a covenantal relationship. The original covenant is between God and the people of God. It is marked by God's faithfulness, and it is a relationship Christians are called to model in their own lives. The language of covenant has been very influential in bioethics, and it would be an unwarranted inference to think that everywhere it is found it reflects a Reformed perspective, but when found in particular thinkers such as Allen Verhey or Lewis Smedes, it clearly finds its roots in Reformed theology.

Third, Reformed theology grounds its understanding of social, political, and ethical matters in a Creation/Fall/Redemption narrative. There are several subsidiary aspects of this narrative. The first is an affirmation of the goodness of creation. All that is created is created in accordance with the will of a good God and is pronounced good at its inception. In the Reformed tradition this is often the basis for two principles: the affirmation of the goodness of life, and a respect for natural orders and processes. We cannot stop with creation, however, or we lose sight of important aspects of the human condition. Creation was created good, but it is now fallen from that state as a result of human sin. The brokenness of creation extends beyond human relationships to the rest of creation. But, again, this is not the final story. Though the world we now live in is broken and burdened, God will not abandon creation and will restore it with the coming of the Kingdom of God. Those who now want to do the will of God in the world should act as agents of that kingdom, acting in ways which bring wholeness and healing to a damaged world (Martin, 1960, p. 55). So, to summarize, the world belongs to God, and all that is created is a part of a good creation, though deeply and ineluctably flawed by the effects of sin. Finally, while the complete instantiation of the Kingdom of God will only occur with the Second Coming of Christ, in the meantime Christians are called to work as partners with God in supporting and developing God's Shalom, or peace through justice, by personal choices and social action.

The fourth theme, developed extensively in the thought of Abraham Kuyper, involves a strong emphasis on worldview and respect for social structures which permit the development and flourishing of alternative communities in society. Influenced by the work of John Calvin and Abraham Kuyper, Reformed thinkers have emphasized the extent to which all our ethical thought takes place within and structured by worldviews, or moral and ontological frameworks, which provide the evaluative and sense-making structure of all our ethical decision-making (Mouw, 1990, pp. 24-25). If ethical thought is always structured by a worldview, then it follows that different worldviews will produce different ethical systems, and so Reformed thought has tended to expect and respect differences of opinion on ethical matters.

Finally, and as a crucial aspect of Reformed reflection, we find the notion of sin as a personal and social force in human life. The Augustinian roots of the Reformed tradition make it impossible ever to be wholly optimistic about the state of human relationships with each other or with the non-human world while in this present life. Humans destroy the integrity of their world, their relationships, and their bodies in myriad ways, and any account of bioethics must be realistic about the depth of brokenness sin creates in the world (Evans, 1999, pp. 77-79). This does not lead to despair, but it should lead to a combination of a realistic understanding of finitude, rejection of utopian thinking, and, importantly, recognition of the need for balances of power and accountability. Recognition of the pervasiveness of sin should lead to an acknowledgement of the need for all humans to be held accountable for their actions and to a suspicion of any human exercise of unbridled authority. It also can contribute to humility in the pronouncements by both individuals and churches – a Calvinist notion of the extent of human depravity should lead to the recognition that one's own firm convictions may themselves be unwittingly tainted by pride or unwarranted self-love.

III. Topics

A. Bioethics in General

The Reformed tradition is not marked by unanimity in its bioethics perspective. Politically it lacks a central authority and so is unlikely to produce a unified view by authoritative pronouncements. Further, the tradition out of which it has developed is one marked by constant dissent and protest, and it thus reflects its rather contentious roots in its perspective on bioethics. Finally, the Reformed tradition has a long history of respect, first for the individual's freedom and responsibility, and second for the extent to which differing perspectives produce different patterns of reasoning; both of these factors make it difficult to speak of one unified Reformed perspective on bioethics.

But although one cannot point to a specific set of beliefs that comprise Reformed Bioethics, it is possible to point to an array of position papers, Council and Synodical Reports, and pastoral advice developed by various Reformed constituencies concerned about various issues in bioethics. The Presbyterian Church (USA), for example, has developed a number of position papers on issues in bioethics, ranging from justice issues in health care, to abortion, to the testing of contraceptives in Third World countries. Their detailed and extensive writings are probably the most well developed in the North American context, though both the Christian Reformed Church and the Reformed Church in America have developed position papers on some of these issues. In the European context, the Netherlands Reformed Church (*Nederlandse Hervormde Kerk*) and the Reformed Churches in the Netherlands (*Gereformeerde Kerken in Nederland*) have developed both position papers and documents intended to function as an overview and general commentary on issues.

In addition to church position papers, there have been a wide variety of bioethical reflections by individual scholars which fall generally in the Reformed tradition. Much of the theological framework that under-girds the thought of Paul Ramsey has been developed in the Reformed and Presbyterian tradition. Ramsey's covenantal theology is closely connected with the thought of Karl Barth and H. Richard Niebuhr (Smith, 1993, p. 8). Furthermore, the strong emphasis on creation found in Ramsey's thought is likewise a theme that has been particularly influential in the Reformed tradition. His deontological understanding of protestant ethics in general and bioethics in particular is clearly compatible, in many ways, with a Reformed perspective.

James M. Gustafson is another thinker whose theological roots are closely entangled with Reformed theology. Gustafson studied under H. Richard Niebuhr and describes himself as "drawing deeply on the Reformed tradition" (Gustafson, 1981, p. 157-193). Like Ramsey, Gustafson emphasizes themes of creation and communal fidelity. He also, more than Ramsey, emphasizes the finitude and sinfulness of humans. Although both thinkers recognize the tendency for humans to sin, Gustafson, more than Ramsey, emphasizes a critical perspective toward the self and condemns self-righteous absolutism based on a strong theological account of the sinfulness of human nature.

The next generation of Reformed thinkers appears to be as productive as Gustafson and Ramsey and to have an even greater set of bioethical issues to reflect on. Allen Verhey has written extensively on a number of bioethical issues, as has Kenneth Vaux, and both have been influential in developing policies and contributing to bioethical discussion in the churches with which they are affiliated (respectively, the Reformed Church of America and the Presbyterian Church [USA]). On a more popular level, Lewis Smedes has written a number of discussions of general ethical issues, including some bioethical topics, which have provided thoughtful articulations of a Reformed perspective on personal morality.

B. *Professionalism*

Reformed perspectives on professional roles in health care have been formed in many ways by the twin concepts of vocation and covenant. The role of the health care professional is seen as valuable and worthy of honor, in part because of the important role health care plays in carrying out the Christian mandate of care for the suffering and dying. At the very least, this entails that a Reformed view of the health care professions begins with respect and gratitude for those who play these roles; any criticism of health care professionals needs to be seen against this basic framework of value and respect.

The role of health care professional, whether physician, nurse, technician, or researcher, is one to which some are called as part of their mission to image the Kingdom of God to a broken world. This situates the professional/patient relationship in a broader context than simply the contract between two autonomous individuals. Instead, the relationship is formed in the context of a broader community called to faithfulness and justice. Allen Verhey summarizes this as follows:

> The physician who owns her role as a calling, then, will serve life and its flourishing. She will never *intend* death. She will use her knowledge and her skills to serve the cause of God. But she will also realize that victory over death is finally a divine victory..., that God is the faithful savior, and *not* either her or her technology. She will not deny either the limits of her art or the truth of the continuing power of death and pain. She will not deny this truth to either herself or her patients (Verhey, 1984, p. 38).

There are several key notions that Verhey develops here, each of which deserves further explication.

The health care professional, first, cannot treat her or his profession as merely a convenient way to make money. It is a calling, not merely a means to the end of a salary (Bouma & Diekema, 1989, pp. 110, 120). Since the professional holds her or his position as a matter of responsive obedience to God, to be carried out in ways that recognize others as image-bearers of God, the relationship between professional and patient must be marked by respect, care, and loyalty. The regular recourse to language of covenant, found famously in Ramsey (1970, p. xii), as well as in William F. May's work (1975, pp. 29-38), is a reflection of this understanding of the professional's status. Alastair Campbell expresses a similar notion of the high calling of health care professionals in defining professional care-givers as moderators of love (Campbell, 1984, pp. 84-86); the term implies that professionals are called to self-giving love, and also that they see themselves as a conduit through which God's love can manifest itself.

Framing health care as a calling, however, should not be taken as providing a license for exploitation of the professionals who engage in it. Health care professionals carry out work which reflects the Christian mandate of relief of suffering, curing the sick, and remaining with the dying (Verhey, 1997, p. 269), and because of this they deserve respect as well as a fair recompense for their work. Further, the dignity of the professional also entails a respect for the professional's own integrity in terms of deciding what practices she or he can or cannot engage in. So while the notion of health care as a vocation is one that makes high demands of the professional, it also reflects the high dignity of the occupation and respect that professionals deserve from others. This respect, then, provides some justification for claims to professional autonomy. Respect for professional autonomy, however, does not remove the need for accountability. And as William F. May has noted, too strong an emphasis on professional autonomy can lead to problems due to lack of self-regulation in the professions (May, 1983, pp. 132-135). A clear-eyed recognition of human sinfulness and self-preference are a necessary balance to respect for professional autonomy.

The responsibilities of the health care professional are not completely determined by his or her relationship with the patient, however. An issue which was raised in the 16th century debate between Luther and Beza (mentioned in the History section above) concerns the health care professional's responsibility to the broader society, a responsibility which may sometimes be in tension with the responsibility to the patient. Sometimes Reformed discussions of these broader social responsibilities are framed in terms of stewardship of scarce medical resources (Bouma & Diekema, 1989, p. 173), other times in terms of distributive justice and the obligations of the physician (May, 1983, pp. 140-141). The tension this can produce is generally treated as one of the difficult aspects of professional life, not as a moral issue to which there is one absolute answer.

Finally, any discussion of professionalism would be incomplete without some discussion of relationships among professionals. Clearly, based on the previous discussion, an attitude of mutual respect is required, though, as Alastair Campbell notes, this attitude can be destroyed by sexism (particularly in the physician/nurse relationship, given current demographics) and other forms of destructive bias (Campbell, 1984, pp. 35-38). However, apart from Campbell, this aspect of professional relationships is frequently overlooked. This may be due in part to the fact that many discussions of bioethics focus primarily on physicians to the exclusion of other health care providers. A recent increase in discussions of the ethics of nursing practice suggests that more attention will be focussed on such relationships in the future.

C. Reproduction, Abortion, Sexuality and Related Issues

Reformed discussions of sexuality, abortion, and reproductive matters have tended to emphasize two aspects of Christian thought: a creation theology, which affirms the goodness of creation, including sexual being; and an emphasis on the notion of human imaging of God, which produces a strong concern for the protection and sanctity of human life. But while there tends to be fairly general agreement on these principles, there is a wide range of interpretation and application. The issue of abortion, in particular, has been a divisive and contentious one for the various churches, and individual thinkers have developed a similar range of analyses.

The variety of views held on abortion can be quickly demonstrated by a survey of three North American denominations: the Presbyterian Church (USA), the Reformed Church in America, and the Christian Reformed Church. The UPCUSA affirms the right to legal access to abortion while simultaneously recognizing abortion as inevitably an evil, albeit sometimes the lesser of several evil choices. It defends and supports legal access to abortion while also advocating respect for the sanctity of human life. Because the church affirms that there are exceptional conditions that justify abortions and respect individual decisions prayerfully made, it affirms the legal protection of the right to an abortion. At the same time it also affirms the sanctity of life and the moral value of the protection of developing life, so it does not condone abortions of convenience (UPCUSA, 1980, p. 68).

The Reformed Church in America has found abortion a divisive issue. In 1971, the General Synod passed a resolution affirming each individual's right to make an abortion decision. However, in 1988, the General Synod passed a resolution calling for the right to life of the unborn child to be written into the Charter of Rights and Freedoms of the Canadian Constitution. That same Synod, however, rejected an overture to encourage the Canadian government to make abortion a criminal act (Reformed Church in America [a]).

The Christian Reformed Church affirms the unique value of all human life. Based on the sixth commandment, the church's official statements condemn any "wanton or arbitrary destruction of human life at any stage of its development" from conception to the point of death. Induced abortion is only a morally allowable option when the mother's life is genuinely threatened by the continuation of the pregnancy. This position has remained unchanged since 1972, although Synodical decisions in the mid-1990s were made to address specific related issues. These decisions recognized the right of faculty members at a church affiliated college to debate or disagree with the church's official position, condemned the practice of partial birth abortion, strengthened the mandate to churches to minister to those who choose to bear children rather than abort, and rejected all violence against those who perpetrate abortion (Christian Reformed Church [a]).

This spectrum of views found in North America is repeated on a global scale, with some Reformed churches in the Netherlands adopting fairly liberal standards on abortion, while other Reformed denominations in Scotland, New Zealand, and Australia adopt the more stringent anti-abortion stance of the Christian Reformed Church.

Among prominent thinkers in the Reformed tradition this same ambivalence toward the issue of abortion can be found as well. Condemnation of virtually all abortions except those performed to save the mother's life can be found in thinkers such as Karl Barth (1987, p. 401). Views that pay more attention to the complexities of abortion decisions and attempt to develop a casuistry of different types of abortions are developed by thinkers such as Gustafson (1987, pp. 403-412) and an interdisciplinary group of scholars funded by the Calvin Center for Christian Scholarship (Bouma & Diekema, 1989, pp. 224-233). These two latter discussions offer carefully developed accounts of the conditions under which abortion may be permissible. And one also finds thinkers who defend a fairly broad conception of abortion rights, largely arguing that decisions about early abortions should be made by the pregnant woman, though the availability of later abortions should be more limited, and drawing distinctions between conditions where abortion may be advisable, permissible, or proscribed (Vaux, 1989, pp. 91-92). In the case of Vaux, the sanctity of life doctrine is taken both to make abortion always a tragic choice, but also to protect the mother's decisional control over her own life.

Having noted the spread of positions on abortion found in the Reformed tradition, however, one can note certain commonalities as well. All of these discussions broaden the field of ethical considerations beyond the context of a conflict of rights between two individuals to a consideration of the communal, social, and economic situation in which abortion decisions are made. The issue of abortion raises fundamental questions about what sort of community the church understands itself to be, the meaning of marriage (Ramsey, 1978, pp. 11-18), and justice in the context of sexist social situations (Pohl, 1995, p. 213).

This very brief review of Reformed views on abortion sets the stage for other bioethical issues connected with reproduction and sexuality. In discussing issues such as contraception, infertility treatment, and homosexuality, the principles mentioned above are all apparent. Different principles will sometimes come to the fore in different contexts, but respect for the image of God in others (the basis of the sanctity of life doctrine), respect for creation order, and concern for the protection of community are apparent in all of these contexts.

When it comes to contraception, this perspective is a bit more muted, though still present. Paul Ramsey notes that the moral assessment of contraceptive use in *Griswold v. Connecticut* is expressed in overly individualistic language, and that such a moral assessment must take into account the nature of a married couple as responsible to each other (Ramsey, 1978, pp. 13-14). Similar reasoning can be found in the Christian Reformed Church, which adopted an official position against birth control in 1936. Its reasoning is based on the biblical mandate to be fruitful and multiply, and in keeping with this reasoning the church discouraged birth control and encouraged married couples to produce as many children as is compatible with the physical, spiritual, and mental well being of the mother and children (Christian Reformed Church [b]). Experience suggests, however, that this official position is more a historical artifact than a vital moral concern, and the more common understanding of contraception in the Reformed tradition is one of welcome acceptance. Some thinkers go further to suggest a weak mandate to use contraceptives, based on consideration of population pressure in the global context, and with careful sensitivity to issues of eugenics, racism, and violation of other's privacy (Vaux, 1989, pp. 1-21). Again, this is not out of keeping with the general notion of covenantal responsibility.

With respect to IVF and related techniques, one again finds a lack of unanimity in the Reformed tradition. Cautious acceptance of new reproductive techniques is characteristic of many Reformed churches and thinkers in the Reformed tradition, limited by concern about the ways in which reproductive techniques may require the production of embryos that will be discarded, multiple births and the problem of selective abortion techniques, and donation of gametes by individuals outside of a marriage relationship. In 1992, the Reformed Churches in the Netherlands published a report, in conjunction with the Dutch Lutheran church, which represented the culmination of four years of examination of new reproductive techniques. The report was issued as an overview of the subject, and so lacks official synodical status, but it has been accredited by some church synods as a "contribution to the debate" providing it with a higher authority than a mere overview (Boer & Schroten, 1993, p. 5). This report defends a view of all humans as more than merely their biological existence. Humans are constituted, in part, by their relationship to God and to other humans; this relational aspect of human identity makes it morally unacceptable to use human beings as mere objects of use. So in the case of scientific research, research using embryos and pre-embryos must be seen as treading on potentially problematic moral ground. Although such research may be morally acceptable if it aims at the well-being of future generations, it still is morally questionable. Other techniques such as IVF and prenatal diagnosis are welcomed insofar as they offer medical treatment for illness and incapacities. However, again they are practices that must be utilized with full recognition of the wrongness of using one human (embryonic stage or not) for the purposes of another. The document notes, in fact, that the care we owe embryos and fetuses may suggest that a revision is needed in the liberal abortion practices which prevail in the Netherlands (Boer et al., 1993, pp. 9-11).

Sexuality, finally, is a contentious issue in the Reformed tradition, particularly in the North American context. Traditionally, all of the churches in the Reformed tradition taught that sexuality was only expressed properly (morally speaking) within the context of marriage. Differences, when they arose in the past, largely concerned heterosexual relations outside of marriage and whether such relations should be dealt with in pastoral or punitive ways. However, in the more recent past this fairly simple consensus has been challenged in several ways. The most central challenge comes from groups and thinkers in the tradition who believe that the church would be more true to its calling if it recognized the way in which all loving, committed relationships image God's covenantal love. The conclusion drawn is that whether a relationship is heterosexual or homosexual, formed by mutual consent or by a public marriage, is less important that its status as an instantiation of loving mutuality. This challenge is fiercely opposed by those who hold that heterosexual relationships are normative and that mutual faithfulness leaves out the essentially communal aspect of a marriage.

This debate has been fiercest over the status of homosexual practices. On one end of the opinion spectrum we find those, mentioned above, who argue that every committed relationship images God's covenantal love. On this view, there is no normative difference between heterosexual or homosexual relationships. What is significant in evaluating any relationship is the extent to which those in the relationship are living out their commitments with love and integrity. Most of the thinkers and churches in the Reformed tradition do not accept this account of human relationships, and maintain, in contrast, that heterosexual marriage is the norm for human sexual relationships. Within that general framework, there is still room for disagreement, of course. Some thinkers hold that while faithful heterosexual marriage is normative, relationships that fall short of that ideal can still be acceptable, whether they are committed homosexual relationships or remarriage after divorce. Others argue that homosexual relationships are never acceptable, and within this camp there are variations as to how morally wrong homosexuality is understood to be.

All of these variations are affected to some extent or another by recent studies on possible genetic or environmental factors that may affect sexual orientation. Those who reject any negative evaluation of homosexual relationships frequently, though not always, consider a physical basis for sexual orientation to provide some grounding for the claim that homosexual practices are within the norm for human relationships. Those who reject the acceptability of such practices use the same evidence to argue for the claim that homosexuality is a pathological condition and so cannot be normative. It is a vexed question in the Reformed tradition, and appears to be an issue that will continue to be divisive in the coming years.

D. Death and Dying

As I write this essay, the news headlines are blaring that the Netherlands has just become the first nation to legalize euthanasia. Given the profound effect the Reformed churches have had on the culture of the Netherlands, this might lead the reader to assume that the Reformed tradition does not disapprove of euthanasia. However, an astute reader will not be expecting the Reformed tradition to speak with one voice on the issues of euthanasia and physician-assisted suicide, and such a reader would be making an accurate assumption. Many churches and theorists in the Reformed tradition are deeply opposed to euthanasia, and the pro-life Protestant State Reformed Party, which holds two seats in the Dutch parliament, voted against and strongly denounced the change in law (Euthanasia.com, 1999). At the same time, public opinion polls have shown that a fairly strong majority of Dutch citizens favor legalized euthanasia, and this majority holds, though less strongly, among religious believers (Griffiths, Blood, & Weyers, 1998).

Having noted all of this, it remains true that there is a strong bias against interventions leading to death in the Reformed tradition, usually based on two notions: first, the covenantal relationship between physician and patient, and second, the affirmation that the Lord of Creation is a Lord of Life. If the Christian's job is to image a foretaste of the Kingdom of God in a world broken by sin, then presumably the Christian physician should be solidly on the side of life, not death. As Allen Verhey puts it, "We do not, and I think we may not pray for death. Death is not the cause of God. In the good future of God, death will be no more" (Verhey, 1992, p. 26). So death is never, in and of itself, a good thing.

At the same time, Reformed bioethical thought also recognizes the finitude and limitations of human action in the world. It would be a presumption of God's authority to claim to have a perfect knowledge or absolute control over anything. So the physician is also counseled to accept the limitations of human finitude and refrain from inappropriately heroic measures at the end of life; ultimately life is in God's hands. There comes a time when the caring physician turns to palliative care and comfort measures, not because death is a good thing, but because we live in this present, imperfect world, and death has not yet been banished.

This general framework seems relatively standard in Reformed thought, but, within that context, there is room for disagreement. And where Reformed thinkers find room for disagreement, they are sure to disagree. Paul Ramsey argues that the very language of euthanasia must be rejected because the term has come to mean choosing death. What we can legitimately choose, he writes, is *how* we will live while dying, whether we choose multiple medical interventions or the removal of feeding tubes. But in either case we must understand that we make choices among the goods of life (length versus comfort, for example), not choices which exercise dominion over life itself (Ramsey, 1978, pp. 146-148). Within the framework of proper human authority, however, he recognizes a broad spectrum of personal freedom to choose or reject medical treatment.

As an interesting side note, Ramsey's formulation of "choosing how to live while dying" is almost the reverse of how many early Calvinist thinkers would have framed the issue. In the late 16th and early 17th centuries, David Harley notes the "godly were expected to 'Study and exercise daily the Art of dying'" (Harley, 1993, p. 107). In contrast to Ramsey's prohibition on ever choosing death, Kenneth Vaux has argued that, under exceptional circumstances, there may be a place for active euthanasia as an act of mercy, though it would need to be carefully circumscribed and perhaps taken out of the medical context (Vaux, 1992, pp. 44-45). His suggestion that the church might properly take on the role of delivering the *coup de grâce*, however, is unlikely to find large support in many churches in the Reformed tradition.

An issue closely related to euthanasia, though often treated separately, is the question of appropriate neonatal care for the severely handicapped infant. When babies are born with such severe defects that their future survival will be either doubtful or severely diminished, how should we respond to them in ways that best reflect the calling of the caregivers? Thinkers in the Reformed tradition, as in other traditions, have drawn careful distinctions between the sorts of handicaps that might be at issue in such a case. The precipitating case for much of this reflection, that of Baby Doe, concerned an infant with Down Syndrome, some congenital heart defects, and an esophageal blockage. The parents and physician together chose not to surgically correct the esophageal blockage, and, since the infant could not take food by mouth, he died after some time. The case galvanized public opinion, and many opinions were written on it. One salient feature of the case, however, was the fact that the infant's handicap, Down syndrome, is not a life-threatening condition and seems compatible with living a rich and satisfying life. A general consensus has arisen among most thinkers in the Reformed tradition that failing to protect the life of a child of this sort is morally unacceptable (see, for example, Verhey, 1987, p. 485). So distinctions are drawn. Some thinkers distinguish conditions that are completely incompatible with life (anencephaly) from conditions one can foresee will lead to a very short painful life (Tay Sachs, Lesch Nyhan) from conditions that will lead to a relatively lengthy life, but one marked by sharply diminished quality of life (severe retardation).

Not surprisingly, given the general Reformed stance toward end of life issues, hospice care has been strongly supported by churches and thinkers in the Reformed tradition. Some churches have made specific requests of their respective governments that hospice care receive adequate funding (Reformed Church in America [b]).

Another related topic is that of the ethics of pain management. The recognition that pain has not always been managed well in the medical context, and that patient fear of prolonged suffering is one of the forces which contributes to the pressure to legalize physician assisted suicide, has resulted in an increase of concern about pain management, but the issue has not generated anything comparable to the debates over abortion and euthanasia. Generally, the Reformed tradition has been in favor of the relief of suffering, so pain management as a practice is not controversial; ethical issues arise in this context over questions of funding, standards of care, and the like.

E. Access to Health Care

Issues concerning access to health care are generally treated as justice issues. They include concern about the provision of health care, either through a national health service or via some system of insurance, as well as issues of different levels of care being offered to various groups of people. In all these areas, the Reformed tradition has taken on the issues. The Presbyterian church (USA) has called for the establishment of a national health service to provide universal insurance coverage to everyone in the United States, arguing that health care is such a basic necessity that it should be provided to all (Presbyterian Church USA, 1990, p. 2). Likewise, the authors of *Christian Faith, Health, and Medical Practice* consider some system of universal medical coverage a moral requirement. This discussion also develops an analysis of the various trade-offs involved in any solution to provision of health care. Systems which strive for universal coverage tend to face problems of stagnation (one of the ways to limit the costs of universal coverage is to not invest in new technologies and research), while those systems which provide the highest quality of care and research in new medical technologies generally exclude some portion of the population from coverage (Bouma & Diekema, 1989, pp. 355-361). There seems no easy way to resolve this dilemma – it is driven by the inevitable constraints of economic and resource limitations – but the authors call for a system that recognizes the moral responsibility of any nation to provide some level of health care for all its members.

In addition to the concern for structural justice issues in the delivery of health care, the Reformed tradition has also always had an active concern for the delivery of health care as a part of their mission of relief work. This has been an aspect of the church's perceived duty since early times. So we find, for example, the Puritan Robert Boyle in the 17th century arguing that, in emulation of Christ's healing ministry, Christians ought to see the provision of medical care as an essential part of Christian charity. Boyle included, in fact, the free dissemination of scientific and medical knowledge under this duty (Hunter, 1996, pp. 247-248). In the contemporary world, the provision of health care as a part of the Christian mission has marked many churches in the Reformed tradition, and it is rare to find one without some form of relief organization incorporated as a part of the church's ministry.

Finally, an issue, which straddles the categories of reproductive and access concerns, has arisen in the context of the UPCUSA in connection with the provision of certain aspects of health care systems managed by the Catholic Health care system. Given Catholic teachings, Catholic systems of health care prohibit or severely limit access to abortion and contraception. The UPCUSA has argued that it is important to maintain access to these legal medical procedures and is beginning to discuss how access to them can be safeguarded under conditions of contemporary health care delivery (UPCUSA General Assembly Policy Statement, 1992).

F. Ethics Committees

The Reformed tradition has relied heavily on study groups, committees, and the like for coming to agreements about bioethical issues. This is a natural course of action for a tradition that has been characterized by a relatively egalitarian structure from its inception. Further, the Reformed tradition has always valued expertise and has seen part of the vocation of those who are knowledgeable as involved in making that knowledge accessible to others in the community who do know much about that subject. So all of the North American Reformed churches regularly commission study committees on bioethical issues, many of which produced the reports from which parts of this essay were written. A similar pattern is found in the European, African, and Australasian Reformed churches.

Given that commitment, it is not surprising that the general concepts of ethical committees exercising either oversight or advisory roles in the bioethical context has been a natural one for many Reformed thinkers. As an expression of this, the UPCUSA has advocated representation of its views on local hospital advisory boards. However, there has been some disagreement in the Reformed tradition over questions of the proper mode of influence on health care. Some thinkers have advocated the creation of a separate health care system which would give expression to a Reformed worldview in its structure and method of health care delivery (Bouma & Diekema, 1989, p. 114), while other thinkers advocate working within the existing systems instead.

G. *Other Issues*

The Reformed tradition has also been concerned with issues raised by disabilities. Several churches consider themselves to have a mandate to work for the fullest possible inclusion of individuals with disabilities into the life of the church and the broader society (Pathways to Promise). This again is a natural extension of a strong notion of the sanctity of human life, coupled with a strongly Calvinist notion of calling. If each human is called to serve God in her or his unique capacity, then there can be no moral justification for considering some lives "more worth living" than others. The lives of individuals who have disabilities, whether physical, mental, or emotional, must be respected and valued. This does not mean that those in the Reformed tradition close their eyes to the suffering disabilities can cause. Rather it requires a response of support and assistance, where appropriate, consciousness of access issues, and a firm commitment to the value of all human lives.

The Reformed tradition is also in the early stages of coming to grips with the ethical issues that are posed by new genetic technologies. This is just beginning to raise moral questions in the context of medicine about the use of genetic techniques to deal with cancer and some genetic disorders; the potential for the genetic manipulation of human embryos, either to avoid genetic defects or for genetic enhancement; and most sensationally, the issue of cloning human beings. These questions are guaranteed to become more and more contentious as scientific and technological advances continue. In addition, the use of genetic manipulation in agriculture and animal husbandry is becoming a matter of moral attention among Reformed thinkers.

In both of these areas, the Reformed notion of creation will become a crucial and contested issue. We cannot adequately assess the moral status of proposed (or actual) genetic manipulation without some sense of the value of the created order's integrity and humility about human intervention into that order, as Dieter Hessel argues in a discussion of theology and genetic engineering (Hessel, 1996, p. 630). And with increasing pressure to perform any techniques that are economically beneficial, it will become increasingly important for traditions such as the Reformed to speak publicly about values other than economic which should guide our thinking on such matters.

IV. Conclusion

A. *Future Challenges*

One of the largest challenges to a Reformed bioethics in the future will be a response to central questions about sexuality, its place and purpose in human life, and proper moral and religious responses to various ways of expressing sexuality. One of the reasons abortion has been and continues to be so enormously controversial within the Reformed communities is its inevitable connection with women's bodies, sexuality, and conceptions of gender roles. One indication of this is the markedly different response of various Reformed theological bodies to issues of euthanasia. While euthanasia and physician-assisted suicide are clearly of moral concern, neither issue has generated the animus of abortion nor the extensive and constant stream of dispute that has arisen in the abortion context. Both euthanasia and abortion deal with much the same sorts of issues about a stance of protection of life, concern for balancing complex human relationships and the like, so the difference in tone and level of debate on the two topics is rather remarkable.

It seems plausible that what accounts for some of the difference is the fact that abortion is inherently tied to issues of sexuality and gender roles. Like debates over women holding ecclesiastical office and debates over the status of homosexuality in the church, debates over the moral status of abortion are deeply tied to disagreements over the place of sexuality in human nature, the proper roles of men and women, and the nature of autonomy. This is a debate that will be enormously difficult and divisive. The Reformed tradition of splitting denominations will likely be resorted to in many cases over these issues, and it seems probable that the debate will be conducted with a fair amount of invective and rancor on all sides.

A second issue that is moving to the forefront of ethical thought, both in the global setting and in the Reformed tradition of reflection, is that of AIDS/HIV. Like many religious traditions, some in the Reformed tradition have taken the world-wide occurrence of AIDS to be evidence of God's punishment on homosexuality, but the official teachings of most churches and the reflective writings of most theorists have rejected this understanding of the epidemic. The need to address the complex of issues posed by a rapidly spreading disease, which can only be managed by a complex and expensive medical regimen in the context of a global economic situation marked by astronomical disparities in wealth, is overwhelming. As with the issues mentioned above, the spread of AIDS challenges traditional silences on difficult sexual matters, and will certainly require churches to face the disparity between the abstinence or sexual fidelity within marriage that they officially teach and the actual sexual practices of their members. And it will also pose new challenges to the church's mandate of providing health care to the most needy, since the needs it is generating are so overwhelming.

B. Future of Reformed Bioethics

The contentious issues I have been discussing indicate that we are not likely to face any shortage of bioethical questions in the future. The Reformed tradition offers a valuable resource to the development of bioethical reflection for a number of reasons. One of the most important reasons is the very plurality and diversity of opinions within the tradition itself. As a tradition which lacks a single centralized authority, it has demonstrated the ways in which people committed to a tradition can disagree heartily about the application and development of the principles which inform that tradition. If, as some thinkers have proclaimed, we are now living in a post-modern world, without any single source of moral guidance, the Reformed community may find itself peculiarly suited to speaking to living in that world without losing sight of the need to engage in careful and principled moral reasoning.

But, in addition to its internal diversity, the Reformed tradition also offers an important source for contemporary moral reflection due to its long and rich theological tradition and its consistent historical commitment to practical action. The combination is a potent one. It holds the potential for great evil when misused, but a parallel potential to mobilize enormous resources for good when channeled appropriately.

Bibliography

Barth, K. (1987 [1961]). The protection of life. In: S. Lammers & A. Verhey (Eds.), *On moral medicine: Theological perspectives in medical ethics* (p. 401). Grand Rapids: Eerdmans.

Boer, T. & Schroten, E. (1993). Bioethics in protestant continental Europe. In: B. Lustig (Ed.), *Bioethics yearbook, volume 3* (p. 5). Dordrecht: Kluwer Academic Publishers.

Bouma III, H. & Diekema, D. (1989). *Christian faith, health and medical practice.* Grand Rapids: Eerdmans.

Campbell, A. (1984). *Professional care: Its meaning and practice.* Philadelphia: Fortress Press.

Christian Reformed Church [a]. *Position: Abortion* [On-line]. Available: http://www.crcna.org/cr/crbe/crbe_pos_abortion.htm

Christian Reformed Church [b]. *Position: Birthcontrol* [On-line]. Available: http://www.crcna.org/cr/crbe/crbe_pos_birthcontrol.htm

Euthanasia.com. (1999) *Dutch government to legalize euthanasia* [On-line]. Available: http://www.euthanasia.com/dutch99.html

Evans, A. (1999). *Redeeming marketplace medicine: A theology of health care.* Cleveland: The Pilgrim Press.

Griffiths, J., Bood. A., & Weyers, H. (1998). *Euthanasia and law in the Netherlands.* Amsterdam: Amsterdam University Press.

Gustafson, J. (1981). *Ethics from a theocentric perspective: Volume 1: Theology and ethics.* Chicago: University of Chicago Press.

Gustafson, James M. (1983). A Protestant ethical approach. In: S. Lammers & A. Verhey (Eds.), *On moral medicine: Theological perspectives in medicine* (pp. 403-412). Grand Rapids: Eerdmans.

Harley, D. (1993). Spiritual physic, providence, and English medicine, 1560-1640. In: O. Grell & A. Cunningham (Eds.), *Medicine and the reformation* (pp. 101-117). London: Routledge.

Hessel, D. (1996). Now that animals can be genetically engineered: Biotechnology in theological-ethical perspective. In: R. Gottleib (Ed.), *This sacred earth: Religion, nature, environment* (pp. 620-633). New York: Routledge.

Hunter, M. (1996). The reluctant philanthropist: Robert Boyle and the 'Communiction of secrets and receits in physick'. In: O. Grell & A. Cunningham (Eds.), *Religio medici: Medicine and religion in seventeenth-century England* (pp. 247-272). Aldershott: Scolar Press.

Jonsen, A. (1998). *The birth of bioethics.* New York: Oxford University Press.

Jonsen, A. (2000). *A short history of medical ethics.* New York: Oxford University Press.

Kuyper, A. (1981 [1931]). *Lectures on Calvinism.* Grand Rapids: Eerdmans.

Martin, B. (1960). *The healing ministry in the church.* Richmond: John Knox Press.

May, W. (1975). Code and covenant or philanthropy and contract? *Hastings Center report, 5(6),* 29-38.

May, W. (1983). *The physician's covenant: Images of the healer in medical ethics.* Philadelphia: The Westminster Press.

Mouw, R. (1990). *The God who commands: A study in divine command ethics.* Notre Dame: University of Notre Dame Press.

Pathways to Promise. *Ministry and mental illness: Faith group: Organizations and networks* [On-line]. Available: http://www.pathways2promise.org/resources/faithgroup.htm#crcia

Pohl, C. (1995). Abortion: Responsibility and moral betrayal. In: J. Kilner, N. Cameron, & D. Schiedermayer (Eds.), *Bioethics and the future of medicine: A Christian appraisal* (pp. 212-223). Grand Rapids: Eerdmans.

Presbyterian Church (USA), 202nd General Assembly. (1990). *Universal Access to Health care: An Emerging Issue Paper Commended to the Church for Study and Comment.* Louisville: PCUSA Office of the General Assembly.

Ramsey, P. (1970). *The patient as person.* New Haven: Yale University Press.

Ramsey, P. (1978). *Ethics at the edges of life: Medical and legal intersections.* New Haven: Yale University Press.

Reformed Church in America [a]. *Summary of General Synod statements on abortion* [On-line]. Available: http://www.rca.org/churchlife/advocate/issues/abortion.html

Reformed Church in America [b]. *RCA: Perspective on physician-assisted suicide* [On-line]. Available: http://www.rca.org/churchlife/advocate/issues/suicide.html

Smith, D. (1993). On Paul Ramsey: A covenant-centered ethic for medicine. In: A. Verhey & S. Lammers (Eds.), *Theological voices in medical ethics* (pp. 7-29). Grand Rapids: Eerdmans.

Vaux, K. (1989). *Birth ethics: Religious and cultural values in the genesis of life.* New York: Crossroad.

Vaux, K. (1992). *Death ethics: Religious and cultural values in prolonging and ending life.* Harrisburg: Trinity Press International.

Verhey, A. (1984). Biomedical ethics: A Protestant perspective. In: P. Sigal (Ed.), *Biomedical ethics: Three theological perspectives* (p. 46). Grand Rapids: Ahavas Israel Congregation.

Verhey, A. (1987). Mongolism, parental eesires, and the right to life. In: S. Lammers & A. Verhey (Eds.), *On moral medicine: Theological perspectives in medicine* (pp. 475-488). Grand Rapids: Eerdmans.

Verhey, A. (1992). The practice of piety and the practice of medicine: Prayer, scripture, and medical ethics. *The Stob lectures of Calvin College and Seminary.* Grand Rapids: Calvin College and Seminary.

Verhey, A. (1997). Bioethics in the reformed tradition. In: B. Lustig (Ed.), *Bioethics yearbook, 5* (pp. 269-282). Dordrecht: Kluwer Academic Publishers.

Southern Baptists and Bioethics

C. Ben Mitchell

The Southern Baptist Convention is America's largest Protestant religious denomination, with nearly 16 million members in over 40,000 churches nationwide. While the largest concentration of Southern Baptists is in the South, they are found in every state. The denomination sponsors approximately 5,000 domestic missionaries serving in the United States, Guam, and the Caribbean as well as 4,000 international missionaries in 126 nations.

In order to understand how Southern Baptist positions and policies on bioethical issues are made, one must understand the polity and doctrine of the Southern Baptist Convention.

I. Southern Baptist Polity and Doctrine

The Southern Baptist Convention was formed in 1845 in Augusta, Georgia. From the beginning, Southern Baptists have valued congregational government of local churches and an associational model of affiliation with other churches and with the denomination as a whole. Southern Baptists do not have a magisterium or denominational hierarchy. Given their ecclesiological form, they are categorized as part of the "free church" tradition. James Sullivan, who for twenty-two years served as president of the Baptist Sunday School Board, the publishing arm of the Southern Baptist Convention, observed:

> To keep from evolving into a hierarchical structure, the denomination has developed a system enabling churches to work together voluntarily for "eliciting, combining, and directing" the energies and resources of the churches in the spread of the gospel to the ends of the earth. This cooperation does not lessen any individual or church freedoms (Sullivan, 1983).

Local Southern Baptist congregations may choose to cooperate with other Southern Baptists on any one, or all, of three separate levels. First, a Southern Baptist congregation may cooperate with another Southern Baptist congregation, and each church retains its autonomy or self-governing polity. When they cooperate on a mission project, for example, they are restricted by their cooperation only insofar as they have mutually agreed to be so bound.

Second, Southern Baptist congregations may choose to cooperate with an association of Southern Baptist congregations within given geographical boundaries. For example, in the South, where there are many Southern Baptist congregations, local Southern Baptist congregations may form an association of churches within a county. In parts of the country in which Southern Baptists are more dispersed geographically, an association may encompass more than one county, perhaps an entire state. Again, even when congregations choose to cooperate on an associational level, each local congregation preserves its autonomy or its right to self-government. Local church autonomy is only voluntarily restricted by the terms of cooperation with other congregations. Just as each local church retains its autonomy, each association is a self-governing entity and may act autonomously.

The oldest Baptist association in America, the Philadelphia Baptist Association, founded in 1707, was founded with the purpose of (1) serving as an advisory council for individual churches; (2) disciplining its churches, including withdrawing fellowship from disorderly churches; (3) ordaining ministers and disciplining individual ministers; (4) adopting a confession of faith; (5) encouraging the education of ministers; and (6) providing a community or fellowship among churches of similar doctrinal convictions (Gillette, 1851; Torbet, 1944). The Philadelphia Association became the paradigm for Baptist associationalism. This pattern was duplicated in the first Baptist association in the South, the Charleston Baptist Association (1751) which, like the Philadelphia Baptist Association, predates the Southern Baptist Convention. Oliver Hart, formerly a minister in the Philadelphia association, was a primary initiator of the founding of the Charleston Baptist Association (Baker, 1974).

A congregation's membership in an association is generally conditioned upon a request by the congregation and approval of the other member churches. Examination typically consists of an affirmation of the association's statement of faith and practice as well as a commitment to mutual cooperation. It is important to underscore that each congregation within an association remains autonomous and each association remains similarly autonomous. As a self-governing body, a congregation may choose to reject the statement of faith and practice agreed upon by the other churches in the association or otherwise divorce itself from the association at any time. An association, likewise, may choose, as an expression of its autonomy, to discipline or disfellowship a church. Both actions are consistent with the Southern Baptist model of associationalism. Contemporary Southern Baptists maintain this model of associationalism as a paradigm for polity.

Local churches may also cooperate at the state level. Southern Baptists have over 30 state conventions of churches. A local Southern Baptist congregation may choose to cooperate with the Southern Baptist congregations in a given state either by being a part of an association of churches in that state or by giving money to that state's mission program. Again, the local congregation and the state conventions retain their individual autonomy. A congregation may choose, at any time, to remove itself from the state convention of churches, or a state convention may censure or disfellowship a church by refusing to seat those persons she sends as "messengers" to the state's annual meeting. "Messengers" (as opposed to "delegates") may be sent from the churches to the annual meetings to help conduct the business of the state convention. These messengers have voting power only during the annual meeting. Afterward, messengers have no authority or power in the operation of the state convention.

Finally, local churches may cooperate at a national level. Many local Southern Baptist congregations send messengers annually to the Southern Baptist Convention. The Convention meets in a different American city each year. Once again, local congregations may send messengers to the annual meeting to vote for officers of the Convention, address the business matters of the Convention, and consider Convention resolutions. Technically speaking, therefore, the Southern Baptist Convention exists for purposes of conducting its business only during those few days each summer during which it meets. In the interim, the Executive Committee of the Southern Baptist Convention conducts and coordinates the work of the Convention, except in those areas assigned to other SBC agencies.

The Southern Baptist Convention is, therefore, a voluntary association of local congregations and not a Church in the sense in which one may speak of the Roman Catholic Church, the Evangelical Lutheran Church of America, or the United Methodist Church. As James Sullivan explains, "The term 'the Southern Baptist Church' is never correct when referring to the denomination as a whole. There are only Southern Baptist churches" (Sullivan, 1983).

This understanding of the nature of associationalism arises from a prior commitment to a particular theological epistemology. Those who identify with the Southern Baptist Convention at the national level confess an evangelical faith of a relatively conservative variety. The *Baptist Faith and Message 2000* is the most recent doctrinal affirmation of the Southern Baptist Convention. In order to understand Southern Baptist statements on bioethics and on other matters, one must understand that for the vast majority of Southern Baptists the scriptures of the Old and New Testaments are regarded as the only authoritative guide for faith and practice. Historically speaking, the Southern Baptist Convention claims, along with other Reformation churches, *sola Scriptura* (scripture alone) in matters of faith and practice. Philosophically speaking, the Southern Baptist Convention's ethical theory is a form of divine command ethics (Henry, 1974). Thus, Article I of *The Baptist Faith and Message 2000* says:

> The Holy Bible was written by men divinely inspired and is God's revelation of Himself to man. It is a perfect treasure of divine instruction. It has God for its author, salvation for its end, and truth, without any mixture of error, for its matter. Therefore, all Scripture is totally true and trustworthy. It reveals the principles by which God judges us, and therefore is, and will remain to the end of the world, the true center of Christian union, and the supreme standard by which all human conduct, creeds, and religious opinions should be tried. All Scripture is a testimony to Christ, who is Himself the focus of divine revelation. Exodus 24:4; Deuteronomy 4:1-2; 17:19; Joshua 8:34; Psalms 19:7-10; 119:11,89,105,140; Isaiah 34:16; 40:8; Jeremiah 15:16; 36:1-32; Matthew 5:17-18; 22:29; Luke 21:33; 24:44-46; John 5:39; 16:13-15; 17:17; Acts 2:16ff.; 17:11; Romans 15:4; 16:25-26; 2 Timothy 3:15-17; Hebrews 1:1-2; 4:12; 1 Peter 1:25; 2 Peter 1:19-21.

Since most Southern Baptists affirm that the Bible is authoritative, the scriptures provide the normative foundation for discussions of moral and ethical issues. Furthermore, Southern Baptists affirm the necessity of social and cultural engagement. Article XV of *The Baptist Faith and Message 2000* on "The Christian and the Social Order" says,

> All Christians are under obligation to seek to make the will of Christ supreme in our own lives and in human society. Means and methods used for the improvement of society and the establishment of righteousness among men can be truly and permanently helpful only when they are rooted in the regeneration of the individual by the saving grace of God in Jesus Christ. In the spirit of Christ, Christians should oppose racism, every form of greed, selfishness, and vice, and all forms of sexual immorality, including adultery, homosexuality,

> and pornography. We should work to provide for the orphaned, the needy, the abused, the aged, the helpless, and the sick. We should speak on behalf of the unborn and contend for the sanctity of all human life from conception to natural death. Every Christian should seek to bring industry, government, and society as a whole under the sway of the principles of righteousness, truth, and brotherly love. In order to promote these ends Christians should be ready to work with all men of goodwill in any good cause, always being careful to act in the spirit of love without compromising their loyalty to Christ and His truth. Exodus 20:3-17; Leviticus 6:2-5; Deuteronomy 10:12; 27:17; Psalm 101:5; Micah 6:8; Zechariah 8:16; Matthew 5:13-16, 43-48; 22:36-40; 25:35; Mark 1:29-34; 2:3ff.; 10:21; Luke 4:18-21; 10:27-37; 20:25; John 15:12; 17:15; Romans 12-14; 1 Corinthians 5:9-10; 6:1-7; 7:20-24; 10:23-11:1; Galatians 3:26-28; Ephesians 6:5-9; Colossians 3:12-17; 1 Thessalonians 3:12; Philemon; James 1:27; 2:8.

Southern Baptists seek to address bioethical and other issues from a perspective which reflects the normative priority of the biblical witness, the priesthood of all believers, the primacy of the local congregation, and the necessity of social and cultural engagement.

II. Southern Baptists's Ethical Voice

There are two primary vehicles by which Southern Baptists address ethical issues from a national perspective. First, Southern Baptists attending the annual meeting may address ethical issues through the process of framing and affirming resolutions. The Bylaws of the Southern Baptist Convention provide for a

> Committee on Resolutions [that is charged with the responsibility] to prepare and submit to the Convention resolutions which the Committee deems appropriate for adoption, and to report on all matters submitted to it by the Convention, with or without recommendation or amendments ... Only registered messengers to the Convention are eligible to submit resolutions (Bylaws §22).

Southern Baptists have adopted resolutions since they began meeting over 150 years ago. Resolutions committees work long hours before and during the annual meeting to evaluate, draft, and recommend resolutions for consideration by the full body present at the Southern Baptist Convention annual meeting. Resolutions have covered everything from the mundane – such as showing appreciation to the city hosting the convention – to the momentous – such as lamenting the racist beginnings of the denomination.

The second vehicle Southern Baptists use to express their views on moral, social, and religious liberty issues is the Ethics & Religious Liberty Commission (ERLC). The ERLC has a long history, and both its name and its assignment have changed over the years. What began in 1908 as the Standing Committee on Temperance became the Christian Life Commission in 1953 and the Ethics & Religious Liberty Commission in 1997 (Hefley, 1997). The ERLC is governed by trustees elected by the Convention who represent the geographical diversity of the denomination. According to its mission statement, "The Ethics & Religious Liberty Commission exists to assist the churches by helping them understand the moral demands of the gospel, apply Christian principles to moral and social problems and questions of public policy, and to promote religious liberty in cooperation with the churches and other Southern Baptist entities" (Bylaws of the Ethics & Religious Liberty Commission, adopted 1997). The ERLC has two basic responsibilities: to educate and to advocate. On the one hand, the ERLC exists to educate and equip the churches to understand and address moral, social, and religious liberty issues. Through the publication of books, pamphlets, and other resources, the ERLC speaks directly to the churches of the Southern Baptist Convention. The ERLC also speaks to the various branches of national government to express to lawmakers and policymakers Southern Baptist convictions as they relate to moral concerns, public policy, and religious liberty. The ERLC has offices in Nashville, Tennessee, and Washington, DC.

The ERLC has convened a number of conferences and consultations on bioethics related topics. Most notably, at its 26th annual seminar in 1993, the ERLC (then the Christian Life Commission), held a conference called, "Life at Risk: Crises in Medical Ethics" in Nashville, Tennessee. Among the speakers were Richard D. Land, president of the Commission, Francis Collins, head of the National Center for Human Genome Research, the late Thomas Elkins, chair of the obstetrics and gynecology department at Louisiana State University's medical school in New Orleans, Thomas Harris, chair of the department of biomedical engineering at Vanderbilt University, Gary Crum, deputy director of policy for the Ohio Department of Health, Franklin E. Payne, Jr., associate professor of family medicine at the Medical College of Georgia, Nigel Cameron, founding editor of the journal *Ethics & Medicine: An International Journal of Bioethics*, and Joe S. McIlhaney, Jr., an obstetrician and gynecologist and founder of the Medical Institute for Sexual Health in Austin, Texas. The conference covered topics including abortion, fetal personhood, RU-486, human genetics, patient autonomy, euthanasia and assisted suicide, sexually transmitted diseases and abstinence education, faith and science, and the future of medicine and the biosciences.

The ERLC also publishes a series of pamphlets and other materials on bioethical issues. Much of the material is produced in-house and is written by Southern Baptists; some of it is available commercially. Pamphlet topics include bioethics, infertility and the new reproductive technologies, euthanasia, advance directives and living wills, genetic engineering, embryo research, abortion, alternatives to abortion, and why violence against abortion providers is wrong. Furthermore, the ERLC has published the papers from its 1993 bioethics conference under the title, *Life at Risk: The Crises in Medical Ethics* (Land & Moore, 1995).

The ERLC is often called upon to participate in dialogues and discussions with policymakers on bioethical issues. For example, in 1992, the director of biomedical and life issues for the ERLC spoke at a public forum on assessing genetic risks sponsored by the Institute of Medicine in Washington, DC.

On January 18, 1994, following the announcement that the Clinton administration was going to undertake healthcare reform, the ERLC convened a special Southern Baptist Consultation on Health Care in Washington, DC. Held in the Dirksen Senate Office Building, the consultation focused on the ethical, legal, and social implications of the Health Security Act proposed by the administration under the impetus of Mrs. Hillary Clinton, the wife of the President of the United States. Participants in the consultation included members of the ERLC board and staff as well as special invitees. Among the presenters at the consultation were Nigel Cameron, a British bioethicist familiar with England's National Health Service, Scott E. Daniels, director of the ethics and health policy project for the

Family Research Council, James T. Herod, senior vice-president of the Annuity Board of the Southern Baptist Convention, and John F. Kilner, director of the newly formed Center for Bioethics and Human Dignity. From this consultation, a statement on health care reform was drafted: "Health Care Reform: A Moral Preamble." The statement is built around seven affirmations: (1) We believe as citizens of the Kingdom of Jesus Christ, the Great Physician, we are called to participate in the current dialogue on health care reform; (2) We believe all persons find themselves in need of medical care at various times in their lives; (3) We believe there is a need for revision in the health care delivery system; (4) We believe the key elements in any successful health care reform include reducing unnecessary medical care and costs (with attendant tort reform), liberalizing access to health insurance and providing medical assistance to those truly in need; (5) We believe the benefits of health care should extend to all of humanity, including the elderly, the chronically ill, the disabled and the unborn; (6) We believe the Hippocratic tradition of medicine, especially as it subsequently has been enriched by the Christian ethos, represents the noblest advance of the healing arts; and (7) We believe the promotion of good health habits is a worthy goal of preventive health care.

On January 26, 1994, the director of biomedical and life issues for the agency, gave testimony on "Health Care Reform: Women's Health," before the Subcommittee on Health and Environment of the Energy and Commerce Committee of the U.S. House of Representatives. In 1995, Richard Land, president of the ERLC, signed a statement along with almost 300 religious leaders "in vigorous opposition to the patenting of human genes and genetically engineered animals," arguing that "humans and animals are creations of God not humans, and as such should not be patented as human inventions" (Appleyard, 1998).

Finally, the ERLC often joins *amicus curia* briefs on legal issues related to bioethics. Recent briefs include *Stenberg v. Carhart*, with the United States Catholic Conference on partial-birth abortion; *Washington v. Glucksberg* and *Vacco v. Quill*, with the United States Catholic Conference on physician-assisted suicide; *Madsen v. Women's Health Center*, with the Christian Legal Society on pro-life speech; and *Planned Parenthood v. Casey*, with the United States Catholic Conference on state restrictions on abortion.

III. Reproduction

A. Abortion

Like some other religious groups, Southern Baptists' first significant foray into bioethics was in response to the practice of abortion. While the convention would modify its position on abortion almost immediately, its first resolution on abortion in 1971 was consistent with what was later codified as law in *Roe v. Wade* (1973) and its companion ruling *Doe v. Bolton* (1973).

> WHEREAS, Christians in the American society today are faced with difficult decisions about abortion; and
>
> WHEREAS, Some advocate that there be no abortion legislation, thus making the decision a purely private matter between a woman and her doctor; and
>
> WHEREAS, Others advocate no legal abortion, or would permit abortion only if the life of the mother is threatened;
>
> Therefore, be it *Resolved*, that this Convention express its belief that society has a responsibility to affirm through the laws of the state a high view of

> the sanctity of human life, including fetal life, in order to protect those who cannot protect themselves; and
>
> Be it further *Resolved*, That we call upon Southern Baptists to work for legislation that will allow the possibility of abortion under such conditions as rape, incest, clear evidence of severe fetal deformity, and carefully ascertained evidence of the likelihood of damage to the emotional, mental, and physical health of the mother.

While the resolution invokes a "high view" of the sanctity of human life as its guiding theological principle, at the same time it allows for what would be regarded by subsequent Conventions as overly expansive exceptions. The 1974 Convention essentially reconfirmed the previous resolution, but in 1976, significant nuances were added.

> WHEREAS, Southern Baptists have historically held a biblical view of the sanctity of human life, and
>
> WHEREAS, Abortion is a very serious moral and spiritual problem of continuing concern to the American people, and
>
> WHEREAS, Christians have a responsibility to deal with all moral and spiritual issues which affect society, including the problems of abortion, and
>
> WHEREAS, The practice of abortion for selfish non-therapeutic reasons destroys fetal life, dulls our society's moral sensitivity, and leads to a cheapening of human life,
>
> Therefore be it *Resolved*, that the messengers to the Southern Baptist Convention meeting in Norfolk in June, 1976, reaffirm the biblical sacredness and dignity of all human life, including fetal life, and
>
> Be it further *Resolved*, that we call on Southern Baptists and all citizens of the nation to work to change those attitudes and conditions which encourage many people to turn to abortion as a means of birth control, and
>
> Be it further *Resolved*, that in the best interest of our society, we reject any indiscriminate attitude toward abortion, as contrary to the biblical view, and
>
> Be it further *Resolved*, that we also affirm our conviction about the limited role of government in dealing with matters relating to abortion, and support the right of expectant mothers to the full range of medical services and personal counseling for the preservation of life and health.

By 1977, Southern Baptists were becoming more sensitive, articulate, and conservative on the issue of abortion. The 1977 resolution on abortion not only reaffirmed word-for-word the 1976 resolution, but added the following prefatory clause: "Resolved, that this Convention reaffirm the strong stand against abortion adopted by the 1976 Convention, and, in view of some confusion in interpreting part of this resolution we confirm our strong opposition to abortion on demand and all governmental policies and actions which permit this." Resolutions on abortion continued to evolve, including resolutions in 1978 and 1979, until, in 1980, the Convention adopted a resolution favoring legislation prohibiting abortion "except to save the life of the mother." In 1982, abortion, infanticide, and euthanasia were linked in a resolution that claimed that "Social acceptance of abortion has begun to dull society's respect for all human life, leading to growing occurrences of infanticide, child abuse, and active euthanasia" and calling for "legislation and/or a constitutional amendment which will prohibit abortions except to save the physical life of the mother" and "legislation which will prohibit the practice of infanticide." The decade from 1973 to 1983 was marked by landmark bioethics cases and literature, which affected all Americans, including Southern Baptists.

Southern Baptist attitudes toward abortion and abortion-related policy continued to grow more conservative. The 1984 convention resolution on abortion opined that abortion was "a national sin" and that an unborn child is "a living individual human being," while the 1988 resolution affirms that "Human life, from fertilization until natural death, is sacred and should be protected, not destroyed." Every subsequent resolution on abortion to date extends that assertion. For instance, in 1993 Southern Baptists passed a resolution against the Freedom of Choice Act and another resolution criticizing President Clinton's abortion policies. In 1995, the Convention passed a resolution against the nomination of Dr. Henry Foster as Surgeon General of the United States. The next year, Southern Baptists passed resolutions favoring the Partial-Birth Abortion Ban and a resolution requesting all political parties to include a pro-life platform.

In addition to the resolutions passed by the SBC, polling data also provide an indicator of Southern Baptist attitudes regarding abortion. There are several studies worth noting. First, sociologist Nancy Tatom Ammerman conducted a scientific poll of Southern Baptists in 1985 and found that among 1200 clergy and 1800 laypersons, 11% thought abortion should never be permitted, 29% thought it should only be permitted to save the life of the mother, 50% thought abortion should only be permitted when the life of the mother was at risk or in cases or rape or incest, and 10% thought women should be free to choose (Ammerman, 1990). In 1990, the Southern Baptist Convention's publishing and data-gathering arm, the Baptist Sunday School Board, found that 14% of those self-identified Southern Baptists polled thought abortion should always be illegal, 69% said it should be legal only in certain circumstances, and 14% said it should be legal regardless of the circumstances. Finally, in an unscientific poll taken at the Sanctity of Human Life booth at the 1994 Southern Baptist Convention annual meeting, 97% said that God gives human beings a spirit at conception, 90% supported abortion to save the physical life of the mother, and 85% said abortion should not be legal. At the same time, 32% said they approved of abortion in cases of rape and 30% supported abortion in cases of incest (*The Current*, 1994).

Based on decades of resolutions and the available polling data, it is safe to say that, judged by most relevant indicators, and with the caveat that there is considerable diversity among individual Southern Baptists, the SBC is pervasively pro-life on the matter of abortion. The foundation of the argument that abortion is wrong in most cases is based on the belief that human life is sacred and inviolable from conception to natural death and may only be taken for just causes. Those causes would include self-defense, and for most but by no means all Southern Baptists, just war and capital punishment.

B. Genetic Technology and Cloning

The doctrine of the sanctity of human life also informs other issues related to reproduction. In 1997, the year that Dolly the sheep was cloned, the Convention meeting in Dallas, Texas, passed a resolution "On Genetic Technology and Cloning." The resolution acknowledges the potential benefits of genetic technology for the treatment of disease, but laments "the hideous potential of increasing the numbers of abortions through the use of prenatal genetic screening, the creation of human embryos for the purpose of experimental research, the cloning of whole human beings, and discrimination against individuals based upon their genetic information." The resolution lauds genetic research "which has as its goal the treatment or cure of genetic illnesses and debilitating genetic conditions," but opposes prenatal genetic testing for abortion decisions, destructive research using human embryos, human cloning, and genetic discrimination.

In 1999, the Southern Baptist Convention meeting in Atlanta, Georgia, passed a very strongly worded resolution against human embryonic stem cell research that requires the destruction of human embryos. The resolution is grounded in the belief that "human beings are made in the image and likeness of God (Gen. 1:27; 9:6) and protectable human life begins at fertilization..." The resolution also points to what it calls Southern Baptists' "decades-long opposition to abortion except to save the physical life of the mother and their opposition to destructive human embryo research."

IV. Death and Dying

Southern Baptists have addressed euthanasia and assisted suicide through their resolutions process. A resolution "On Assisted Suicide" was passed in 1996. The resolution begins by citing recent developments in law and social practice related to assisted death, including two U. S. Courts of Appeals decisions to strike down laws prohibiting assisted suicide, Jack Kevorkian's persistent assistance in the suicide of his patients, and the erosion of the medical consensus against assisted death. It then offers Biblical support for condemning assisted suicide and euthanasia (e.g., Exodus 20:13) and

> that we the messengers of the Southern Baptist Convention, meeting in New Orleans, Louisiana, June 11-13, 1996, affirm the biblical and Hippocratic prohibitions against assisted suicide; and
>
> Be it further RESOLVED, that we commend and encourage medical science in it efforts to improve pain management techniques, thus removing one major impetus toward assisted dying; and
>
> Be it further RESOLVED, that we call upon physicians, nurses, hospice workers, individual Christians and local churches to make emotional, psychological, and spiritual care of suffering patients a priority, thereby relieving the sense of isolation and abandonment some dying patients feel; and
>
> Be it further RESOLVED, that we vigorously denounce assisted suicide as an appropriate means of treating suffering; and
>
> Be it finally RESOLVED, that we call on federal, state, and local governments to prosecute under the law physicians or others who practice assisted suicide.

V. Fetal Tissue Research and Gene Patenting

Through Convention resolutions, Southern Baptists have also spoken on fetal tissue research, trafficking in human tissues, and the commodification of human and animal genes. Fetal tissue research came to the minds of Southern Baptists in 1992 when the United States Congress was considering legislation that would overturn the federal moratorium on the use of fetal tissue from induced abortions in tax-funded transplantation research. The "Resolution on Fetal Tissue Experimentation" adopted in Indianapolis in 1992 contained only four brief paragraphs. Southern Baptists at that Convention resolved to call on Congress to sustain the President's federal moratorium and to affirm their opposition to "the unethical practice of using fetal tissue from induced abortions in experimental research, whether privately or publicly funded."

At the sesquecentennial meeting of the Convention in 1995, in Atlanta, Georgia, Southern Baptists passed a resolution against the patenting of "animal and human tissues and genetic sequences." The resolution is explicit in its rationale for rejecting this practice, namely, "The scriptures of both the Old and New Testaments plainly teach that God alone is creator and owner of all he has made (Genesis 1:1; Colossians 1:15-16)" and "Human life is uniquely made in the image and likeness of God (Genesis 1:27)." Moreover, the resolution encourages the development of genetic technologies "which contribute to the treatment and cure of genetic illnesses;" calls for "a national dialogue about the merits and liabilities of patenting animal and human genes;" and enjoins "the President, the Congress, the National Institutes of Health, and the United States Patent Office to place an immediate moratorium on the patenting of animal and human tissues and genetic sequences until a full and complete discussion has occurred."

VI. Organ Donation and Transplantation

Southern Baptists passed a resolution encouraging organ donation at the 1988 meeting in San Antonio, Texas. The resolution points both to the critical need for transplantable organs and to the view that "the values of a godless society promote self-sufficiency to such a degree that people are indifferent to the needs of others, as seen in resistance to organ donations." While acknowledging that the decision to donate one's organs is a matter of personal conscience, the resolution encourages "voluntarism regarding organ donations in the spirit of stewardship, compassion for the needs of others, and alleviating suffering." The resolution also affirms the "validity" of living wills, donor cards, and the right of next of kin to make decisions regarding organ donation. The final paragraph of the resolution contains the caveat that "nothing in the resolution be construed to condone euthanasia, infanticide, abortion, or harvesting of fetal tissue for the procurement of organs."

Over a decade later, against the backdrop of reports that a few companies were selling human fetal body parts for research, the Southern Baptist Convention meeting in Orlando, Florida, in 2000, adopted a resolution strongly denouncing the practice. In a lengthy resolution, the Convention mentioned by name the Anatomic Gift Foundation and Opening Lines as companies "found to traffic (sic) in human fetal body parts – buying, dissecting, and selling those tissues." In addition, the resolution states that "The growing industry of buying and selling human fetal organs, tissues, and cells represents a grisly practice that converts human body parts into a commodity to be bought and sold in the marketplace." Earlier, in the 1995 resolution on gene patenting, the problem of commodification of human body parts was invoked. Here the problem of commodification is extended beyond patenting to support the prohibition of sales of human tissues. Particularly problematic for the SBC is that many of the tissues at stake are procured through elective abortion and "Elective abortion is an act of violence against unborn human beings, and the sale of their tissues is an assault on the biblical truth that all human beings are created in the image of God (Genesis 1:27; Psalm 139:13-16)." The consistent thread running through almost all of the resolutions of the SBC on bioethics is that human beings are created in the image of God and that this requires that we respect and protect human life from conception to natural death. This message is found in most if not all SBC resolutions regarding human life issues, and the Convention routinely delivers this message to elected officials.

VII. Public Health and Access to Health Care

Whether it is an advantage or liability, one reality of the resolutions process in Southern Baptist life is that resolutions address timely issues. In fact, for most of the SBC resolutions on bioethical issues one could, as it were, hold a newspaper in one hand and the resolution in the other. That is to say, Southern Baptists have used resolutions to speak to what they believe are the most pressing moral, social, and bioethical issues of the moment. This has been the case throughout the history of the Southern Baptist Convention. For example, in 1910 the SBC passed a resolution supporting a Senate bill that would establish a national Department of Public Health. The resolution states that "the enactment of this bill into law would go far toward conserving the health of the American people, thus carrying out the highest and most beneficent function of government, at the same time creating conditions that will promote morality and religion." During this era Southern Baptists and others were working hard for prohibition. At the annual Convention meeting that year in Jacksonville, Florida, Maldon Browning Adams, representing the Temperance Committee, the forerunner of the ERLC, said, "The kingdom of God stands face to face with an aggressive, vicious, and unscrupulous enemy, the legalized liquor traffic. We cannot avoid giving battle if we would. Our Christian civilization demands ...[that] [t]he saloon must go. It must die as slavery died, and witchcraft and dueling" (cited in Hefley, 1997).

More recently, the SBC addressed issues of health care reform in 1994 when the debate regarding the Clinton Health Security Act reached its zenith. The Southern Baptist Convention acknowledged the importance health care has for human life, that health care is a ministry through which we demonstrate compassion for others, and that the present health care system in the United States leaves some without access to care such that some form of health care reform was necessary. It also pointed to morally objectionable aspects of the Clinton plan, including the access it provided to abortion and to contraceptives for minors without parental consent. The resolution passed also expressed concern that the Clinton plan did not have an adequate conscience clause such that some physicians and health care organizations could be forced to participate in morally objectionable practices. In light of these difficulties, the SBC resolved

> That while our Baptist heritage of insistence on limited government causes us to believe the need for reform does not mandate a government-controlled,[sic] health care system, we, the messengers to the Southern Baptist Convention meeting in Orlando, Florida, June 14-16, 1994, nevertheless encourage the President and Congress in their attempt to reform America's health care system; and
>
> Be if finally RESOLVED, That we oppose any health care reform legislation that includes any of the aforementioned morally objectionable provisions.

VIII. Conclusion

There is every reason to think that Southern Baptists will continue to address issues in bioethics by considering the impact they have on human life and evaluating the ways in which we show respect and disrespect for human life given the premise that humans are created in the image of God. The Ethics & Religious Liberty Commission of the Southern Baptist Convention will continue to speak prophetically regarding biotechnological advances, including pharmacogenetics, proteomics, xenotransplantation, stem cell research, nanotechnology, and robotics. The agency will continue to speak forthrightly against violations of the sacredness of human life, including abortion and euthanasia. Moreover, Southern Baptists will continue to address bioethics-related issues in their resolutions process. Given the polity of the Southern Baptist tradition, this is an effective means of making the voice of Southern Baptists heard on significant issues. At the same time, local congregations, state conventions, and mission agencies will continue to engage in ministry which applies their convictions to serving God and their neighbors.

Bibliography

Ammerman, N.T. (1990). *Baptist battles: Social change and religious conflict in the Southern Baptist convention*. New Brunswick, NJ: Rutgers University Press.

Appleyard, B. (1998). *Brave new worlds: Staying human in the genetic future*. New York: Penguin Books.

Baker, R.A. (1974). *The Southern baptist convention and its people 1607-1972*. Nashville: Broadman Press.

Bylaws of the ethical and religious liberty commission. Available online www.erlc.com

Bylaws of the Southern baptist convention. Available online www.sbc.net/aboutus/legal/bylaws.asp

(1994). Moral concerns newsletter of the First Baptist Church of Orlando. In: *The Current*. Florida.

Doe v. Bolton (70-40) 410 U.S. 179 (1973).

Gillette, A.D. (Ed.) (1851). *Century minutes of the Philadelphia baptist association: 1707-1807*. Philadelphia: American Baptist Publication Society.

Henry, C.F.H. (1974). The good as the will of God. In: W.K. Frankena & J.T. Granrose (Eds.), *Introductory readings in ethics* (pp. 95-99). Engelwood Cliffs, NJ: Prentice-Hall.

Hefley, J. (1997). *Conscience of a People*. Unpublished manuscript history of the Ethics & Religious Liberty Commission. Nashville: Ethics & Religious Liberty Commission.

Land, R. & Moore, L. (Eds.) (1995). *Life at risk: The crises in medical ethics*. Nashville: Broadman and Holman.

Madsen v. Women's Health Center (93-880) 512 U.S. 753 (1994).

Planned Parenthood v. Casey (91-744) 505 U.S. 833 (1992).

Roe v. Wade (70-18) 410 U.S. 113 (1973).

Southern Baptist Convention Resolutions (1910, 1971, 1974, 1976, 1977, 1978, 1979, 1980, 1982, 1984, 1988, 1992, 1993, 1994, 1995, 1996, 1997, 1999, 2000). Available online at www.sbc.net

Stenberg v. Carhart (99-830) 192 F.3d 1142 (2000).

Sullivan, J.L. (1983). *Baptist polity as I see it*. Nashville: Broadman Press.

The Baptist faith and message 2000 (2000). Available online at www.sbc.net

Torbet, R.G. (1944). *A social history of the Philadelphia baptist association 1707-1940*. Philadelphia: Westbrook Publishing Company.

Vacco v. Quill (95-1858). 117 S. Ct 2293, 138 (1997).

Washington v. Glucksberg (96-110) 117 S. Ct. 2258, 138 L.Ed 2d 772 (1997).

Authority and Agency: Policies and Principles in Latter-day Saints Bioethics

Courtney S. Campbell

I. Introduction

The Church of Jesus Christ of Latter-day Saints (LDS), whose members are known as the Mormons, was founded in 1830 under the direction of Joseph Smith, Jr. Smith claimed that he had received visitations from God, Jesus Christ, and biblical prophets of antiquity, giving him authority to restore the gospel and organization of the apostolic Christian church. Beginning with Joseph Smith, his successors in ecclesiastical leadership have been designated "prophets, seers, and revelators" by the LDS community. They act to reveal divine truth for the community, and ultimately the world, in a manner that is portrayed as analogous to the role of the Hebrew prophet Moses.

Through belief in doctrines, performance of rituals, and the living of Christian discipleship, LDS members perceive the church to be the earthly mediator of the saving grace of Jesus. However, since in LDS teaching the "soul" is comprised of a union of spirit and body, the ecclesiastical emphasis on the salvation of souls necessarily encompasses matters of physical and bodily health. Thus, within three years of organizing the LDS church, Smith promulgated to his followers a code of health, known as the "Word of Wisdom" (*Doctrine*, 1981, pp. 175-176). The health code requires LDS members to abstain from wine, strong drinks, tobacco, and hot drinks, while commending the use of herbs, grain and fruit, and the moderate consumption of flesh for nutrition. Those persons who adhere to the "Word of Wisdom" are promised divine blessings such as health, physical strength and vitality, wisdom and knowledge, and protection from illness.

The "Word of Wisdom" is often cited in LDS discourse and writing as an example of a prophetic health ethic within the LDS tradition that anticipates, warns, and instructs. However, this anticipatory approach has become suffused with ambiguity upon the advent of biomedical technology in the middle and late 20th century. Indeed, with respect to questions of bioethics, the precedents for a "prophetic" ethic seem often to give way to a procedural approach. Procedural questions about who decides, at both the level of the scientific and biomedical research agenda, and at the level of clinical application, have tended to create an ethic that is now more reactive than anticipatory. Scientific developments in biomedicine and biotechnology largely have an ecclesiastical *carte blanche*, unless they directly involve terminating pre-natal life (abortion) or prematurely ending adult life (euthanasia or medical assistance in suicide). With respect to the many other issues that comprise the terrain of academic bioethics–reproductive issues, including fertility technologies and contraception; medical research on human beings; genetic testing, gene therapy, and genetic engineering; the allocation of health care resources; organ transplantation; the definition of death; and issues in the care of the dying, such as the withdrawal of life-sustaining treatment – the pattern of the LDS tradition has largely been to let the scientific advances and social questions play themselves out without direct ecclesiastical commentary.

If this scientific and social process eventuates in innovative clinical treatments for patients, the general tendency of LDS ecclesiastical leaders has been to belatedly acknowledge the new options, often only when they have emerged as issues in clinical interactions between practitioners and patients. Ecclesiastical discourse directed to a public audience offers very generalized substantive guidance for members of the LDS community, while affirming and deferring to the integrity of a collaborative decision-making process between medical professionals and the family (or the patient and the patient's family). Ultimately, LDS teaching emphasizes that the final responsibility for making a decision on matters such as whether or not to use reproductive technologies, or participate in research, or donate organs, or forgo life support, is a matter between the individual (or couple) and God. With the exceptions of abortion and euthanasia noted above, bioethical decision-making is not ecclesiastically mediated in the LDS community. LDS bioethics is most frequently a matter of praxis rather than substantive discourse.

This essay seeks to advance a more substantive discussion of LDS bioethics. It begins with a brief overview of ecclesiastical authority in the LDS tradition, which is an important background condition for assessing perspectives on bioethics addressed by LDS teaching. I then turn to an analysis of those questions in bioethics that have been the subject of ecclesiastical commentary or instruction. This topical analysis lends itself to the construction of a continuum of ecclesiastical policy conclusions, depending on such matters as social context, moral gravity, ecclesiastical interests, and personal moral responsibility. Since these policy positions are seldom issued with any supporting rationale, my conclusion seeks to identify some principles in LDS teaching that seem to be presupposed in ecclesiastical judgments.

II. Ecclesiastical Resources: Patterns and Problems

The administrative responsibility and direction of the LDS polity is developed by two central organizations. The presiding ecclesiastical body is known as the "First Presidency," which is comprised of a president and (traditionally) two counselors. A "Quorum of Twelve Apostles" acts under the direction of the First Presidency. It is these fifteen individuals who are collectively recognized as "prophets, seers, and revelators" within the LDS community (*Doctrine*, 1981, p. 217).

The administrative, pastoral, and hortatory guidance provided by these ecclesiastical leaders is derived ultimately from LDS canonized scripture. The tradition recognizes four books of "scripture," the *Bible* (Old and New Testament), the *Book of Mormon*, the *Doctrine and Covenants*, and the *Pearl of Great Price*, which are collectively referred to as "the standard works." The personal and communal actions of LDS members are held up to the normative "standards" articulated in these canonized books of scripture.

The canonical scriptures provide minimal content with respect to "standards" for bioethics issues and decisions. While they do not offer direct instructions or stipulations, the scriptural writings do provide an indispensable *indirect* influence for LDS bioethics, serving as the embedded source of general principles, such as moral agency or the sanctity of human life, that shape ecclesiastical perspectives on issues of medical ethics. Moreover, specific policies that have been formulated by presiding ecclesiastical authorities on topics of bioethics are held by the community to ultimately derive from some scriptural foundation, even if this foundation is not explicitly delineated in the policy statement itself.

Inevitably, then, LDS bioethics requires hermeneutics and interpretation of canonical stories and embedded principles. Yet, neither the stories, principles, or interpretative process are delineated in the primary resource for LDS bioethics positions, a set of policies promulgated by the presiding ecclesiastical authorities through the administrative guidebook known as the *Church Handbook of Instructions* (*Church*, 1998, pp. 155-160). As noted subsequently, current policies are an outgrowth of an ecclesiastical document developed in 1976, which formulated "attitudes" of the LDS Church on nineteen "medical problems," some of which are directly relevant to questions in bioethics. The current *Church Handbook* (1998) contains eleven "medical and health policies" and sixteen "policies on moral issues." Among these twenty-seven policies, some sixteen are relevant to analyses of bioethics within the LDS tradition. An inquiry regarding the LDS "position" on a certain question in bioethics will invariably consult the *Handbook* policies, with the canonized scriptures providing an implicit theological context and rationale for the position. At the same time, since these policies, unlike the canonical scriptures, are not given canonical status, their change and revision (often in conjunction with advances in medical science and biotechnology), at times makes it possible to examine innovative developments in ecclesiastical perspectives on bioethics. This methodology is developed more fully in the subsequent analysis.

Other than the presiding ecclesiastical authorities, the LDS Church has no paid clergy. It has moreover no formal training for "theologians." Thus, the scholarly locus and pastoral forums for advancing discussion of bioethics issues in many religious denominations are not available within the LDS polity. As physician-historian Lester E. Bush formulates the point: "One way in which individual Mormons, at any level, have *not* contributed appreciably to the development of church teachings is through an influential body of reflective medical-ethical literature. ...LDS medical ethics is finally still largely limited to the everyday application of the First Presidency's succinct behavioral guidelines" (Bush, 1993, p. 201).

One such guideline affirms procedural ethics by acknowledging the validity of personal moral agency and accountability. Thus, a third authoritative resource for LDS bioethics is personal decisions, at least insofar as such decisions are deemed "inspired" by God or as an answer to prayers for divine guidance. In theory, at least, personal inspiration should not contravene the basic "standards" or principles of the LDS canonized scriptures; however, the specific personal, familial, or institutional context within which the question is asked may lead to different applications and decisions. Personal inspiration in a specific clinical setting cannot be generalized as guidance for the entire ecclesiastical body. While the deference of the presiding ecclesiastical leadership to personal inspiration does exemplify how fundamental the moral agency and accountability of responsible decision-makers, including professionals, patients, and families, is taken to be in LDS thought, this deference to procedure also displays a refusal to generalize expertise from the ecclesiastical office to the vocations of scientific research or medicine.

There are, to be sure, important consequences of this ecclesiastical reliance on procedural ethics. The first consequence is that the LDS community has no real prophetic voice or tradition in bioethics, and indeed, more commonly than not, finds itself to be the recipient of a biomedical *fait accompli*. The agenda and priorities of contemporary biomedicine and the options available in its clinical applications are seldom questioned from any perspective commanding ecclesiastical authority. Thus, the bioethical issue with the greatest social scope – the re-orientation of health care allocation to ensure basic access for all citizens – has never been addressed in LDS discourse. At the same time, a scientific research priority involving high technology but very few individuals – the development of the artificial heart – received praise from some ecclesiastical leaders (Fox & Swazey, 1992). The social problem with this posture of ecclesiastical deference is that issues of greater urgency and scope are neglected while the scientific and medical communities are permitted to set their own agenda for society. The theological problem with this posture is that it very much suggests that the divine will is contingent on the current state of research and biomedical technology.

The second important consequence is that "new developments" in general LDS thought on the subjects of biomedical ethics are very rare. The controversy over the prospect of human cloning is a case in point. While the actual birth of a human clone will unquestionably require re-thinking of several important claims in LDS theology, the issue has yet to warrant ecclesiastical attention (Campbell, 1998). While it is possible to identify some historical changes and evolution in thinking on questions of bioethics, in general this process occurs at a slow, almost glacial, pace.

With these ecclesiastical patterns and problems as the context for LDS bioethics, I now to turn to an analysis of ecclesiastical instructions on substantive bioethical questions.

III. Ecclesiastical Horizons of Medical Ethics

The LDS engagement with contemporary medical ethics can be traced to a document prepared by James O. Mason, LDS Church Commissioner of Health, in June, 1974, in the aftermath of *Roe v. Wade* and promulgated in the wake of *Quinlan*. Entitled "Attitudes of The Church of Jesus Christ of Latter-day Saints Toward Certain Medical Problems," Mason submitted the paper to the presiding ecclesiastical authorities, including the First Presidency, and the document was subsequently presented to special gatherings known as "solemn assemblies" in 1976 (Bush, 1979, p. 97). The document, which provides short statements of ecclesiastical attitudes on nineteen such "problems," soon became an authoritative basis for local ecclesiastical leaders seeking to provide pastoral care on practical matters faced by members of their congregations. Thus, any developments in LDS medical ethics really must be measured against this document.

I will here present a short overview of these guidelines on ten questions of general concern in bioethics. I will also present the major modifications in focus and wording since the formulation of the original policies in 1976. This analysis will be organized through six categories (although not all attitudes or policies incorporate all six categories):

Attitude: the ecclesiastical position articulated in 1976;

Rationale: the theological, scriptural, social, or scientific reason(s) offered for the ecclesiastical position;

General Application: what this position means for lay members faced with a medical ethics situation;

Practical Exceptions: whether any exceptions to the general position or attitude are permitted;

Decision-making Procedure: how a decision on the issue should be made, and who should be involved;

Policy Modifications: developments on the topic since the formulation of the attitude that have been formalized in the *Church Handbook*.

A. *Beginning of Life*

A.1. *Abortion*

Original Attitude: The LDS Church is opposed to abortion.

General Application: LDS members are not to submit to, perform, or assist in an abortion. That is, the prohibition applies not only to pregnant women, but health care professionals, and depending on the nature of "assistance," family members or counselors. Participating in an action to which the church is "opposed" may carry with it ecclesiastical discipline, such as suspension of certain privileges of membership or even ex-communication.

Practical Exceptions: An "exception" to the prohibition of abortion may occur in circumstances where (1) medical prognosis confirms that continuation of the pregnancy places the life or good health of the mother in serious danger, or (2) the pregnancy is a result of rape and the mother is experiencing serious emotional distress as a result of this violation of her body.

Decision-making Procedure: The decision-makers (whether a couple or a single woman) should consult with a local ecclesiastical leader about their impending decision, and if a determination is made to seek an abortion, "divine confirmation" of this decision should be made through prayer.

Policy Modifications:

1) Attitude: The current version of the *Church Handbook* (1998) indicates that the LDS Church "opposes elective abortion for personal or social convenience," a potentially more open-ended perspective depending on the content given to "personal" and "social convenience."

2) Theological Rationale: The attitude on abortion articulated in 1976 did not include an explicit rationale, but the LDS tradition has long held that abortion violates the divine prohibition of the killing of human beings and is contrary to the value of the sanctity of human life. This rationale is more explicit in a recent ecclesiastical statement, which includes a reference to LDS scripture: "Thou shalt not kill, ... nor do anything like unto it" (*Doctrine*, 1998, p. 108). Thus, abortion is not considered the moral equivalent of killing an innocent human being, but its religious and moral gravity approximates or is "like" such killing.

3) Exceptions:

a) Incest leading to pregnancy is now considered a possible exception to the general prohibition, having the same status as pregnancy through rape. In addition, the antecedent involuntary sexual act that creates pregnancy is now by itself a sufficient ground to consider an exception; that is, the mother no longer needs to be experiencing emotional distress to request an abortion.

b) In the late 1980s, in the wake of advances in genetic testing, a third ground for an exception was ecclesiastically sanctioned: that is, an abortion may be permissible upon a medical finding that "the fetus has severe defects that will not allow the baby to survive beyond birth." These circumstances are not specified, but, since a baby who cannot survive beyond birth is stillborn, by definition this genetic exception will have rare applicability.

A.2. Artificial Insemination

Original Attitude: Artificial insemination with donor sperm (AID) is not approved by the LDS Church. No formal stance on artificial insemination with the sperm of the husband (AIH) was articulated.

Theological-Cultural Rationale: The performance of AID may create "problems related to family harmony."

General Application: As delineated subsequently, the language of "not approved" is less conclusive for LDS members than the language of "opposed" used in the context of abortion. The language of "non-approval" is not coupled with the prospect of ecclesiastical discipline for non-compliance.

Decision-making Procedure: The responsibility for resort to AIH or even AID should be determined by the married couple. Indeed, even while stating that AID is not approved, ecclesiastical authority acknowledges that use of AIH and/or AID is a "personal matter between husband and wife."

Policy Modifications:

1) Attitude: AID is now "strongly discouraged," language that is yet a further step down the scale of ecclesiastical concern.

2) Rationale: Ecclesiastical discourse does not provide a theological rationale for the current position. The concern about disruption of family harmony that provided the original rationale is likely empirically unsupportable given the widespread use of AI technology in the United States and other countries.

3) General Application: In response to a possible application of reproductive technology that was not contemplated in the 1970s, ecclesiastical discourse in the past decade has made it clear that AID for single women "is not approved."

A.3. Contraception

Original Attitude: It is contrary to LDS teaching to artificially curtail or prevent the birth of children.

Theological Rationale: Contraception violates the divine command to "multiply and replenish the earth." A practice of birth control will ensue in "disappointment" for the couple. It is not clear whether a practice (i.e., systematic use of contraception throughout a marriage) is distinguished from an act (e.g., use of contraception for any act of sexual intercourse, or for purposes of spacing the birth of children).

General Application: All LDS members are subject to the divine command to multiply and replenish promulgated in Genesis, and are expected to fulfill what may be considered a "procreative imperative" (Campbell, 1991, p. 25).

Practical Exceptions: The procreative imperative may be suspended in the following circumstances:

1) The couple does not enjoy health and vigor; in particular, the husband should make the health and strength of his wife his primary consideration.

2) Sexual union may risk generating genetic anomalies that could be transmitted to children.

Decision-Making Procedure: The couple should exercise "self-control" in their intimate relationships, and as noted above, the husband has an additional obligation to be considerate of the health of his spouse.

Policy Modifications: Of any LDS ecclesiastical teaching on medical ethics, the "attitude" and "rationale" regarding contraception have undergone the most extensive revision.

1) Attitude: The prior ecclesiastical condemnation has been fully withdrawn. In its place is a statement that affirms the moral agency of the couple: "The decision as to how many children to have and when to have them is extremely intimate and private and should be left between the couple and the Lord." As with other religious traditions, this revision may reflect in part an ecclesiastical concession to what couples were in fact already practicing.

2) Rationale: LDS teaching on birth control is now rooted in theological anthropology rather than a timeless scriptural injunction. In this theological view of the embodied self, it is a "privilege" of married couples, rather than a divine imperative, "to provide mortal bodies for the spirit children of God."

3) Decision-making Procedure: Contemporary teaching focuses neither on self-control nor on the duty of consideration of the husband toward the wife, but rather reconfigures the purposes of marital sexuality, such that procreation is not seen as the sole or primary purpose of sexual relations. Ecclesiastical guidance recognizes, to draw upon terminology from Roman Catholic teaching, the significance of the "unitive" dimension of marital sexuality, that is, sexual relations constitute a "means of expressing love and strengthening emotional and spiritual bonds."

A.4. Sterilization

Original Attitude: As with contraception, sterilization is also conceptualized within the divine command imposed on all Latter-day Saints to "multiply and replenish the earth." The procreative imperative implies general opposition to sterilization.

General Application: The procreative imperative applies to all LDS members, except as noted below.

Practical Exceptions: Rare medical conditions could warrant sterilization to protect the health of the mother.

Decision-making Procedure: The exceptional situation in which there is a medical indication (protecting the health of the mother) for sterilization must be determined by competent medical judgment, and the procedure must comply with relevant laws. A request for a sterilization procedure cannot legitimately be initiated by a couple.

Policy Modifications:

1) Attitude: The concept of sterilization has been clarified somewhat, in part reflecting new medical methods of reversible sterilization such as Norplant. Thus the general topic is now "surgical sterilization," which in most circumstances refers to procedures that are generally irreversible. The context for policy has also shifted away from the procreative imperative and towards appropriate methods of contraception. Thus, current ecclesiastical policy affirms: "The Church strongly discourages surgical sterilization as an elective form of birth control."

2) General Application: This policy is applicable to both genders, but makes special mention of vasectomy. This gender difference acknowledges that there are medical indications for a hysterectomy, whereas a vasectomy is commonly a personal choice. The language of "strong discouragement" does, however, remove a non-compliant choice from the scope of ecclesiastical discipline.

3) Practical Exceptions: Surgical sterilization is a consideration only in circumstances of (1) medical conditions that seriously jeopardize life or health, or (2) persons who are mentally incompetent and not responsible for their actions owing to a birth defect or serious trauma.

4) Decision-making Procedure: Compared with the formulation of the 1970s, the procedural standard is more demanding in that new criteria have been added to those of medical competency and legal compliance. In addition, the responsible persons (parents or spouses) must (1) consult with each other, (2) consult with their local ecclesiastical leader, and (3) pray to receive divine confirmation that sterilization is a warranted option in the circumstances.

B. Medical Progress: Experimentation and Research

Original Attitude: The LDS Church recognizes the need for carefully conducted and controlled experimentation.

Scientific Rationale: The justification is a matter of the integrity of scientific research and medical application, that is, that research on humans is required to assess the safety and efficacy of pharmaceuticals and medical procedures.

Decision-making Procedure: Two procedural controls are considered necessary to sound research: (1) protection of the moral agency of the subject through informed consent procedures and (2) peer review of the research project to determine its scientific necessity, design adequacy, and risk imposition.

Policy Modifications: No current ecclesiastical statement exists on research ethics. The advent of Institutional Review Boards (IRBs) in the mid-1970s arguably provides the procedural protections on consent and risk delineated above.

C. End of Life

C.1. Cremation

Original Attitude: The LDS Church believes that burial is the appropriate method for disposition of the bodily remains of the deceased. Cremation is discouraged.

Social Rationale: The rationale offered for preference for burial is "custom."

Practical Exceptions: Disposition of the body needs to comply with laws of the locale.

Decision-making Procedure: The family and loved ones of the deceased are entrusted with the final decision regarding disposition.

Policy Modifications:

1) Attitude: Currently, cremation is "not encouraged," a more permissive approach than the prior provision of being ecclesiastically "discouraged." This means that if cremation is a legal option, it may be an option for an LDS family in any country.

2) Rationale: Both custom and law in certain countries make cremation legally mandatory.

3) Decision-making Procedure: The family is the decision-maker about cremation and must consider the legal status of cremation and burial in its relevant jurisdiction.

C.2. *Dissection and Autopsy*

Original Attitude: In its original form, the attitude toward autopsies was framed by the absence of a prohibition. The ecclesiastical instruction stated the LDS church "does not object" to performance of autopsies, with two procedural provisions noted below.

Decision-making Procedure: The two presuppositions of legitimate autopsy are: (1) compliance with applicable law and (2) consent of the deceased's loved ones or family. These provisions are retained in contemporary ecclesiastical guidelines.

Policy Modifications:

1) Attitude: The contemporary ecclesiastical attitude is framed in terms of "permission" rather than the absence of objection: "Autopsies may be performed" provided the procedural guidelines are fulfilled.

C.3. *Euthanasia*

Original Attitude: In its original formulation, the tone of the LDS position on euthanasia was somewhat mild, especially in comparison with the language of "opposition" to abortion or "strong disapproval" of AID: "The Church does not look with favor upon any form of mercy killing." The milder tone may indicate that immediately in the aftermath of the *Quinlan* decision permitting the refusal of a life-sustaining ventilator, the question of forgoing life support had not, unlike the issues of abortion and AID, directly affected the LDS community.

Theological Rationale: The primary rationale invoked is the "dignity of life."

Decision-making Procedure: In certain circumstances, LDS members are called upon to apply faith in God and in medical science to reverse life-threatening conditions, rather than presumptively seeking to hasten death by medical means.

Policy Modifications:

1) Attitude: Even as civil and professional society has become more tolerant of euthanasia and physician-assisted suicide, the ecclesiastical attitude has become more rigid. First, the term "mercy killing," which intimates that love or compassion motivated the medical killing, has been discarded and replaced by a definition of euthanasia: deliberately putting to death someone suffering from an incurable condition or disease. This definition is deemed applicable to "so-called assisted suicide" as well. This shift directs ethical attention to the nature of the act and not simply to the intention of the agent.

2) Theological Rationale: The rationale for opposition to euthanasia has shifted from a general value, the dignity of life, to that of divine commandments. To resort to euthanasia is considered to "violate the commandments of God," although ecclesiastical instruction does not specify which commandments are indeed contravened. If the policy were rooted in the prohibition of killing, then moral consistency would seem to require ecclesiastical discipline for participation. Lacking disciplinary sanction, it seems that the prohibition of euthanasia is grounded in commandments other than or in addition to the prohibition of killing.

3) Decision-making Procedure: While the ecclesiastical *conceptualization* of euthanasia focuses on the action, the ecclesiastical *prohibition* is directed more at agent-morality than at act-morality. That is, the commandments of God are violated by "a person who participates in euthanasia" (as well as in assisted suicide). This emphasis on agent-"participation" substantially broadens the scope of prospective complicity beyond the physician-patient relationship, to other professional caregivers and even family members.

C.4. Transplantation
Original Attitude: The donation of bodily organs for post-mortem transplant or research is a matter for individual conscience.

Theological Rationale: While no rationale is stated, a decision of conscience would be consistent with the LDS doctrine of personal moral agency.

Decision-making Procedure: Those considering donation should (a) familiarize themselves with the benefits and risks of donation, (b) pray to God for guidance, and (c) act in such a way as to experience peace and comfort.

Policy Modifications:

1) Attitude: Current ecclesiastical teaching distinguishes donations of one's own organs or tissues for general medical purposes (presumably encompassing transplant, research, or education) from donations made on behalf of a deceased family member.

2) Decision-making Procedure: The three criteria for decision-makers (either the individual or family) to consider delineated above are no longer explicitly stipulated.

C.5. Treatment Termination
Original Attitude: In the social context of *Quinlan*, the Church of Jesus Christ of Latter-day Saints did not take a formal stand on treatment termination, but rather affirmed a qualified commitment to the dignity of life. By omission, the social meaning of a "right to die," in particular, the liberty to choose the timing, circumstances, and method of death, was rejected.

Theological Rationale: A foundation for a theology of dying is invoked: in contexts where it is determined that "dying is inevitable," the dying process should be seen as a "blessing" and an opportunity to experience the meaning of mortality.

General Application: Faith in God and the ministrations of medicine should be utilized to reverse the course of life-threatening conditions.

Practical Exceptions: The unstated implication of the theology of dying is that in those circumstances in which dying is inevitable, resort to all medical interventions to prolong life is not required.

Decision-making Procedure: Perhaps because of the *Quinlan* context, and the lack of legal validity or precedent, no procedure or decision-makers are designated.

Policy Modifications:

1) Attitude: What was previously implicit has now become ecclesiastically explicit: there is no obligation to "extend mortal life by means that are unreasonable."

2) Decision-making Procedure: The family of the dying person may engage in prayer and fasting to receive divine guidance, as well as consult with professional caregivers, regarding end-of-life decisions. While there is no explicit ecclesiastical direction on the subject of advance directives, both the silence on the subject and the LDS cultural attitude that preparation alleviates fear suggest there may be appropriate mechanisms for members facing such issues.

IV. In Medicine's Wake: Additions and Omissions

Despite the ongoing advances of biomedicine and their clinical application over the past quarter century, contemporary ecclesiastical policy has developed additional instructions on only three specific questions in bioethics, all of which are sub-issues of the general topic of reproductive technology. The three issues are *in vitro* fertilization (IVF), sperm donation, and surrogate motherhood. Despite the technical complexity and social controversy over these procedures, the ecclesiastical guidance is minimal. On each question, ecclesiastical teaching "strongly discourage[s]" such actions. Only on *in vitro* fertilization (IVF) is there any further exposition, but the wording of the policy on IVF is almost a verbatim reiteration of the teaching on AID, with the obvious difference that a donor egg might be involved in IVF. Thus, the policy, which was first formulated in 1989, instructs: "*In vitro* fertilization using semen from anyone but the husband or an egg from anyone but the wife is strongly discouraged." The decision-making process with respect to AI also is the model for IVF: "However, this [i.e., gamete donor IVF] is a personal matter that ultimately must be left to the judgment of the husband and wife, with responsibility for the decision resting solely upon them" (*General Handbook*, 1989, p. 4).

With respect to sperm donation and surrogate motherhood, the question is addressed succinctly in one-sentence statements that express strong discouragement. However, these statements do not acknowledge decision-making latitude on the issue, such that the act could be a "personal matter" as is the case with AID and IVF.

Just as significant as the addition of these new topics, current ecclesiastical instructions omit any direction on such staples of bioethical concern as medical research on human subjects, genetic screening or gene therapy, health care allocation, and the determination of death. The following brief analysis of the rationale for such omissions must be understood as relying on conjecture and inference.

A. *Research on Human Subjects*

As indicated above, pre-IRB policy statements did contain guidance on research issues, recognizing a need to validate medical treatments and drugs through testing on human beings. However, advancements in medical knowledge were constrained by protection of human subjects from harm and by respect for their right to informed consent. It could be argued that the implementation of IRB oversight of research provides these protections, and the ecclesiastical leadership therefore has decided to entrust research ethics to the oversight and integrity of the medical profession.

However, this is arguably a shortsighted approach. There are certain kinds of questions that do not fall within IRB purview or for which IRB assessment may be erroneous. For example, IRB review and approval was provided for human research on artificial heart technology that occurred at the University of Utah in the early 1980s. Although there was certainly no ecclesiastical endorsement of the research, sociologists Fox and Swazey indicated that a general pro-research ethos of LDS culture was an important catalyst for scientists to proceed with such studies in humans (Fox & Swazey, 1992).

In addition, some federally-supported research studies clearly have implications for related bioethical questions on which there is ecclesiastical direction. Recent studies of the efficacy and risks of RU-486 could well be interwoven with the discussion of abortion. Similarly, scientific studies that disaggregate intact human embryos for purposes of embryonic stem cell research raise significant questions about the moral status of the human embryo and of prenatal life. It is thus not so clear that the ecclesiastical posture of deferring questions of research ethics to the supervision of the scientific and medical communities, or of appointed procedural oversight boards, is theologically consistent or compelling.

B. Genetics

Genetic screening has in the past decade become part of the landscape of clinical medicine. Prenatal genetic diagnosis is widely used to identify malformations in the fetus prior to birth. Given that prenatal genetic screening has moved beyond the research stage and is a routine clinical option, it is somewhat puzzling that ecclesiastical guidance has been so minimal in this regard. As Bush has observed, "Ironically, while abortions are *not* condoned even when the fetus is known to be malformed, the Church has taken no stand on the subject of performing or undergoing amniocentesis as an antenatal check on the status of the fetus – a procedure for which there is virtually no justification if abortion is not considered an acceptable alternative" (Bush, 1979, p. 100).

Gene therapy, by contrast, is still in the early research stages and thus may be subject to the ecclesiastical entrustment described above regarding human research in general. Nonetheless, gene therapy has been described, often with hyperbole, as the future of medicine in the 21st century, and it is difficult not to see at least somatic cell gene therapy as a clinical option for patients suffering from various ailments in the near future. Somatic cell therapy may well prove to be a further example in the LDS community of ecclesiastical instruction being deferred until the technical scientific and medical questions about feasibility, safety, and efficacy have been answered to a level of satisfaction within the research and policy communities and until the public has been educated on the subject.

C. Health Care Access

The most conspicuous moral failure of the American health care system is its porous safety net, as over 40 million citizens lack access to coverage for basic health care services. Many religious denominations have issued prophetic statements decrying this situation and recommending some radical change in the health care system, including advocacy of a single-payer system for health care with the intent to ensure universal access. However, this issue has never engaged LDS ecclesiastical discourse or the LDS community in general. Almost certainly, this neglect is because the issue of access is deemed to be a "political" or "social" question that is peripheral to the fundamental ecclesiastical goals of proclaiming salvation of the soul.

It should be noted that the LDS church has a well-organized and generously funded welfare program for the basic living needs of its members. Should a member require assistance with regard to a fundamental health care need, it is quite possible that the internal welfare program would be used to provide such assistance. However, this resource is extended to members only in extreme circumstances, and, on the basis of scriptural injunctions to take care of the needs of one's own first, would in all likelihood not be made available to persons who are not members of the LDS faith community regardless of their need.

D. The Determination of Death

There is a rather well understood conceptual definition of biological death within the LDS community: biological death occurs upon the separation of the spirit and the body

(Campbell, 2002, p. 189). However, parallel to the LDS ecclesiastical policy indicating "there is no direct revelation on when the spirit enters the body," there is a similar agnosticism regarding the timing of the separation of the spirit and body that is called "death." Religious definitions of death that draw upon metaphysical claims are not helpful when practical decisions with a temporal dimension – such as when to forgo or cease medical treatment, or when organ removal may be permitted – have to be made. The metaphysical criterion of death as separation provides neither a locus of death, that is, a bodily organ (such as heart or brain) that could be examined to determine the absence of spirit, or tests by which such absence could be definitively established.

In the context of ecclesiastical agnosticism about the determination of death, the LDS church appears to have implicitly accepted the current legal and medical conventions as to the adequacy of heart-lung and/or whole brain criteria. That is, this issue might also be considered a political or scientific/medical question to which the church does not speak, despite the fact that determining death could well have practical complications for stopping medical treatment or for organ retrieval. If current philosophical support for a higher brain or neocortical standard of death were to generate momentum for a change in public policy, it could well impact current LDS teaching on end-of-life issues. A proposal for changing the criterion of death to reflect neocortical criteria would seem to either necessitate ecclesiastical re-thinking of the current teaching, or explicit advocacy of the current heart-lung and/or whole brain policy. The latter scenario seems more probable.

V. Ecclesiastical Policy Judgments: A Continuum

As illustrated by the above analysis, LDS ecclesiastical policy judgments on bioethics rely on several categories. The development of different categories reflect matters of vital ecclesiastical interests, the moral gravity of the act, social policy, and moral agency and accountability. It is possible then to develop a continuum of ecclesiastical judgments that reflect a range of prohibitions and permissions. I will begin with the most restrictive.

A. Ecclesiastical Opposition

The judgment that the LDS Church is "opposed" to a bioethical practice is reserved for only one issue: abortion. This judgment reflects both the ecclesiastical view of the morally serious nature of abortion decisions and the prospect that certain decisions – those made for reasons of "convenience" and that do not fall within the acceptable exceptions – can bring on a variety of forms of ecclesiastical discipline. Although (and perhaps because) the legal right to abortion is largely unrestricted, the LDS view is that a legal choice does not entail an appropriate exercise of moral agency.

A second question concerning ending life, that of euthanasia, does not prompt application of the language of ecclesiastical opposition as such, but is rather assessed within a framework of "violation" of divine commandments. Nor is ecclesiastical discipline proposed for participants in euthanasia. This does not necessarily signify a more permissive ecclesiastical expectation. Rather, it reflects the different context of social policy. Unlike abortion, euthanasia remains illegal in almost all jurisdictions. A professional participant in euthanasia would likely confront discipline as mediated through the law and through professional associations. However, recent trends to legalize medically-assisted suicide or euthanasia could well prompt a change in ecclesiastical judgment that would bring policy on euthanasia in close conformity to that of abortion. A position rooted in violation of religious commandment would certainly not be adequate should euthanasia become a permissible choice under social policy.

B. Ecclesiastical Disapproval

The ecclesiastical language of "not approved" pertains to issues in the creation of life. It has been applied to two bioethical practices, donor insemination in the "attitudes" articulated in 1976, and donor insemination requested by unmarried women in current policy. Thus, while the taking of human life prompts an ecclesiastical sanction of opposition, the perception of disruption of the kind of human life the LDS tradition believes is of paramount soteriological importance – family life – evokes a less dogmatic but still serious ecclesiastical judgment.

A recent proclamation issued by ecclesiastical leadership, a document similar in ecclesiastical significance to a papal encyclical, asserted: "Children are entitled to be born within the bonds of matrimony" (*Proclamation*, 1997). This seems to provide the rationale for holding out the prospect of ecclesiastical discipline in the situation of AID in single women, while a different category of judgment (without discipline) is applied to IVF with donor gametes.

C. Strong Ecclesiastical Discouragement

A third category of ecclesiastical judgment is expressed in the language of "strong discouragement." This is applied in the context of nearly all new reproductive technologies where procedures involve the mixing of gametes from non-related sources. Thus, AID, IVF, surrogate motherhood, and sperm donation are all addressed through this category. In addition, surgical sterilization for non-medical reasons is also strongly discouraged.

This approach may be differentiated from the previous categories because of different assumptions about the relevant values at stake: (a) social policy on reproductive technologies (like abortion, but unlike euthanasia) is permissive; (b) the moral gravity of the act is serious because it involves the creation, nature, or intentional disruption of family life; (c) despite the moral seriousness of reproductive technologies, ecclesiastical discipline is not considered for participants; and (d) the ultimate decision for resort to these procedures is (unlike abortion) left to the moral agency of the concerned couple.

D. Ecclesiastical Discouragement

A less restrictive category of "discouragement" has historically been adopted on certain questions dealing with body disposition such as cremation. The language of "discouragement" suggests an ecclesiastical presumption, for example, in favor of burial, but the general presumption may be overridden in light of cultural values, legal issues, and personal moral agency. This category is not used in current ecclesiastical discourse.

E. *Refraining from Ecclesiastical Objection*

The preceding four categories all express various degrees of ecclesiastical opposition to a bioethical practice. The fifth category expresses "neither prohibition nor permission." The only current procedure in this category is dissection of the body and autopsy. This is coupled with procedural guidelines about legal compliance and familial consent such that social policy and moral agency are the values that are ecclesiastically determinative.

F. *Ecclesiastical Silence*

There are certain bioethical issues on which there are no ecclesiastical instructions or positions. As noted above, these include human experimentation, AIH, access to health care, genetic technologies, and the definition of death. The reasons for ecclesiastical silence may differ. On some issues, it may be deemed that there is a relatively settled social consensus (for example, human research ethics and definition of death), as mediated by social policy or professional guidelines or procedures, such that ecclesiastical guidance is not needed. In cases where there is little social consensus, such as access to health care, ecclesiastical silence may reflect a judgment that the social question is beyond the purview of central ecclesiastical interests. On still other controversial questions, such as genetics and human cloning, ecclesiastical judgments may be deferred pending the comprehensive assessment of scientific and technical questions.

G. *Ecclesiastical Deference to Procedure and Personal Conscience*

On almost all bioethical questions that do not directly address the creation or termination of life, the LDS ecclesiastical approach is to defer decisions to matters of procedural ethics. This means that the action is permissible, insofar as it is not forbidden or discouraged, so long as certain procedural guidelines are followed.

This procedural ethic includes in almost all cases familial discussion because the locus of moral decision-making is the family. In only one circumstance, that of organ and tissue donation, is individual choice considered a sufficient decision-making resource. As deemed necessary, familial authority may be supplemented with ecclesiastical consultation and/or medical assessment. Local ecclesiastical leaders, such as a bishop (the LDS equivalent of a parish priest), may be involved in decisions to help couples and spouses think through the options and ramifications of their impending choice from a religious-moral perspective. Medical authorities, by contrast, are not considered to have moral authority but they do provide the necessary factual basis, in terms of diagnosis and prognosis, that helps constrain some options and facilitate others. In addition, decisions made either by the family or in collaboration with others presume legal compliance, a procedure that is at times stated explicitly and at times assumed.

A further procedural presumption of LDS bioethical decision-making is the request for and receipt of divine confirmation. Personal or collaborative openness to divine guidance or inspiration involves common LDS spiritual disciplines, including reading scriptures, fasting or abstention from food for short periods of time, and prayer. Underscoring the LDS emphasis on personal moral agency and accountability, a prayer typically does not request that God make the decision or instruct the family as to the right decision. Rather, LDS scripture and discourse encourage the family to exercise their moral agency and make their decision based on their values, as well as ecclesiastical support, and medical assessment, and then seek out the divine will to "confirm" the decision (*Doctrine*, 1981, p. 16). A confirmation is often thought to have been received by an emotional feeling of peace, comfort, and serenity, while a decision that does not receive such validation may prompt confusion and anxiety.

VI. Filling the Gaps: Principles of LDS Biothics

I have described the LDS approach to most bioethical questions as "procedural," as distinguished from substantive or prophetic. This perspective is displayed most prominently in ecclesiastical instructions in the *Church Handbook* (1998), in which general conclusions or statements of policy are presented, with some direction as to the appropriate decision-making procedure on the issue for persons or families faced with a practical question. However, there is virtually no reference to the religious and moral values upon which the ecclesiastical position is based. That is, the ecclesiastical policies are primarily conclusions for which no supporting claims derived from theological teachings are offered. This risks permeating both the substantive conclusions and the procedural instructions with arbitrariness. In concluding this essay, I wish to try to fill in the gaps between bioethical question and ecclesiastical position by suggesting some principles that LDS discourse seems either to presume, or without which the ecclesiastical claim seems incoherent. These principles function as moral *presumptions*, rather than absolutes that can never be overridden or maxims that can be used or discarded as deemed appropriate by the decision-maker(s). A moral presumption identifies a relevant value that must be taken into account, but can be overridden in certain situations where it comes into conflict with other moral presumptions (Beauchamp & Childress, 2002, pp. 14-23). A determination of which presumption should be followed is in part a matter of human decision and in part a matter of divine inspiration.

A. *Agency and Accountability*

A fundamental principle of both mortal and eternal existence in LDS teaching is that of moral agency. This is deemed to be inviolable even by God. All human beings are given the capacity to recognize and choose between both religious truth and falsehood, and between moral good and evil (*Doctrine*, 1981, pp. 199-200). It is recognized that this capacity is more or less fully actualized according to the developmental and social circumstances of the person. Thus, agency is only embryonic at birth, and, in the normal course of childhood development, is nourished and cultivated by parental instruction. At a certain period of psycho-social development (the LDS initiation rite of baptism is set at 8 years old), persons are considered morally mature enough to be responsible for their own actions. Even so, the rest of one's mortal life provides many opportunities to expand and deepen one's agency. In particular, choices in conformity with divine standards of right action enable a fuller actualization of agency, while choices contrary to such standards result in compromising and restricting agency.

The LDS tradition also recognizes that for various reasons, certain persons are unable to be held responsible for their actions, including children in the early stages of life, persons with debilitating mental impairments or illness, or the onset of senescence. In such circumstances, it is appropriate for others, most commonly family members, to act as proxies for those who cannot make decisions with a minimal level of agency.

The emphasis on procedural ethics illustrates that the principle of agency is central to all decisions on bioethics by members of the LDS church. A couple of implications must be noted here. First, moral agency in the LDS tradition should not be confused with the secular principle of autonomy. Moral agency is not a sufficient condition of ethical decision-making. Moreover, moral agency is inextricably connected to a concept of accountability before the community; this community may encompass family, local ecclesiastical leaders and community, and ultimately God. Accountability sets constraints on agency in a way not accommodated by the secular principle of autonomy.

Second, the principle of moral agency in LDS teaching typically presumes that the good or right course of action is known; within this framework, the central moral issue is the motivation to do what is known to be good. However, most bioethical questions offer a different paradigm of moral dilemma, in which the right course is uncertain, or conflicting courses of action with apparent equal moral validity may present themselves. That is, the principle of moral agency often presumes a base of epistemic knowledge that may not be available in the specific circumstances of bioethics decision-making. In part, the point of the procedural emphasis in LDS ecclesiastical instruction is to acknowledge this diminished epistemic base and to suggest ways to compensate and supplement what may be the limited horizons of the person or family.

B. *Embodiment*

The LDS tradition presents distinctive teachings on the question of embodiment, or the body-self relation. Rather than positing a materialistic metaphysics in which body and self are identical, or a dualistic metaphysics that views the body as either an adversary of the self or subordinated to the self, the teaching of the tradition is that the human "soul" is comprised of an integration of body and spirit (Campbell, 1993). A central purpose of human mortality is to obtain bodily experience, and human happiness is conditioned upon a harmonious rather than dysfunctional body-self relationship. An unembodied or disembodied self cannot obtain a "fulness of joy" (*Doctrine*, 1981, p. 182).

The body thus has an elevated moral significance in LDS discourse and practice. The theological rationale for the "Word of Wisdom" (1833/1981), the LDS code of health issued in 1833, has often invoked the concept of the body as a "temple" or "tabernacle," a sanctuary of the self that possesses its own intrinsic sacred nature. A more recent ecclesiastical concern, adornment of the body by piercing or tattooing, has been theologically maneuvered into the domain of "health" rather than "fashion" by invoking the image of the body as temple. This has provided grounds for fairly harsh condemnations of both piercing and tattoos.

The principle of embodiment also is relevant in LDS teachings pertaining to pre-marital and marital sexuality. Abstinence prior to marriage and chastity within marriage are prescribed in part because of the sacredness of the body and its powers of life-generation.

The traditional presumption against contraception relied upon responsible sexuality as a means of providing "mortal bodies" for God's spirit children. The recent revision of ecclesiastical teaching on contraception in favor of respect for the moral agency of the marital partners also promotes an expanded vision of the human goods of sexual relationships besides procreation, including love and emotional and spiritual relationality.

Ecclesiastical teaching about bodily disposition must also be situated in the theological-moral context created by the principle of embodiment. In the early years of transplantation, LDS members were informed they should not donate organs out of concern that donation might compromise the integrity and intactness of the resurrected body (Bush, 1993, p. 106). This restriction has gradually evolved to a position of personal or familial agency, a modification that has been consonant with the increasingly safe and beneficial results for the recipient, including greater longevity and improved quality of life.

However, the sacred integrity of the body continues to be an important theme in ecclesiastical discourse not only about sexuality, but also with respect to transplantation and disposition of the body, including questions of cremation, dissection, and autopsy. Like Jewish teaching, the LDS perspective is concerned that the embodied remains of the person not be desecrated.

C. *Family Integrity*

The LDS tradition has emphasized that the family is not only the basic form of social organization, but also a community with eternal potential. Much of LDS bioethics is intelligible, particularly in matters having to do with the creation of life and contraception, with the recognition that the family, rather than the autonomous self of secular bioethics, is the basic locus of authority for moral decision-making.

The principle of family integrity has several important dimensions or implications. Integrity as a moral concept often refers to "wholeness" or "completeness." One way of assuring this wholeness in the context of a marital relationship is through bringing children into the world. Indeed, LDS teaching indicates that men and women realize the fullness and measure of the creation through raising children in the context of marriage (*The Pearl*, 1981, p. 12). Even though ecclesiastical instruction is now more open to contraceptive practice as decided by the couple, the tone of ecclesiastical discourse continues to emphasize that human wholeness is achieved through marriage and procreation.

The principle of family integrity also is embedded in LDS teaching on most reproductive technologies that may involve mixing of gametes from sources external to the marriage. Family wholeness is viewed as complicated or compromised in the context of gametes from non-related sources; indeed, past ecclesiastical teaching cited disruption to family harmony as the rationale for opposition to AID. And the access of single women to reproductive technologies continues to be severely proscribed, possibly bringing on the sanctions of ecclesiastical discipline. In such a circumstance, a child would be brought into the world without an intact biological family, thus making the achievement of spiritual and emotional wholeness for both the mother and the child a much more difficult task. Thus family integrity encompasses efforts to keep the family intact.

Finally, the presumption in LDS bioethics to defer to the family as the locus for decision-making authority reiterates the necessity of family integrity and wholeness. Without an intact family, the difficult nature of many bioethical decisions will create more personal and collective anguish.

D. *Protection of the Vulnerable*

Those persons who lack full moral agency often need protection from those who may misuse their agency, or exercise what the tradition refers to as "unrighteous dominion" upon others (*Doctrine*, 1981, p. 242). In LDS scriptural teaching, the principle of protection of the vulnerable is most often invoked to focus special attention to the plight of the poor, the widowed, and the homeless. That is, persons who have social, economic, or religious power are required to provide special care for those who may be vulnerable due to their physical or social circumstances, and whose voice may otherwise be neglected by members of the religious community.

In the context of LDS bioethics, the application of this principle involves two steps. First, those in power are reminded of their own vulnerability and dependency. They are, in company with those on the social margins, to understand themselves as "beggars before God" (*Book of Mormon*, 1981, p. 156). This should prompt among those with full moral agency and the capacity to exercise it a sense of fellow-feeling, solidarity, and empathy towards the vulnerable.

Second, the vulnerable must be identified and cared for appropriately. In bioethical matters, this has often meant ensuring the protection of women (especially mothers), children, the unborn, and the dying. Ecclesiastical teachings on contraception, abortion, and the forgoing of life-prolonging measures require this kind of principle.

This principle is thus an important adjunct to the principle of moral agency. However, it questionably runs the risk of imposing religious paternalism on persons who may already be subjected to the encroachments of medical beneficence and the general patriarchal structure of LDS culture. Normatively, the principle should be used to protect those persons subject to exploitative power and to enhance the capacity for their own exercise of moral agency. In practice, however, those offering care and protection may be tempted to substitute their own judgments and values for those deemed incapable of exercising their agency fully.

E. *Sanctity of Human Life*

The ecclesiastical opposition to bioethical practices that terminate life (such as abortion, euthanasia, medically-assisted suicide, or suicide) presumes a principle of the sanctity of human life and a more specific rule prohibiting killing of innocent human beings. The endings of human life are, in these situations, determined to be decisions appropriate to divine will and immune from the vagaries of human fallibility. However, the principle of the sanctity of human life cannot be considered an absolute and exceptionless principle in LDS bioethics for at three reasons.

First, there is a question of what entities bestowed with life can be designated as "human." This issue surfaces most prominently in the question of abortion. Ecclesiastical teaching has never formally adopted a position on the matter of ensoulment, or when in the course of pre-natal development the spirit and the body are united. It is possible to find ecclesiastical leaders defending a time frame of thresholds of humanness at conception, or birth, or any period in between. The theological problematic is manifest in the current ecclesiastical view of abortion, in which abortion is considered analogous to ("like unto") but not the moral equivalent of paradigm cases of killing human life. This different moral status of abortion is reiterated in the recognized ecclesiastical exceptions to the prohibition of abortion. This means that other principles besides the sanctity of life must be relied on to ground the opposition to abortion. In particular, the principle of protection of the vulnerable from exploitation and misuse of power must be invoked.

Secondly, the sanctity of human life may be subordinated to the protection of communal quality of life or the enhancement of spiritual life in certain defined circumstances. The LDS defense of human life at its beginning and end in morality has not culminated in a "seamless web" of protection or a "consistent ethic of life" that has been prominent in recent Roman Catholic moral teaching. LDS ecclesiastical leaders have supported capital punishment and participation in warfare for a variety of theological, social, and civic reasons. The tradition also acknowledges certain instances, albeit extremely rare, in which mortal life may be "sacrificed" to achieve certain goods of spiritual life.

Finally, in some circumstances, a dynamic between the principles of agency and sanctity may issue in a refusal to attribute blameworthiness to a person even though the act of taking life is still opposed. The most evident bioethics example of this refusal to transfer judgments about the act to judgments about the agent is ecclesiastical teaching on suicide. This position has undergone significant evolution in the past two decades. Prior to the 1980s, an act of suicide was thought to consign the actor to an eternal life separated from the presence of God. However, an approach that leavens the sanctity principle with compassion has prevailed in recent teaching. Even though there remains a general prohibition of the act of suicide, the intent and motives of the person who takes his life are believed to be inscrutable to all but God. Thus, diminished capacities of subjective moral agency may constrain judgments when the sanctity of human life principle is objectively violated.

F. Stewardship

The principle of stewardship is the more benevolent face of the principle of protection from harm. The latter seeks to prevent harm from occurring to the vulnerable, while stewardship requires seeking occasions to enhance their welfare and promote their good. The steward is in a fiduciary relationship with God to care for others and is accountable to divine authority for his or her actions.

There are two exemplary illustrations of the stewardship principle in LDS bioethics. I have noted the stress ecclesiastical instructions lay upon pastoral consultation on many bioethical issues. This is because local ecclesiastical leaders are considered to have been entrusted with a stewardship responsibility to ensure the temporal and spiritual welfare of members of their religious community. In addition, much LDS discussion and instruction on care for the dying presupposes a familial and communal stewardship responsibility. A decision to forgo medical life-support for example should not prompt abandonment but rather stewardly expression of care, respect, and presence. It can also be claimed that the LDS ecclesiastical opposition to physician euthanasia follows not only the commandment of not killing, but also the principle of responsible stewardship by the person and professionals who should have made a commitment to caring presence.

It is the case, however, that the stewardship principle has not been extended to encompass vocations in the world, including such matters as access to health care or education, or the prioritization of social resources. This is rather unfortunate, given that recently many interesting theological innovations in medical ethics, biotechnology, and environmental bioethics have been developed out of a stewardship paradigm.

VII. Future Prospects

The last decade of the 20th century witnessed developments in biomedicine and bioethics that are unprecedented in scope and significance. Physician-assisted suicide and euthanasia were legalized in some jurisdictions, as competing scientific groups rushed to complete genome mapping, research on genetic therapy was initiated, human embryonic stem and germ cells were successfully cultivated, and human cloning moved from the realm of science fiction to scientific possibility. Yet, this ferment in bioethics had virtually no notice in the LDS community, at least as reflected in ecclesiastical instructions or in academic writings. Unless and insofar as a bioethical issue directly touches on matters of central ecclesiastical interest, or the underlying principles, the LDS tradition seems content to let biomedical science and research set the moral agenda of contemporary medicine.

Bibliography

Beauchamp, T.L. & Childress, J.F. (2001). *Principles of biomedical ethics* (5th ed.) New York: Oxford University Press.

The Book of Mormon (1981). Salt Lake City, Utah: The Church of Jesus Christ of Latter-day Saints.

Bush, L.M. (Ed.) (1979). Mormon medical ethical guidelines. *Dialogue 12(6)*, 97-106.

Bush, L.M. (1993). *Health and medicine among the Latter-day saints: Science, sense, and scripture.* New York: Crossroad Publishing.

Campbell, C.S. (1991). Sounds of silence: The Latter-day Saints and medical ethics. In: B.A. Lustig (Ed.), *Theological developments in bioethics: 1988-1990* (pp. 23-40). Dordrecht, The Netherlands: Kluwer Academic Publishers.

Campbell, C.S. (1993). Embodiment and ethics: A Latter-day Saint perspective. In: B.A. Lustig (Ed.), *Theological developments in bioethics: 1990-1992* (pp. 43-68). Dordrecht, The Netherlands: Kluwer Academic Publishers.

Campbell, C.S. (1998). Prophecy and citizenry: The case of human cloning. *Sunstone 21(2)*, 11-15.

Campbell, C.S. (2002). Eschatological passage: Death as progress in LDS tradition. *Ultimate reality and meaning 25(3)*, 185-202.

Church handbook of instructions (1998). Salt Lake City, Utah: The Church of Jesus Christ of Latter-day Saints.

The Doctrine and Covenants (1981). Salt Lake City, Utah: The Church of Jesus Christ of Latter-day Saints.

Fox, R. & Swazey, J. (1992). *Spare parts: Organ replacement in American society* (pp. 155-169). New York: Oxford University Press.

General handbook of instructions (1989). Salt Lake City, Utah: The Church of Jesus Christ of Latter-day Saints.

Harris-Abbott, D. (1995). *The Latter-day Saints tradition: Religious beliefs and health care decisions.* Chicago: Park Ridge Center.

The pearl of great price (1981). Salt Lake City, Utah: The Church of Jesus Christ of Latter-day Saints.

Proclamation on the family (1997). Salt Lake City, Utah: The Church of Jesus Christ of Latter-day Saints.

Word of wisdom (1833/1981). Salt Lake City, Utah: The Church of Jesus Christ of Latter-day Saints.

Jewish Bioethics

Harvey L. Gordon and Mark Washofsky

I. Introduction

"Jewish bioethics," as a descriptive title for our subject, is something of a misnomer. This does not mean that Judaism has nothing to say concerning ethical issues that arise in the context of medical practice and the provision of health care. On the contrary, the historical Jewish tradition boasts a rich and sophisticated body of teachings to address these questions. It means rather that these teachings do not exist in Judaism as an autonomous discipline, separated by a firm academic or theoretical boundary from other forms of Jewish moral inquiry. It means, too, that this body of teaching should not be construed, as is the case with "bioethics" generally, as a sub-field of philosophy. Jewish thought on matters of medical ethics partakes of the tradition of *halakhah*, of Jewish law. "Jewish bioethics" is thus no more and no less than the discourse of *halakhah* as it is applied to moral issues related to medicine and health care. The law-centered nature of Jewish discussions on matters of medical practice accounts for some of the significant differences between "Jewish bioethics" and bioethics in general, in both process and substance. For example, if general bioethics posits the centrality of patient rights and autonomy, Jewish law speaks of obligations, of the duty of all, including patient and caregiver, to follow the dictates of the Torah. An "obligation," to be sure, is often a right in reverse: the duty to provide medical care to a patient implies what other systems would define as a person's right to medical care. Still, language is important, because it implies a value orientation, a particular way of looking at the world. When we refer in this article to "Jewish bioethics," therefore, we have in mind that aspect of *halakhah*, rather than an intellectual discipline separate and distinct from it.

II. History

For these reasons, we cannot speak of "Jewish bioethics" without first saying something, however brief and cursory, of the history of Jewish law, or *halakhah*, as the predominant mode of Jewish moral and religious discourse.[1] *Halakhah* is best perceived as an ongoing tradition of text and argument, out of which emerges Jewish teaching on all matters of religious and moral practice. In the traditional Jewish narrative, the history of *halakhah* begins with God's revelation of the Torah to Moses at Sinai. This Torah (a word that means "authoritative instruction") consisted of two elements: a written Torah – generally associated with the five Biblical books of Moses – and an oral Torah. The latter comprised a large body of laws (*halakhot*) that expand upon, modify, and supplement the legislation of the written Torah. (Academic historians identify the "oral Torah" with the numerous traditions, interpretations, and ordinances of long standing that, over the course of centuries, achieved canonical status.) In addition to these *halakhot*, the Rabbis (or "the Sages," the teachers of this two-fold Torah tradition during the first five centuries of the Common Era) expounded other genres of legal material: interpretations of Biblical and earlier Rabbinic texts, legislative acts (*takanot* and *gezerot*) promulgated by the Rabbis in order to accomplish specified social or religious ends, the customary law (*minhag*) of various Jewish communities, and the acts, rulings, and behaviors of particular Sages (*ma'asim*) whose lives and wisdom were seen as worthy of emulation. This literary product was redacted in books that comprise the classic library of Jewish law. These include the *Mishnah*, the basic compilation of the Oral Torah; the *midrashim*, collections of legal interpretations of Scripture; and the Talmuds, which comprise generations of analysis of and debates over the written and oral Torah, Jewish custom, legend, theology, and all other matters that concerned the Rabbis. One Talmud was produced by the Rabbinic scholars of Palestine (*Eretz Yisrael*), the other in the academies of Babylonia. It is this latter work, redacted ca. 500-650 C.E., that over time won acceptance as the authoritative source of the *halakhah*. This authority lies in the fact that all statements and decisions of Jewish law must ultimately find their justification in the texts of the Babylonian Talmud. For fifteen centuries, rabbis (halakhic scholars who take their title from that of the great Talmudic Sages) have studied and argued over those texts to derive authoritative legal judgment from them. These arguments and decisions fill a massive literature of post-Talmudic *halakhah* that assumes several genres: commentaries to the Talmud and other legal texts, codes or systematic compilations of Jewish law, and responsa, answers by rabbis to questions submitted to them by individuals or communities on matters of law and practice.

The halakhic *literature* just described forms the textual basis of the halakhic *process*, the modes and procedures utilized by rabbis to answer questions of law and practice. If the answer to a question is not clear or obvious – if it cannot be resolved to general satisfaction by reference to a particular text or to the consensus understanding of the literary sources as a whole – a rabbi will endeavor to derive a response by way of halakhic reasoning. This reasoning, much like "legal reasoning" in the common law tradition, is largely casuistic in nature. It proceeds inductively, seeking sources, cases, and prior rulings upon which to draw analogies to the issue at hand. To the extent that the halakhist relies upon these earlier texts it is proper to call them "precedential." We should note here that the *halakhah* does not recognize a doctrine of binding precedent, the idea that some previous decision or line of decisions determines the answer that a rabbi will give to the present case. The rabbi is entitled to rule as he sees fit, so long as he can support his decision by means of persuasive argumentation based upon the sources; "the judge," as we are told, "can only follow the evidence before him" (*Talmud, Bava Batra* 131a). In practice, however, the cumulative weight of centuries of halakhic decision will exert an enormous and usually decisive influence upon the ruling of the contemporary authority. If and when a certain interpretation establishes itself as the consensus view among the rabbinical community (and, just as importantly, if and when that interpretation is accepted in practice by the community to which it is addressed), we can say with some accuracy that "the" *halakhah* accords with that ruling. This is especially true of halakhic practice among

Orthodox rabbis, although by no means is it *always* true. Scholars representing the more liberal Jewish denominations are more likely to depart from the consensus understandings of the *halakhah* and to issue innovative rulings.

This halakhic process is not centered in any particular institution. No single body of rabbinical authorities enjoys the power to decide the "official" *halakhah* for the entire Jewish community and to impose its interpretations upon the individual rabbi. This emphasis upon freedom of decision would seem to make for unpredictability and idiosyncrasy in Jewish law, yet the opposite is in fact the case. *Halakhah*, in other words, is expressed not only through the working of individual minds but through institutions, loci of authority that promote stability and continuity within the halakhic process. The halakhic consensus, noted above, is such an "institution." This consensus is largely shaped by the opinions of a relatively small number of outstanding scholars who, by dint of their prodigious learning and reputation for religious probity, attain the status of *posek* (plural, *poskim*), a decisor whose rulings command the respectful attention of large portions of the observant community. Some of these *poskim* develop a particular expertise in the area of medical *halakhah*.[2] In addition to actual rulings, these and other rabbis publish articles[3] and monographs (see the Bibliography) specifically devoted to Jewish bioethics that do much to define the parameters of the field.

The above description addresses the halakhic process as it takes place within Orthodox Judaism. Matters differ somewhat within the liberal Jewish denominations. For example, the Conservative and Reform movements have established committees of rabbis to issue rulings that help to establish the denomination's stance on bioethical issues.[4] In the Reform movement, committees made up primarily of laypersons supplement rabbinical guidance in this area.[5] While Conservative rabbis explicitly declare their stance within the traditional halakhic process, Reform authors tend to rely upon and appeal to contemporary moral sensitivities as a guide to ethical decision-making independent of *halakhah*. Yet Reform rabbis do write responsa, and in any case, virtually all substantive Reform Jewish bioethical teaching is based upon and informed by the Jewish legal tradition.

III. Topics

A. *Bioethics in General: The Commandment to Practice Medicine*

Although Jewish legal discourse is casuistic in nature, general principles will guide the discussion in specific areas of the *halakhah*. Jewish medical law, for example, is founded upon an affirmation that human life is a gift of God and remains the property of God as long as the human being, as steward of that life, possesses it. Life itself, in this view, becomes the paramount value and its preservation the apex of all responsibilities that the human being owes to God. The central Rabbinic expression of this doctrine is based upon an interpretation of Leviticus 18:5, "You shall keep My laws ... by the pursuit of which a man shall live," to which a *midrash* (Rabbinic interpretation of Scriptural text) adds: "and he shall not *die* by the pursuit of them" (*Talmud Yoma* 85b and parallels). Thus, virtually every other commandment (*mitzvah*) of the Torah is set aside if its observance would endanger human life.[6] This notion is conveyed by the halakhic concept *pikuach nefesh*, "the preservation of human life." On the basis of this concept, the Rabbis teach that medicine is itself a *mitzvah* (a religious duty),[7] an aspect of the duty to save life, deriving this *mitzvah* from the Torah even though Scripture never explicitly enjoins humankind to practice the healing arts.[8]

To call the practice of medicine a *mitzvah* is to imply a number of moral duties on the part of the patient, the health-care professional, and the community as a whole. It is the responsibility of each person to seek medical treatment in time of illness. To refuse life-saving treatment out of a misplaced sense of religious devotion or for the sake of observing another religious obligation is the act of a "pious fool." The physician, in turn, bears an obligation to provide medical care to those who call upon him. He has no right to refuse: the physician "who withholds himself from practicing medicine is guilty of shedding blood" (*Shulchan Arukh Yoreh De'ah* 336:1). Although like all other workers he may demand fair compensation for his labor, the fact that his labor is a *mitzvah* places some significant limitations upon his personal economic freedom. The community, for its part, is the ultimate guarantor of the provision of medical care. Medical practice is therefore a public responsibility, not merely a private contractual matter between providers and consumers, a fact that will bear relevance to our discussion of "access to health care" below.

B. *Professionalism*

Although the mitzvah of *pikuach nefesh* is incumbent upon the entire community, only those who are knowledgeable and experienced in the healing arts may practice medicine. Even an "expert" physician (*rofe baki*) must be licensed to practice by the appropriate legal authorities. This license protects the physician from monetary liability for unintentional damages he may cause the patient, save for those that result from clear and outright negligence. Some authorities hold that despite this exemption, the physician bears the moral responsibility to compensate the patient for damages caused in the course of medical treatment. Others, however, excuse her from moral responsibility as well: so long as the physician is not negligent and takes all accepted precautions, the fact that she is engaged in the performance of a commanded act exempts her from all culpability, financial or otherwise (Washofsky, 2001, pp. 229-232; 447).

The physician is thus an expert who performs an act that is obligatory upon him and the patient alike. As such, the patient in most circumstances has no morally defensible choice but to heed the doctor's advice. For example, when the physician declares that the observance of the fast of the Day of Atonement (Yom Kippur) might endanger a patient already suffering from medical complications, the patient must eat; he has no right to observe the fast against the doctor's orders.[9] Indeed, as noted above, since Jewish law tends to express itself in the language of duty and covenantal obligation, it is difficult to say that the patient enjoys any "rights" at all. This includes the so-called "patient's right to know." The codified *halakhah* holds that a person whose condition is grave should not be informed of that fact, lest the "bad news" cause her to despair and give up hope of recovery, thus hastening her death. The *mitzvah* of medicine defines the preservation of the patient's life, rather than concern for her liberty or autonomy, as the paramount concern. This attitude reflects the paternalistic, "doctor knows best" stance that once dominated medical practice. Yet, just as paternalism has in recent decades receded as the prevailing model of the physician-patient relationship, the halakhic attitude has also begun to change. Some (though not all) Orthodox as well as most liberal Jewish thinkers now accept that, as a general rule, a patient ought to be kept fully informed of his medical condition. It is instructive, though, that the reason for this change is not that these thinkers have come to recognize the existence of a patient's "right to know." They base this view rather upon the understanding that this knowledge, by giving the patient a sense of some control over her fate, can boost her morale and therefore be beneficial to her medical condition (Washofsky, 2001, pp. 228-229, 446-447; Avraham, 1985, 2:239; Rosner, 1990, pp. 31-64).

The physician-patient relationship operates under a presumption of confidentiality. That the doctor can be trusted to keep medical and personal secrets encourages the patient to share all relevant information. At the same time, both doctor and patient are obligated to uphold the commandments of the Torah, among them the obligation to rescue those whose lives are in danger (Lev. 19:16; *Talmud Sanhedrin* 73a). On this basis, halakhic authorities have ruled that a physician must reveal information about his patient if the withholding of that information would endanger the life or health – including the emotional health – of others. Accordingly, if a person engaged to be married is afflicted with a serious (even if non-communicable) disease, or if he or she is physically incapable of conceiving a child, the physician is required to reveal this information to the intended spouse. Even when the physician has sworn an oath to maintain the strictest confidence, most opinions require that the oath be set aside in favor of releasing the vital information in question. The operative halakhic theory is that the people of Israel have already sworn an oath at Sinai to uphold the Torah, which commands us to preserve life; any subsequent oath that would bind us to violate that commandment is therefore null and void.[10] On the other hand, in the event that these standards conflict with the civil law in the physician's jurisdiction, *halakhah* would in all probability require the physician to follow the civil law standard. This is based upon the rule *dina demalkhuta dina*, "the law of the state is valid law," the tendency of Jewish law to give full force to the legal arrangements promulgated by the government acting within the scope of its legitimate law-making authority.[11]

C. Reproduction

Jewish ethical thinking on the subject of human reproduction tends to revolve around two fundamental affirmations. The first is that procreation is a *mitzvah*, the fulfillment of a religious duty ("be fruitful and multiply"; Gen. 1:28) and of the divine plan for the world ("God did not create the earth a waste; He formed it for habitation"; Is. 45:18). The second is that the human embryo, though it properly demands our moral concern, is not reckoned as a full legal person (*nefesh*), a status it achieves only upon birth.

C.1. Fertility Technologies

Jewish law differs from some other moral traditions in that it does not approach questions of human sexuality and reproduction primarily on the basis of natural law. Nature is neither sacred nor perfect; it may be improved upon for the betterment of the human condition. Thus, Judaism does not forbid technological intervention into these processes simply because it is "artificial." Nor, according to the preponderant majority of rabbinical opinion, does there exist a specific halakhic prohibition against such intervention. Still, that which is not explicitly prohibited is not on that account necessarily permitted; therefore, one cannot assume rabbinical assent in all cases. Let us consider, for example, the technique of artificial insemination, particularly when the woman is to be impregnated with her husband's sperm (AIH). Most Orthodox authorities presume this procedure to be prohibited, as a departure from "natural" conception. They will waive this prohibition when AIH is necessary to enable the couple to conceive and thereby allow the husband to fulfill the *mitzvah* of procreation, a duty incumbent in Jewish law upon the male and *not* upon the female.[12] Yet according to one reading of the *halakhah*, legal paternity is established only when the child is conceived in the "natural" manner; a child conceived by means of artificial insemination would not, in this view, be the halakhicly-recognized offspring of the semen donor. If this view were to prevail in the law, many rabbis would find it difficult to permit AIH. Moreover, some authorities rule that the extraction of semen for this procedure, if done through masturbation, violates the specific prohibition against the "destruction of seed" (*cf.* Gen. 38-9:10). In the final analysis, most authorities permit AIH, although many Orthodox scholars do so only as a last resort, when the couple can conceive by no other means. Orthodox opinion is virtually unanimous in condemning AID, artificial insemination using the semen of a donor other than the woman's husband. In this case, there is no question that the husband does not fulfill the *mitzvah* of procreation. In addition, assuming that the identity of the biological father remains anonymous, the child might grow up to marry a forbidden blood relative of the semen donor. Finally, many Orthodox rabbis raise moral objections against the insertion of "foreign" semen into the womb of a married woman. (Even so, the preponderance of authorities do not regard AID as an act of adultery.) Liberal authorities, while sensitive to these concerns, tend to permit AID in order to allow the couple to build a family. The wife's desire to have children is of paramount importance, even though she is not traditionally obliged to "be fruitful and multiply" (Washofsky, 2001, pp. 233-236, 447-448; Dorff, 1998, pp. 50-53, 80-97).

In vitro fertilization (IVF) poses some of the same issues as does artificial insemination. The difference is that the entire process of conception takes place outside the womb, a fact that, along with various moral and societal concerns, leads one prominent Orthodox authority to forbid the procedure. Most rabbis, however, permit IVF as a means of helping couples conceive children. If the child conceived through IVF is carried to term in the womb of a woman other than the egg donor, most Orthodox authorities would ascribe maternity to the birth mother. Other opinions recognize the possibility that the egg donor is the mother of the child under Jewish law, so that the matter of maternity remains a debated one (Washofsky, 2001, pp. 236-237, 448; Dorff, 1998, pp. 53-58; Bleich, 1991, pp. 86-88).

C.2. Birth Control

Judaism traditionally emphasizes the *mitzvah* of procreation and the value of large families. And as we have seen, rabbinical thought has looked favorably to a great extent upon the modern technologies that combat human infertility. This does not mean, however, that infertile persons are under a religious requirement to undergo fertility treatments. The invasive nature and expense of some of these procedures, along with their uncertain prospect for success, renders them voluntary rather than obligatory. Nor does Jewish law deny to women and couples the option of birth control to prevent unwanted pregnancy. Orthodox rabbis permit the use of birth control for sufficient cause, particularly when physicians judge that pregnancy would endanger the woman's physical or emotional health. Rabbinical approval is much more likely when her husband has already fulfilled the minimum content of the commandment of procreation (i.e., by fathering a son and a daughter).[13] As to the various methods of birth control, both Orthodox and liberal opinion reject the use of surgery, such as vasectomy or tubal ligation. Orthodox rabbis tend also to reject condoms and other contraceptives used by males. The male, remember, is obligated under the commandment to procreate, so that such devices are seen as a direct frustration on his part of the *mitzvah* as well as the destruction of semen. Most authorities, however, permit the woman to use a diaphragm, an intrauterine contraceptive device (IUD or IUCD), or an oral contraceptive, since she is obliged neither under the *mitzvah* of procreation nor under the prohibition against the destruction of semen. Among these methods, the oral contraceptive seems to pose the fewest halakhic problems from an Orthodox perspective (Tendler, 2000, pp. 117-124; Feldman, 1975, pp. 227-248; Rosner, 2000, pp. 105-115). Again, it must be remembered that the permit is granted "for sufficient cause," a category unlikely to include the desire to limit family size in the absence of substantive health considerations (Tendler, 2000, pp. 117-124; Rosner, 2000, pp. 105-115; Avraham, 1985, vol. 3, 59ff). Liberal rabbis take a more generally permissive view of family planning considerations as a justification for contraception, although they continue to stress the value of procreation for couples and for the future of the Jewish people (Dorff, 1998, pp. 123-125; Washofsky, 2001, pp. 242, 449).

C.3. *Abortion*

As noted above, Jewish law does not regard the human embryo as a *nefesh*, a full legal person. Unwarranted feticide is therefore not construed as murder, for murder is the unlawful taking of the life of a legal person. This is not to imply that Jewish law has no objection to abortion. Far from it: *halakhah* generally understands the termination of pregnancy to be forbidden. Yet since the fetus is not a *nefesh*, this prohibition is waived when there is sufficient cause to justify the abortion. The question just what counts as "sufficient cause" for abortion has been a bone of contention among halakhists for centuries. The discussion begins with a text in the Mishnah that permits the dismemberment of the fetus in a case of dangerous childbirth. On this basis, all authorities agree that abortion is permitted and even required in order to save the woman's life. The disagreement begins with the interpretation of the Talmudic discussion of that Mishnah. According to some commentators, the Talmud understands the abortion to be permitted because the fetus is to be considered a "pursuer" of the mother, threatening her life; like all such pursuers, the fetus may be killed if necessary to save the life of the victim. Other authorities, however, read that Talmud passage in the opposite fashion: the fetus is *not* a "pursuer." The abortion is permitted instead because the mother, as a *nefesh*, takes precedence over the fetus, which lacks that status. This difference in interpretation, in turn, leads to widely differing legal conclusions. Subsequent halakhists who hold that the Mishnah permits or requires the abortion on the grounds that the fetus is a "pursuer" tend to rule in favor of abortion only in cases where it can be convincingly demonstrated that termination of pregnancy is necessary to save the mother from mortal danger. On the other hand, those who read the Mishnah as permitting the abortion on the grounds that the fetus is not yet a *nefesh* will extend that permit to circumstances of less than mortal danger. They will permit abortion, for example, for purposes of the mother's "healing," since the vital interests of the mother, as a full legal person, take precedence over the life of the fetus. "Healing" will often include the mother's emotional as well as physical health. Some twentieth-century halakhic rulings have allowed abortions in cases where the child would be afflicted with severe defects or Tay-Sachs disease and where the mother would suffer great anguish on that account.

The preponderance of Orthodox opinion today sides with the stringent approach: abortion is permitted (that is, required) in cases where childbirth threatens the mother's life, although serious danger to the mother's health is sometimes defined as "danger to life"; outside of that range of cases, abortion is not permitted. Some Orthodox rabbis, along with most Conservative and Reform rabbis, construe the warrant for abortion more broadly, basing themselves upon an expansive understanding of "danger to the mother's physical and emotional health." This is one reason that the more liberal Jewish bodies therefore usually oppose government legislation limiting a woman's access to abortion: such restrictions tend to deny to the woman the opportunity to reach a decision that could be morally justifiable under Jewish tradition. In any case, maternal indications, not fetal indications, are decisive. That a fetus will be born with severe defects or disease is not in and of itself sufficient warrant for an abortion; rather, the procedure may be allowed if it is determined that the birth of such a fetus will have significant deleterious effects upon the mother's emotional health. We should note as well that none of these trends in rabbinical opinion permits abortion "on demand" (i.e., in the absence of sufficient cause), as a method of family planning, or on economic grounds (Dorff, 1998, pp. 128-133, 101-102; Rosner, 2001, pp. 175-204; Feldman, 1975, pp. 251-294; Washofsky, 2001, pp. 242-245, 449-451).

C.4. Pregnancy Reduction

Another important factor in the decision for abortion is the age of the fetus. Jewish law considers the fetus prior to forty days of gestation as unformed, "mere fluid." Some authorities hold that the prohibition of abortion "without sufficient cause" does not apply at all to the fetus until it has developed beyond this initial stage. For this reason, rabbis who generally take a stringent position on abortion may rule more permissively when the fetus has not yet reached the age of forty days. This factor, in turn, is critical in determining the stance of Jewish bioethics on the question of pregnancy reduction, which is sometimes referred to as "fetal reduction" or "selective abortion." This issue tends to arise in connection with fertility treatments. Some fertility drugs that stimulate ovulation may engender the creation of multiple fetuses; in addition, IVF involving the implantation of multiple embryos can result in a multiple gestation. Rabbinical authorities who have considered this problem have tended to permit the reduction of pregnancy – i.e., the abortion of some of the fetuses in a multiple gestation – in order to spare the mother the serious medical complications that can occur in a multiple-pregnancy situation. The halakhic basis for the permit is stronger and surer, however, if the fetal reduction takes place during the initial forty days of gestation, when the Jewish legal objections to abortion are not as serious.

C.5. Stem Cell Research, Cloning, and Genetic Engineering

Abortion, as we have noted, is prohibited without sufficient cause; still, it is not considered murder because the fetus is not a legal person (a *nefesh*) whose life is protected by the laws against homicide. We have seen further that the severity of the prohibition against abortion decreases when the fetus is at less than forty days of gestation. Recent halakhic rulings, moreover, have posited that there is no explicit prohibition in Jewish law against the destruction of an embryo *in vitro*. Although *halakhah* does protect the fetus from wanton destruction, this protection stems from the presumption that the fetus will develop into a person, a *nefesh*. Embryos *in vitro*, particularly the excess embryos developed in the process of IVF, do not enjoy this presumption, since in all likelihood they will never be implanted. For this reason, rabbinical authorities tend to approve the disposal of excess embryos and, by logical extension, the use of such embryos in medical research, even though the derivation of stem cells from the blastocyst (the zygote at the initial stages of its development) results in the killing of the embryo. It remains to be seen whether this permit will be extended to allow the actual creation of human embryos, whether through fertilization or through cloning, in order to harvest stem cells from them (Eisenberg, 2001; CCAR Responsum, 2001).

Similarly, rabbinical authorities have as yet uncovered no explicit halakhic basis upon which to forbid the cloning of human beings. Again, Jewish bioethics does not generally proceed from premises of natural law. As we have seen with respect to the various fertility technologies, a technique for producing children is not forbidden simply because it is artificial. Rabbis are at present more engaged with such questions as the status of the clonee (e.g., who are his/her parents?), the purposes for which cloning might be adopted (might one fulfill the *mitzvah* of procreation thereby? As cloning is asexual, with the entire gene complement coming from a single parent, could it be understood as *replication*, in contradistinction to *procreation*? Might cloned embryos be permitted for medical experimentation?), and the social implications of the development and widespread use of this technology (Loike & Steinberg, 1998).

Many of the same considerations apply to the question of genetic engineering. Again, natural law is not the issue: *halakhah* does not deem the introduction of alterations into the human genetic code to be an unwarranted intervention into the divine order of creation. On the contrary, genetic engineering may be seen as the application of human knowledge for the betterment of the human condition, specifically toward the fulfillment of the *mitzvah* of healing. Rabbinical enthusiasm for genetic engineering is tempered, on the other hand, by the potentially fateful societal implications of this technology. Some Orthodox rabbis have raised objections to screening for genetic conditions such as Tay-Sachs disease, on the grounds that the finding that one person or a couple is a carrier of the gene might predispose them to abort a fetus or to avoid marriage altogether. Most rabbis, however, prefer to counsel these individuals and couples as to available alternatives rather than to forbid screenings of this sort (Rosner, 2001, 205-222; Dorff, 1998, 151-164; Washofsky, 2001, 239-241, 449).

D. *Death and Dying*

D.1. *Euthanasia and Physician Assisted Suicide*

Two general principles run through most Jewish discussion of the treatment of the terminally ill patient. The first of these is the understanding that the dying person "is a living person in all respects": one does not cease to be fully human until the moment of death. The second is the conception of medicine as a *mitzvah*, a religious duty: we administer medical and surgical therapies to the patient precisely because they are therapeutic, a response to disease.

The unlawful killing of the dying person, even for reasons of compassion, is strictly prohibited, just as it is forbidden to murder any living person. Accordingly, physician assisted suicide and other forms of "active euthanasia" find no support in the sources of Jewish law. At the same time, the texts distinguish between the forbidden "active euthanasia" and a range of permitted acts, sometimes termed "passive euthanasia," aimed at removing an artificial "impediment" to the patient's otherwise inevitable death. This distinction would seem to offer an ethical basis on which to judge whether certain therapies in particular circumstances may be withheld or withdrawn from the terminally ill patient. The matter, however, is not so simple. For one thing, in the context of modern medicine it is not always easy to distinguish between the removal of an "impediment" and the introduction of a factor that hastens death. The "impediments to death" of which we read in the traditional texts stem from the realm of what we moderns would label "folklore" or "superstition" rather than *medicine*, and some authorities question whether one can reasonably compare them to today's medical technologies. Additionally, the texts apply this active/passive distinction to the case of the *goses*, the patient whose death is imminent (three days or less, according to rabbinic sources). It is uncertain that the same distinction applies to the patient who is terminally ill but seems able to survive for weeks, months, or even years.

A more useful way of posing the question, then, is this: is it permissible to withhold or withdraw from the terminally ill any of the therapies – drugs, surgery, life-support systems – that are routinely applied in the course of the medical management of the patient? Contemporary rabbinical opinion on this question is divided across a wide spectrum of views, extending from the comparatively stringent to the comparatively permissive. Most Orthodox rabbis hold that the permit to remove an "impediment" to death applies only to the *goses*, who lies at the very threshold of death. Since every moment of life is sacred, the prolongation of life through medicine is the fulfillment of a religious duty. Medical professionals must therefore use every accepted medical means to prolong the life of the terminally ill patient. On the other hand, the prolongation of the process of dying is forbidden. Thus, a patient may be removed from a ventilator if it is clear that the patient meets the criteria of death as defined in Jewish sources.[14] While certain heroic measures need not be undertaken to resuscitate a patient who is clearly, irreversibly ill with no chance of recovery, all routine medical measures, including nutrition, hydration, and antibiotics, along with palliative care must be administered to the terminally ill patient.

A responsum adopted by Conservative rabbis, meanwhile, defines the subject in a crucially different way. The opinion applies the category of *terefah* – a person with an incurable terminal illness, even though he or she may live for months or even years – rather than that of *goses* to describe the end-stage patient. This redefinition allows us to withhold or withdraw useless medical therapy from patients once they are diagnosed as incurable and terminal; we do not have to wait until they are at death's door before disconnecting the machines. The most recent Reform responsum on the subject identifies the *mitzvah* of healing or medical practice as the proper criterion of judgment. It holds that medical therapies may be withheld or withdrawn once it is determined that those measures are no longer "medicine," that is, they no longer serve a legitimate therapeutic function. The responsum therefore permits withholding or withdrawal in a fairly wide range of cases, although its authors readily concede that the definition of "legitimate therapeutic function" is seldom easy to arrive at and must be thoroughly argued and carefully drawn in each individual medical situation (Rosner, 2001, pp. 223-270; Dorff, 1998, pp. 176-220; Washofsky, 2001, pp. 249-254, 451-452).

Do artificial nutrition and hydration qualify as "medical therapies" such that they may be withheld or withdrawn from certain terminal patients? Again, a difference of opinion exists. Virtually all Orthodox rabbis say "no": nutrition and hydration are not medicine and should never be regarded as "impediments to death." Some liberal rabbis agree with this determination; others approve the withdrawal of artificial nutrition and hydration, from some patients, particularly those in persistent vegetative state (PVS) or in the advanced stages of terminal illness, on the grounds that in such cases, these measures should be viewed as medical interventions that are no longer therapeutic (Rosner, 2001, pp. 248-251; Dorff, 1998, pp. 231-271; Washofsky, 2001, pp. 250-251, 452). Rabbinical authorities will permit or even encourage patients to draw up advance directives for health care ("living wills") to convey their wishes to medical professionals and to all who may one day become their legal guardians. These directives are binding from a Jewish point of view only to the extent that *halakhah* permits a patient to make a particular choice for him- or herself. As we have seen, rabbinical attitudes on this subject differ, and those contemplating such directives should consult their own rabbi for counsel. Similarly, Jewish law countenances hospice care for terminally ill patients to the extent that the rabbi consulted agrees that the patient may refuse heroic measures or other forms of aggressive treatment (Dorff, 1998, pp. 168-172).

Although a person is obliged to seek medical treatment during time of illness, Jewish law does not require him or her to seek *all* suggested forms of treatment. The prevailing category here is the concept of *refu'ah bedhukah*, "proven medicine." The commandment to heal covers all medical measures of recognized therapeutic efficacy; it exempts experimental therapies or therapies of uncertain value, on the grounds that such treatments do not qualify as "medicine" with a certainty that would require their application. On the other hand, a patient is entitled to undergo experimental or even risky treatment that might shorten his life if the treatment offers a reasonable prospect of recovery from or control of disease. This is done on the theory that medical treatment, by its nature, always involves *some* element of risk; therefore, so long as the intention is toward a legitimate medical objective, the risky treatment is permitted (Bleich, 2000, pp. 30-36; Washofsky, 2001, pp. 245-256, 451).

D.2. Pain Management

For much the same reasons, Jewish law approves of aggressive medication, including narcotics, to relieve pain, even though the medication is so powerful that it might hasten death. The operative word here is *might*: the drug must not be administered with the intention to kill the patient. So long as these conditions are observed, the alleviation of pain is considered a proper medical objective the achievement of which, like that of all other such objectives, justifies undertaking a significant degree of risk (Rosner, 2001, pp. 248-251; Washofsky, 2001, pp. 248-249, 451).

E. Access to Health Care

Jewish bioethics does not specify the parameters of the ideal health-care delivery system. How a community chooses to distribute its medical resources will depend upon a number of economic, social and cultural factors on which *halakhah per se* is neutral. On the other hand, Judaic texts and the rabbinical authorities who interpret them emphasize certain principles that define the ethical practice of medicine and that ought to govern the health care system of any community that aspires to justice and compassion.

The first of these principles is the fact that medicine is a *mitzvah*, a religious duty, a species of the obligation to save life and to rescue those in danger. Since *pikuach nefesh*, the preservation of human life, is a responsibility that every member of the just society owes to his or her fellow, it follows that the just society is one that guarantees medical care to all, regardless of economic status. For example, we have noted above that the physician is obligated to practice medicine and to treat all who come to him; the physician may not turn away a person in need on grounds of that person's inability to pay for treatment. The same duty would extend to other health care professionals and to the community's medical institutions, since all of these persons and organizations are engaged in the practice of medicine, the saving of human life. At the same time, the physician works for a living and like all other workers is entitled to just compensation. This seemingly obvious point is actually the subject of no little controversy in the classical Jewish sources. The physician, in fact, may not be paid for practicing medicine, since medical practice is a *mitzvah*, a divine commandment; one may not charge a fee for performing an act that God enjoins upon us. *Halakhah* can justify compensation only by means of the legal fiction that the physician receives payment not for the actual practice of medicine but instead for expenses and for time that he or she would otherwise devote to gainful employment. Yet once it is granted that the physician is entitled to compensation, it follows that the community may not penalize the physician by forcing her to care for those who cannot pay for her services.

The conflict between these two principles – the definition of medicine as a religious obligation and the physician's legitimate demand for payment – plays out in rabbinical discussions of labor relations in the healthcare industry. Physicians in some countries have gone on strike against the national health service for (among other things) higher wages. Even if we concede that all workers may withhold their services in the absence of a satisfactory labor contract, can we truly say that a physician is like all other workers, that he may "go on strike" against the divine requirement to save human life? Rabbinical authorities have answered this dilemma by ruling that physicians may *not* refrain from fulfilling this commandment: they must not withhold their services from patients who seek their help. At the same time, physicians are entitled to set a reasonable fee for these services. If some persons cannot afford to pay that reasonable fee, the responsibility lies not with the physicians but with the community or the society, which bears the ultimate responsibility for the well-being of its members.

To formulate this conclusion in specifically Judaic terms, the community is charged with creating an institutional structure that will ensure the proper fulfillment of the *mitzvah* of medical practice. The community, and not the physicians or the health care institutions, bears the ultimate responsibility of seeing to it that medical care is made available to all. Again, this does not mean that Jewish law endorses any particular structure of healthcare delivery but simply that it requires that health care be delivered, since the preservation of life is a duty owed by all to all. Rabbinical authorities are therefore likely to look with favor upon efforts in the public sphere to achieve the goal of universal health coverage, while not dictating the specific forms that those public initiatives must take (Dorff, 1998, pp. 299-310; Washofsky, 2001, pp. 224-226, 446; Rosner, 2001, pp. 513-530).

At the same time, Jewish bioethical thought would not appear to prohibit private individuals from purchasing a greater amount of medical care than that available to others under a fair-distribution scheme. Since Judaism does not object in principle to a free market system, it would not object to individuals using their economic power to purchase a greater amount of health care for themselves. We might learn this by analogy from the classical rules concerning the ransom of captives. Although the law, for obvious reasons of social policy, places limits upon the amount of ransom that the community can be forced to pay to kidnappers and hostage-takers, it also permits wealthy individuals and families to spend as much as they desire to free themselves or their relatives. The same would seem to be true for life-saving medical treatment: an individual may purchase whatever he or she is willing or able to afford, provided that an acceptable level of health care is available to all. Moreover, truly scarce medical resources, such as organs for transplantation, must be allocated on the basis of criteria other than personal wealth (Dorff, 1998, p. 305).

What criteria of allocation are favored in Jewish tradition? The halakhic sources offer support to several different – and conflicting – sets of standards. Some texts suggest that the only fair means of allocation is to ensure that each member of the community receives an equal portion of resources. In the event that the resources are indivisible, they must be distributed on a random basis (first-come, first served, a lottery, etc.). Other texts would have us distribute our resources so as to favor those in closest proximity to us: one's household comes before the residents of one's city, who come before the residents of another city, and so forth. A third set of criteria is based upon an individual's status in a hierarchical society, where those of higher Biblical "caste" or purer lineage take precedence and where knowledge of Torah is the highest degree of all. This specific arrangement, of course, does not offer much guidance for contemporary society, but it is possible to imagine other hierarchies that more closely mirror the value system of such a society. A fourth approach would allocate life-saving resources according to the criterion of medical efficacy: priority in treatment is given to those who are more likely than others to benefit from it. This principle, which corresponds to classical medical doctrine, can be understood as an application of the *mitzvah* of medical practice itself: the best way to fulfill this duty, it might be argued, is to practice medicine in as efficient and successful a manner as possible. Therefore, in the event of more than one potential recipient of an organ for transplantation, the decision would favor the recipient with the best chance for survival following the surgery. This notion might be extended to the societal context as well: a community's medical resources should be allocated in such a way as to save the most lives or to distribute the greatest medical benefit to the widest possible public. Based upon this criterion, a community could justify placing limitations upon its provision of expensive "heroic" technologies that extend the lives of end-stage patients in favor of investment in more economical therapies and measures that would deliver medical and health care benefits to a larger number of persons. Rabbinical opinion seems to favor the standard of medical efficacy as the best criterion for the allocation of resources, although a firm consensus has not yet been established (Washofsky, 1998; Washofsky, 2001, pp. 260-262 and 454; Dorff, 1998, pp. 280-299; Rosner, 2001, pp. 435-450).

IV. The Future of Jewish Bioethics

While it is always risky to deal in predictions, we can safely assume that new developments in medical science and technology will continue to pose new and perhaps undreamed-of challenges to those who seek moral guidance from traditional systems of ethics. Will Jewish bioethics be up to that challenge? To this point, the halakhic process has demonstrated sufficient flexibility to do so, a fact that justifies cautious optimism with respect to the future. Rabbis will simply have to display the same sort of creative reasoning that, through the power of analogy and the openness to change, has kept the ancient and medieval texts of Torah and *halakhah* relevant and up to date. Differences will continue to exist on medical ethical matters, both between the denominations and within the same denominations, on medical ethical matters, and these may well sharpen. Yet the halakhic process, though it has sought consensus as a way of arriving at sure and certain teachings, has also learned to prize *machloket*, dispute, as a powerful dialectical impulse toward the testing of views and the attainment of truth. As the Talmud notes, two contradictory interpretations of Torah may both reflect, in some illogical yet essential fashion, "the words of the living God" (*Talmud Eruvin* 13b). And this affirmation, perhaps, lies at the heart of the Rabbinic dictum that describes better than any other the nature of *halakhah*: "Turn the Torah over again and again, for everything is included therein" (Mishnah Avot 5:22).

Notes

1. The most comprehensive summary of the halakhic tradition and literature is Elon, 1994.
2. Among Orthodox *poskim*, for example, Rabbi Eliezer Yehudah Waldenberg, the author of the responsa collection *Tzitz Eliezer*, is known for this sort of expertise. Steinberg's *Jewish Medical Law* draws heavily upon Waldenberg's rulings.
3. Many of these articles, written from an Orthodox perspective, appear in the Hebrew journal *Assia*, published by The Dr. Falk Schlesinger Institute for Medical-Halakhic Research at Sha'arey Zedek Medical Center, Jerusalem.
4. These include: the Committee on Jewish Law and Standards of the Rabbinical Assembly (Conservative); the Responsa Committee of the Central Conference of American Rabbis (Reform); and the *Va'ad Hahalakhah* of the Israeli Masorati (Conservative) movement.
5. The reference is to the Committee on Bioethics of the Union of American Hebrew Congregations.
6. For example, the prohibition against various forms of work on the Sabbath and the obligation to fast on Yom Kippur are set aside when the preservation of life requires their suspension. The only commandments that are never set aside even to preserve life are the prohibitions against idolatry, specific sexual acts, and murder; *Talmud Sanhedrin* 74a and parallels. Other authorities derive the commandment to practice medicine from the duty to rescue those in danger; *cf.* Leviticus 19:16 ("Do not stand idly by the blood of your neighbor").
7. As such, the obligation to practice medicine must be understood as part of a netwok of *mitzvot* and in relationship to them. Thus, other religious duties exist and are observed, even if these seem on some level to conflict with the duty to heal and to "save life." For example, a Jewish adult is required to fast on certain holy days unless fasting would cause untoward damage to her health; the mere fact that fasting may bring physical pain and discomfort does not in and of itself mean that one should not fast on those days. Similarly, Jewish males are traditionally circumcised at the age of eight days. As a mitzvah, a religious duty, circumcision (*berit milah*) is practiced without consideration of any alleged medical benefit or harm of routine neonatal circumcision, although circumcision is postponed when medical indications suggest that the procedure would be harmful to the health of *this* particular child.
8. The mention of "healing" in Exodus 21:19 is read by the Rabbis as a *permit* to practice medicine and not as a commandment to do so. Indeed, various Biblical and Rabbinic sources speak in

scathing terms of physicians and of those who resort to them. See, for example, II Chronicles 16:12, on King Asa; *Talmud Berakhot* 10b, on King Hezekiah; the prayer cited in *Talmud Berakhot* 60a (human beings committed a serious error when they began to practice medicine, because they should have sought God's mercy as the source of healing; and *Mishnah Kidushin* 4:14: "the best physician is deserving of hell." This attitude, however, is not universally shared. Thus we read that "one who is in pain should go to the physician" (*Talmud Bava Kama* 46b) and that a scholar should not live in a city that has no physician (*Talmud Sanhedrin* 17b).

9. *Shulchan Arukh Orach Chayim* 618. Actually, the patient is heeded if he or she says "I must eat," then "even if one hundred physicians say otherwise, we heed the patient." In this direct conflict between two religious values – ritual observance and *pikuach nefesh* – the *halakhah* goes out of its way to err on the side of the latter. The exception to this rule: when one physician says "he must eat" and the patient and another physician say that he may safely fast. In that case, we do not require that the patient eat until the end of the fast.
10. Jewish tradition does speak of oaths taken by physicians upon assuming medical practice; for a selection, see the article by A. Steinberg in *Sefer Assia* (Jerusalem: The Falk Schlesinger Institute, 1976) 1:248-256. The point is that these oaths cannot obligate a physician to act in contradiction to the responsibilities that the Torah imposes upon her.
11. On the definition and limitations of rule *dina demalkhuta dina* (specifically: just what counts as the "legitimate law-making authority" of a government in the eyes of Jewish law), see the article by Shmuel Shilo in *Encyclopaedia Judaica* (Jerusalem: Keter, 1971) 6:51-55.
12. *Talmud Yevamot* 65b; *Shulchan Arukh Even Ha'ezer* 1:1 and 1:13.
13. *Shulchan Arukh Even Ha'ezer* 1:5. But see at 1:8: even though a man has already fulfilled this requirement, he should engage in the *mitzvah* of procreation.
14. Whether Jewish law accepts "brain death" (i.e., the "Harvard criteria," originally published in *Journal of the American Medical Association* 205 [1968], 337-350) as a proper criterion of death is the subject of a fierce controversy in the Orthodox halakhic world; compare Rosner, 2001, 287-301, to the articles by Bleich and Soloveitchik in Rosner and Bleich, 2000, 297-338. Liberal rabbis tend to accept the Harvard criteria; see Dorff, 1998, 213, and Washofsky, 2001, 256-257 and 453.

Bibliography

Avraham, A.S. (1985). *Nishmat Avraham*. 6 volumes. Jerusalem: Schlesinger Institute.

Bleich, J.D. (1991). *Kevi'at zeman ha-mavet le-or ha-halakah/me-et Yehudah David Bleikh*. New York: Z. Berman Publishing Co.

Bleich, J.D. (2000). In: F. Rosner & J.D. Bleich (Eds.), *Jewish bioethics, augmented edition*. Hoboken: Ktav.

CCAR (Central Conference of American Rabbis). (2000). *Responsum*, no. 5761.7. [On-line] Available: http://ccarnet.org/cgi-bin/respdisp.pl?file=7&year=5761

Dorff, E.N. (1998). *Matters of life and death: A Jewish approach to modern medical ethics*. Philadelphia: Jewish Publication Society.

Eisenberg, D. (2001). Stem cell research in Jewish law. [On-line] Available: http://jlaw.com/Articles/stemcellres.html

Elon, M. (1994). *Jewish law: History, sources, principles*. Philadelphia: Jewish Publication Society.

Feldman, D. (1975). *Marital relations, birth control, and abortion in Jewish law*. New York: Schocken.

Loike, J.D. & Steinberg, A. (1998). Human cloning and Halakhic perspectives. *Tradition 32(3)*, 31-46.

Rosner, F. (2001). *Biomedical ethics and Jewish law*. Hoboken: Ktav.

Rosner, F. (Ed.) (1990). *Medicine and Jewish law*. Northvale: Jason Aronson.

Rosner, F. & Bleich, J.D. (Eds.) (2000). *Jewish bioethics, augmented edition*. Hoboken: Ktav.

Rosner, F. (2000). *Encyclopedia of medicine in the Bible and the Talmud*. Northvale: Jason Aronson.
Tendler, M.D. (2000). In: F. Rosner & J.D. Bleich (Eds.), *Jewish bioethics, augmented edition* (pp. 117-124). Hoboken: Ktav.
Washofsky, M. (1998). Is old age a disease? The elderly, the medical system, and the *Halakhah*. In: W. Jacob & M. Zemer (Eds.), *Age and aging in the Halakhah* (pp. 43-82). Tel Aviv and Pittsburgh: Freehof Institute of Progressive Halakhah.
Washofsky, M. (2001). *Jewish living: A guide to contemporary reform practice*. New York: UAHC Press.

Jewish Perspectives on Embryo and Stem Cell Research

Aaron L. Mackler

In this paper I present an overview of traditional Jewish thinking concerning embryo and stem cell research. I begin by noting two values central to these deliberations: a powerful mandate to heal, and a commitment to demonstrate appropriate respect for fetal life. I then examine briefly the traditional interplay between these values in the context of abortion, as well as in the more limited literature regarding *in vitro* embryos. Finally, I review some positions that have been articulated with regard to recent challenges raised by stem cell research, and offer my appraisal.

I. General Values

The mandate to heal is a powerful imperative in Jewish ethics. This mandate flows in part from an appreciation for the value of human persons and for life as a blessing and a gift from God. Each human being has intrinsic dignity and value in God's eyes. This view of the human person provides a basis for the notion that one has the responsibility to care for oneself and seek medical treatment in the effort to recover. One should help others receive healing as well. This commitment entails responsibilities to provide health care, and to improve means of healing through biomedical research (Feldman, 1986, pp. 15-21).

Over the centuries, some have noted a theoretical tension between this active human role in health and healing, and respect for divine sovereignty, for the Bible depicts God as purposefully causing illness, famine, and other forms of human suffering. While various explanations have been offered for the mysteries of theodicy and divine providence, the overwhelming consensus of the tradition is that God has entrusted humans with the power and responsibility to feed the hungry, comfort the afflicted, and heal the sick. One classical narrative depicts two rabbis as offering medical advice, only to have the patient accuse them of interfering with God's will for God made the patient ill. The rabbis asked the man, a farmer, why he interfered with the God-given state of his vineyard by fertilizing and weeding. When he responded that crops would not grow well without human care, the rabbis replied: "Just as plants, if not weeded, fertilized, and plowed, will not grow and bring forth fruits, so with the human body. The fertilizer is the medicine and the means of healing, and the tiller of the earth is the physician" (*Midrash Temura*, in Feldman, 1986, p. 16).[1] The authority and responsibility to heal has been understood to be grounded in biblical mandates to heal the injured (Exodus 21:19); to restore that which has been lost, construed to include lost health and function (Deuteronomy 22:2); and to love one's neighbor as oneself (Leviticus 19:18). The mandate to help those in need becomes especially powerful when it is possible to save a life (*pikuah nefesh*). Saving a life justifies virtually any action that is otherwise prohibited by Judaism.[2] Furthermore, violating provisions of Jewish law in order to save a life is not only permitted, but required. One has an obligation to help others in need and especially to save life.

Jewish ethics also mandates appropriate respect for the life of an embryo (or fetus), but it understands the implications of this mandate very differently than do many Christian views. Traditional Jewish law values the embryo or fetus as a miraculous divine creation and potential human person, but does not ascribe the status of full personhood until birth. A traditional support for this understanding is found in the Book of Exodus (21:22-23): "When men fight, and one of them pushes a pregnant woman and a miscarriage results, but no other misfortune ensues, the one responsible shall be fined ... But if other misfortune ensues, the penalty shall be life for life." Feticide (at least generally) is wrong, but it is not homicide. The status of the embryo or fetus is significant, but less than that of a born, full person.

II. Abortion

In the Jewish tradition, the most extensive discussion of the status of embryonic and fetal life, and its relation to healing, occurs in the context of abortion. In keeping with the understanding of fetal status seen above, abortion is religiously and ethically prohibited in most cases. Abortion is not considered homicide, though, and abortion to preserve the life and health of the woman is warranted. The third-century Mishnah (*Oholot* 7:6) provides a clear mandate to sacrifice fetal life for the sake of the woman's: "If a woman is having [life-threatening] difficulty giving birth, one dismembers the fetus within her and brings it forth limb by limb, because her life comes before its life. Once the greater part has emerged, one may not touch it, for one may not set aside one life (*nefesh*) for another."

Jewish thinkers differ with regard to how far this paradigm should extend. It is generally agreed that to preserve a woman's life, abortion is mandatory. According to most thinkers, abortion is permitted to protect a woman from a serious threat to her health. But differences are found regarding how severe the threat to health must be to justify abortion, and how decisive the woman's own evaluation should be. For some, respect for fetal life is almost as powerful as respect for the woman's life, and only a direct threat to her life would justify abortion. For others, even a "slim reason," including virtually any health-related concern, would suffice to justify abortion. In addition, some authorities maintain that abortion can be justified to save the woman from severe suffering, even when the pregnancy does not directly threaten her health. See Feldman (1998, pp. 251-294) and Mackler (2000, pp. 193-231).

III. *In Vitro* Embryos

The status of *in vitro* embryos is generally understood to be somewhat less than that of those *in utero*. Some Orthodox halakhic authorities have ruled that *in vitro* embryos, at least those that are not intended to be transferred, have no significant status and may be discarded. Rabbi Hayyim David Halevi, for example, holds that "all ova that are fertilized *in vitro* do not have the legal status of an embryo; one does not violate the Sabbath on their behalf, and it is permissible to discard them if they were not chosen for transfer, since the law of abortion only applies to [an embryo] in the womb ... *In vitro*, there is no prohibition whatsoever" (Halevi, 1990, p. 15). Rabbi Mordechai Eliyahu, while less categorical, agrees: "Fertilized ova that have been designated for transfer to a woman's uterus should not be destroyed, since a live fetus will develop from them, but fertilized ova that have not been designated for transfer may be discarded" (Eliyahu, 1991, pp. 272-273).[3] In contrast, Rabbi J. David Bleich objects that "there are no obvious grounds for assuming that nascent human life may be destroyed simply because it is not sheltered in its natural habitat, i.e., its development takes place outside the mother's womb." He suggests that *in vitro* embryos that are viable should not be destroyed (Bleich, 1991, p. 97).

My own position would fall somewhere in between. The view of Halevi seems overstated, reflecting perhaps an overly narrow or positivist reading of legal sources. The values and sources of Jewish ethics suggest that the early embryo should be accorded a significant degree of respect and sanctity. It would seem implausible to claim that traditional Jewish understandings of and responsibilities with regard to *in utero* embryos and fetuses are simply irrelevant because of the embryo's location. At the same time, the fact that the embryo is *in vitro* does make its potential development more complicated and less likely. Unlike *in utero* embryos, it is not on a natural trajectory in which development would occur, and an *in vitro* embryo would require active intervention to have a chance at development. An additional consideration is that embryos *in vitro* can only reach the stage of a week or so of development. They remain a mass of undifferentiated cells, which has not yet individuated and can give rise to two or more embryos. This scientific picture fits relatively well with the traditional halakhic category of "mere fluid" (*maya b'alma*) found in the Talmud in connection with the early embryo (*Yevamot* 69b).[4]

The use of embryos for non-therapeutic research, in order to gain scientific knowledge but without the expectation that the embryo would be transferred for gestation, is a topic of controversy in the United States and other countries. Some have suggested that *in vitro* embryos that a couple does not wish to implant could be used for research under certain conditions. One example of such a case would be one in which the information is important and could not be gained in any other way, the experiment has been appropriately reviewed, and embryos are not maintained beyond the fourteenth day of development (American Fertility Society, 1994, pp. 78S-80S; Feldman & Rosner, 1984, p. 51). Allowing an embryo to be observed for scientific research does not seem intrinsically more objectionable than simply discarding the embryo. On the other hand, using an embryo for research becomes more troubling as the embryo reaches further points of development. Additional concerns also are raised by the creation of an embryo specifically for the purpose of research, a prospect beyond the scope of this paper.

IV. Stem Cell Research

Great attention has been given recently, in the United States and other nations, to one particular area of research involving embryos, stem cell research. Stem cells are capable of reproducing indefinitely, and are pluripotent, capable of giving rise to any type of human cell (though not able to develop into an embryo and person). Research with stem cells could provide scientists with valuable knowledge about cell growth and development, knowledge that could help in fighting diseases such as cancer. Stem cells could give rise to tissues that could be transplanted to a patient. For example, in one experiment, nerve cells derived from stem cells were transplanted into a mouse that had been paralyzed. Under the influence of the new tissue, nerve cells were regenerated and neural activity increased, so that the mouse regained the ability to walk (Gearhart, 2001; NBAC, 1999).

The derivation of stem cells, however, poses ethical problems. Stem cells have been derived by removing the inner cell mass from a blastocyst of an early embryo, several days after fertilization. (These are referred to as embryonic stem cells, or ES cells.) This process entails the destruction of the embryo. Stem cells with similar properties have been derived from tissue (primordial germ cells) from fetuses that had been aborted after five to nine weeks of development (embryonic germ cells, or EG cells). Stem cells also have been derived from adult tissue, but these cells do not appear to be pluripotent, and have different properties than those derived from embryos. For example, nerve cells that developed from embryonic stem cells led to nerve regeneration in the experiments involving paralyzed mice; nerve cells that developed from adult stem cells did not show this capacity (Gearhart, 2001; NBAC, 1999).

Comparing stem cell research to precedents regarding abortion reveals analogies and disanalogies. Both areas reflect tension between central values of healing and respect for embryonic or fetal life. One difference is that abortions done to save the mother's health or life involve a direct threat to the health of an identifiable individual. Stem cell research has the potential to improve health and save lives, but it does not respond to a direct threat, making it somewhat more difficult to justify. On the other hand, precedents regarding abortion concern a developing fetus *in utero*. The derivation of stem cells entails the destruction of a very early *in vitro* embryo, or indirect material cooperation with a woman's choice to abort, making stem cell research somewhat easier to approve.

Stem cell research has received overwhelming support from Jewish ethicists. This support reflects in part the lesser weight given to the embryo, relative to many Roman Catholic and other Christian views. In part, though, this support reflects positively the great power of the imperative to heal. Conservative rabbi Elliot Dorff, for example, has argued: "We both may and should take the steps necessary to advance stem cell research and its applications in an effort to take advantage of its great potential for human healing. We may and should engage in such research for two reasons: First, we have a duty to heal and, as a corollary to that, to develop our means to heal; and second, ... embryos outside the womb lack the status of a person or even" that of an *in utero* fetus (Dorff, 2001, p. 25).

Orthodox rabbi Moshe Tendler holds that the early embryo does not have significant status in Jewish law, supporting the derivation and use of ES cells. With regard to EG cells, he reasons that while complicity with abortion raises concerns, these give way to the value of stem cell research: "In stem cell research and therapy, the moral obligation to save human life, the paramount ethical principle in biblical law, supersedes any concern for lowering the barrier to abortion by making the sin less heinous" (Tendler, 1999, p. H-4).

Laurie Zoloth likewise argues that stem cell research is supported by the Jewish commitments to healing, and in particular the imperative to save life. She acknowledges the need for thoughtfulness and caution, since blind pursuit of technology can lead to persons being treated as things. Developments must be consistent with justice and society's responsibility to support the vulnerable. Regulation is needed to avoid abuses, and to correct for the frequent failures of the unrestrained marketplace to care for the needy. At the same time, ethicists are called "not only to worry about possible abuses of power, but also to raise concerns about unwarranted fears that might unduly block research" (Zoloth, 2001).

My own judgment is cautiously to join this developing consensus in support of stem cell research. This research offers the potential to promote the healing of human persons, which can outweigh concern for the early embryo. At the same time, even the earliest embryo has potential to develop into human life, mandating caution and thoughtfulness. Ethically, there should be oversight and safeguards to ensure that stem cells would be used only when they would contribute in an important way to research with clear value.

To address an issue of public controversy in the U.S., I believe that government funding of stem cell research would help to foster such ethical oversight. Such funding would also help to diminish somewhat the dominance of the commercial profit motive in the field. It could also lessen the proliferation of patent claims and commodification. Government funding would not automatically guarantee the ethical conduct of research or the ethical use of research discoveries. This would require the careful and ongoing work of scientists, ethicists, patent attorneys, policy analysts, and others. Government funding would, however, help to increase the possibility and likelihood of effective ethical oversight and guidance. Government funding both would help to foster progress of stem cell research, and increase the extent to which the benefits of this research spread to include the poor and disadvantaged. This course of action would be supported by the Jewish mandate to pursue justice, as well as the mandate to heal.[5]

Notes

1. See similarly Bleich, 1979.
2. The Rabbis of the Talmud (*Yoma* 85b) found a basis in a passage from the Book of Leviticus (18:5), "You shall observe my statutes and rules, which a person should do, and should live by them." As the Talmud interpreted: one should live by the commandments, and not die by them.
3. See similarly Feldman & Rosner, 1984, p. 51.
4. See Feldman, 1998, p. 266. The Talmudic term is applied to the first forty days of development. Given the current state of scientific knowledge, it may be less plausible to see as "mere fluid" later stages of embryonic and fetal development, especially beyond the fourteenth day. On this issue, my position would have much in common with others such as the American Fertility Society Ethics Committee (1994) and McCormick (1991). These contrast with the Vatican's position that "the human being must be respected – as a person – from the very first instant of his existence" – i.e., the moment of conception (Congregation for the Doctrine of the Faith, 1987, p. 12).
5. An earlier version of this paper was presented at a meeting of the Society of Jewish Ethics, meeting in conjunction with the Society of Christian Ethics, Vancouver, Canada, January, 2002.

Bibliography

American Fertility Society Ethics Committee (1994). Ethical considerations of assisted reproductive technologies. *Fertility and Sterility 62 (Nov., suppl.)*, 13S-14S, 30S-31S.

Bleich, J.D. (1979). The obligation to heal in the Judaic tradition: A comparative analysis. In: F. Rosner & J.D. Bleich (Eds.), *Jewish bioethics* (pp. 20-28). New York: Sanhedrin.

Bleich, J.D. (1991). *In vitro* fertilization: Questions of maternal identity and conversion. *Tradition, 25(4)*, 82-102.

Congregation for the Doctrine of the Faith (1987). *Instruction on respect for human life in its origin and on the dignity of procreation: Replies to certain questions of the day [Donum vitae].* Washington, DC: United States Catholic Conference.

Dorff, E. (2001). Stem cell research, paper for the Committee on Jewish Law and Standards of the Rabbinical Assembly, Draft #3, 25.

Eliyahu, M. (1991). Destroying fertilized eggs and fetal reduction. *Tehumin 11*, 272-73.

Feldman, D.M. & Rosner, F. (Eds.) (1984). *Compendium on medical ethics* (6th ed.). New York: Federation of Jewish Philanthropies of New York.

Feldman, D.M. (1986). *Health and medicine in the Jewish tradition.* New York: Crossroad.

Feldman, D.M. (1998). *Birth control in Jewish law* (rev. ed.). Northvale, NJ: Jason Aronson.

Gearhart, J. (2001). Embryonic stem cell research. Presentation to the American Association for the Advancement of Science, International Jewish Discourse Project on Religion and Ethics at the Frontier of Genetic Medicine, December 10. Washington, DC.

Halevi, H.D. (1990). On fetal reduction and the halakhic status of *in vitro* embryos. *Assia no. 47-48*, 15.

Mackler, A.L. (Ed.) (2000). *Life and death responsibilities in Jewish biomedical ethics.* New York: Jewish Theological Seminary of America, Finkelstein Institute.

McCormick, R.A. (1991). Who or what is the preembryo? *Kennedy Institute of Ethics Journal 1*, 1-15.

National Bioethics Advisory Commission [NBAC] (1999). *Ethical issues in human stem cell research (Vol. 1).* Rockville, Md.: NBAC. Archived at: http://bioethics.georgetown.edu/nbac/pubs.html

Tendler, M. (1999). Testimony for the National Bioethics Advisory Commission, May 7. In: NBAC, *Ethical issues in human stem cell research, vol. 3* (H-4). Rockville, Md.: NBAC. Archived at: http://bioethics.georgetown.edu/nbac/pubs.html

Zoloth, L. (2001). The ethics of the eighth day: Jewish bioethics and research on human embryonic stem cells. In: S. Holland, K. Lebacqz, & L. Zoloth (Eds.), *The human embryonic stem cell debate: Science, ethics, and public policy* (pp. 95-111). Cambridge: MIT Press.

Islamic Bioethics

Abdulaziz Sachedina

I. Introduction

Islam, as a comprehensive religious-moral system, does not divide the public space in terms of spiritual and secular domains with separate jurisdictions. Its comprehensive ethical deliberations cover all areas of human activity and are founded upon moral realism touching the lives of ordinary people. Ultimate questions connected with human suffering through illness and other afflictions, reproduction and abortion, death and dying, are within the purview of its religiously based ethics. Human beings are essentially God's creatures, and, hence, their total welfare related to this and the next world is God's concern.

Historically, there has been much interest among Muslims in medical ethics (*adab al-tabib*) dealing with practical morals and professional ethics connected with both patient and physician (Bakar, 1986; Burgel, 1973, 1926; Masoom, 1992). The Hippocratic oath and other similar documents derived from Persian sources were part of the classical Arabic literature that sought to inculcate proper manners and correct procedures among physicians and patients. However, the case of biomedical ethics is different. Biomedical ethics evolved in the context of rapid changes in the biological sciences and in health care around the middle of the twentieth century. As a field of inquiry dealing with the moral obligations of health professionals and society in meeting the needs of the sick and injured, modern biomedical ethics provides a framework for moral judgement and ethical decision-making in the wake of phenomenal advancements in medicine. In recent years, Muslim religious scholars have produced legal and ethical responses to the majority of the questions raised by these developments. In major centers of Islamic learning like Cairo, Egypt, and Qumm, Iran, prominent scholars of Islamic law and ethics are engaged in providing ethical decision on all sorts of questions that have arisen in the last three decades (see, e.g., Assad, 1971; Giorgis, 1981). Before we begin to assess Islamic resources for modern reflection on the relationship between the professional and patient, let us understand Islamic tradition in its general outline. This information will enable the reader to grasp the adequacies and the inadequacies of Islamic tradition in providing solutions to contemporary problems in the biological sciences, medicine, nursing, and other modes of health care (Sachedina, 1996a, 1996c; *Islamic Medical Wisdom*, 1991; Plessner, 1974).

II. Historical Background

Islam, the last of the Abrahamic religions, literally means "submission to God's will." It was proclaimed by Muhammad (born 570 C.E.), the Prophet of Islam and the founder of

Islamic public order in the seventh century C.E. in Arabia. The beginning of Islam in 610 C.E. was marked by a struggle to establish a monotheistic faith and create an ethical public order embodying divine justice and mercy. Muhammad as a statesman instituted a series of reforms to create his community, *umma*, on the basis of religious affiliation.

Within a century following Muhammad's death in 632 C.E., Muslim armies had conquered the region from the Nile in North Africa to the Oxus in Central Asia up to India. This phenomenal growth into a vast empire required an Islamic legal system for the administration of the highly developed political systems of the conquered Persian and Byzantine regions. Muslim jurists formulated a comprehensive legal code, using the ethical and legal principles set forth in the *Qur'an*, the collected revelations of Muhammad, and the precedents set by the Prophet and the early community, in addition to the customary law found in the conquered regions.

Differences of opinion on certain critical issues emerged as soon as Muhammad died in 632 C.E. The question of succession to Muhammad was one of the major issues that divided the community into the *Sunni* and *Shi'a*. Those supporting the candidacy of Abu Bakr (d. 634), an elderly associate of the Prophet as a *caliph* (political successor), formed the majority of the community, who gradually came to be known as the Sunnis; those who acclaimed 'Ali (d. 660), Muhammad's cousin and son-in-law, as the *Imam* (religious and political leader) designated by the Prophet, formed the minority group, known as the *Shi'a* ("partisans"). The dispute had profound implications beyond the political. The paradigmatic nature of prophetic prestige in the community, established both in the *Qur'an* through persistent admonition to obey him and through his personal exercise of discretionary power in shaping the public order, meant acknowledgement of an authority whose decisions in all spheres affecting Muslim life would be binding for the posterity (Hodgson, 1974).

III. Fundamental Teachings: The Five Pillars

The two authoritative sources of Islamic teachings are the *Qur'an*, regarded by Muslims as the "Book of God," and the *Sunna*, the exemplary conduct of the Prophet. The *Qur'an* consists of the revelations Muhammad received intermittently from the time of his call as the prophet in 610 C.E. until his death in 632 C.E. Muslims believe that the *Qur'an* was directly communicated by God through the archangel Gabriel, and accordingly, it is regarded as inerrant and immutably preserved. It has served as the source for ethical and theological doctrines and principles for the public organization. The *Sunna* (meaning "trodden path") has functioned as the elaboration of the Qur'anic revelation, providing details about each and every precept and deed, purportedly traced back to the Prophet's own precedent. The narratives that carried such information were designated as *hadith*. In the ninth century, Muslim scholars developed an elaborate system for the theological and legal classification of these *hadith*-reports to deduce certain beliefs and practices.

The tradition describes the Muslim creed and practice as "The Five Pillars of Islam."

The First Pillar is the *shahada*, the profession of faith: "There is no deity but God, and Muhammad is the messenger of God." Belief in God constitutes the integrity of human existence, individually and as a member of society. The *Qur'an* speaks about God as the being whose presence is felt in everything that exists; everything that happens is an indicator of the divine. Faith in God results in being safe, well-integrated, sound, and at peace.

Life is the gift of God, and the body is the divine trust given to humankind to enable it to serve God as completely and fully as the wonderful creation of God has made that serving possible. The humble origin of humans is established by the Qur'anic reference to their creation from "dry clay of black mud formed into shape" (Q. 15:26). Through the well-proportioned creation of human being in God's image and the perpetual guidance provided to perfect it both spiritually and morally, human beings have been given the trusteeship of their body. On the Day of Resurrection, all parts of the human body will have to account for the actions of the person whose bodily organs they formed. God has set limits on what human beings may do with their own bodies. Suicide, homicide, and torturing one's body in any form are regarded as acts of transgression against God.

The Qur'anic affirmation of bodily resurrection has determined many religious-ethical decisions regarding cadavers. Dead bodies should be buried reverently as soon as possible. Islamic law prohibits mutilation of the cadaver and, thus, cremation. Under certain circumstances, in order to determine the cause of death, autopsy is permitted. Postmortem dissection is permitted, for instance, to retrieve a valuable object belonging to another person that might have been swallowed by a deceased person. There was still doubt about the use of human cadavers for medical research until more recently. The rulings are now well established in regards to the cadavers. If the research for a cure is dependent on the dissection of a Muslim cadaver, then, most of the Sunni and the Shi'ite jurists rule it permissible and as a precautionary measure also require the payment of compensation to the family of the deceased (*Fiqh al-tabib* [Islamic Laws for Physicians], compiled by Drs. Mustafa Najafi, Mas'ud Salihi and Mas'ud Firdawsi, International Congress on Medical Ethics, Tehran, July 14-16, 1993, pp. 159-180). Some recent rulings from the Shi'ite jurists permit research and use of organs for transplantation (Ibid.).

The *Qur'an* affirms reverence for human life in reference to a similar commandment given to other monotheists: "We decreed for the Children of Israel that whosoever killeth a human being for other than manslaughter or corruption in the earth, it shall be as if he had killed all humankind, and whoso saveth the life of one, it shall be as if he saved the life of all humankind" (Q. 5:32). This passage has provided modern Muslim jurists with religious documentation to legitimize medical advancement in saving human lives. It has also served as an incentive to protect humanity against peril by choosing to save oneself and others from perdition and serve humanity as service to God.

The corollary of the belief in God's guidance is human accountability to further divine purposes on earth. The purpose of creation is to allow human beings, created with cognition and volition, to accept freely the responsibility of perfecting their existence by working with the laws of nature grasped by the divinely endowed innate disposition (*fitra*) and understanding principles of causality that regulate their well-being. The *Qur'an* emphasizes God's benevolence, all-forgivingness, and mercy. But it also accentuates God's justice, and stresses that humanity should develop moral and spiritual awareness (*taqwa*) in fulfilling everyday requirements of life.

Human existence is not free of tension and inner stresses caused by rejection of truth (*kufr*) and impairment of moral consciousness. To help humanity, God sends prophets "to remind" humanity of its covenant with God (Q. 7:172). There have been 124,000 prophets from the beginning of history, of whom five (Noah, Abraham, Moses, Jesus, and Muhammad) are regarded as "messengers" sent to organize their people on the basis of the guidance revealed by God.

The Second Pillar is daily worship (*salat*), required five times a day: at dawn, midday, afternoon, evening, and night. These prayers are very short and require bowing and prostration. A Muslim may worship anywhere, preferably in congregation, facing Mecca. Muslims are required to worship as a community on Fridays at midday and on two major religious holidays. The congregational prayer gives expression to the believer's religious commitment within the community. Women are exempt from this obligation of congregational participation, and the tradition recommends that they worship in the privacy of their homes. However, although segregated from men, they have always worshiped at designated areas in the mosque. The *Qur'an* prescribes the state of physical purity for the worshipper through the performance of ablutions and a full washing after sexual intercourse or a long illness prior to undertaking worship. Women are required to perform a full washing after the menstrual cycle and child birth because blood is regarded as ritually unclean. Islamic law prescribes regular cleansing and physical hygiene as expressions of one's faith.

Prayer in Islam is regarded as therapeutic. Besides seeking medical treatment Muslims are encouraged to seek healing, especially in psychological illnesses, by praying to God. Many illnesses, according to the teachings of the Prophet, are caused by psychological conditions like anxiety, sorrow, fear, loneliness, and so on. Hence, prayer restores the serenity and tranquility of the soul.

The Third Pillar is the mandatory "alms-levy" (*zakat*). The Muslim definition of the virtuous life includes charitable support of widows, wayfarers, orphans and the needy. Islamic law includes technical regulations about how much *zakat* is due and upon what property it is to be levied. These legal rulings, which originated in early Islam before the disintegration of the Islamic public order, do not necessarily prevail in contemporary Muslim nations. Although *zakat* has for the most part been left to the conscience of Muslims, the obligation to be charitable and contribute to the general welfare of the community continues to be emphasized.

The Fourth Pillar is the fast of the month of Ramadan, marked according to the Muslim lunar calendar that has been in use since the seventh century. Since the lunar year is shorter by 10-11 days than the solar one, the fasting occurs in different seasons. Ramadan is also regarded as the holy month during which the *Qur'an* was revealed to Muhammad. During the fast, which lasts from dawn to dusk, Muslims are required not only to refrain from eating, smoking, and drinking; they are also to refrain from sexual intercourse and acts leading to sensual behavior. The fasting is meant to alter the pattern of life for a month, and Muslims are required to make necessary adjustments in their normal schedules of work and study. The end of the month is marked by a festival, *'Id al-fitr*, after which life returns to normal. The discipline engendered by Ramadan varies from individual to individual. Although instituted to cultivate individual spiritual and moral self-control, Ramadan also provides a community experience in which families and friends share both fasting and evening meals in the spirit of thanksgiving.

Like prayer, fasting also possesses therapeutic value. Prophetic medical tradition prescribes fasting for different kinds of ailments, including psychological problems caused by fear and anxiety. It was regarded as a remedy for curing excessive sexual drive.

The Fifth Pillar is the annual pilgrimage, the *hajj*, which all Muslims are required to undertake once in their lives, provided they have the financial means. The rituals of the pilgrimage at Mecca are a collective commemoration of the sacrifice story of Abraham and of the lessons to be derived from it. Its spiritual objective is to inculcate a form of asceticism accompanied with renunciation of worldly desires (sexual intercourse, use of perfumes, and so on) and concern with the hereafter. The experience brings together Muslims of diverse cultures and nationalities to achieve a purity of existence and a communion with God that will exalt the pilgrim for the rest of his/her life.

IV. The Shari'a: Islamic Legal Tradition

Islamic jurisprudence (*fiqh*) was developed to determine normative Islamic conduct as detailed in the *Shari'a*, the Sacred Law. The *Shari'a* is the divinely ordained blueprint for human conduct, which was inherently and essentially religious. The juridical inquiry in discovering the *Shari'a* code was comprehensive because it necessarily dealt with every case of conscience covering God-human relations, as well as the ethical content of interpersonal relations in every possible sphere of human activity. Most of the legal activity, however, went into settling more formal interpersonal activities that affected the morals of the community. These activities dealt with the obligation of doing good to Muslims and guarding the interests of the community.

Islamic legal theory recognized four sources on the basis of which judicial decisions could be deduced: the *Qur'an*, the *Sunna*, consensus (*ijma'*) of the early community of the Muslims, and analogy (*qiyas*) which is a method of reasoning from data furnished by the *Qur'an* and the *Sunna* attempting to estimate the unknown from the known ruling. Al-Shafi'i (d. 820), a rigorous legal thinker, systematically and comprehensively linked the four sources to derive the whole *Shari'a* to cover all possible contingencies. The legal precedents and principles provided by the *Qur'an* and Sunna were used to develop an elaborate system of rules of jurisprudence. Human conduct was to be determined in terms of how much legal weight was borne by a particular rule that rendered a given practice obligatory or merely recommended. For instance, if it is deemed that by risking one's life one may be able to save another person from impending death, then the law permits not only donation but also sale of a needed body part or an organ after a careful risk-benefit analysis. Vital organs like eyes are excepted in this ruling because deforming one's countenance was not permissible. Likewise, it had to be decided whether an obligatory act, because of its social relevance and the degree of applicability of a given rule or precedent, was to be enforced by penalties in the courts or left to God's judgment in the hereafter.

All schools, although tending to give the male an extensive prerogative, presupposed a considerable social role for women. The Qur'anic injunction to propriety were stretched by means of the *Sunna* to impose seclusion. The veil was presented simply in terms of personal modesty, the female apartments in terms of family privacy. It was not to become a form of social distinction, as it did with the upper-class women living upon rigorous segregation. Among the latter, it became a mark of a woman of a quality that she was secluded from all men but her own.

Segregation of sexes as required by the *Shari'a* has led to numerous problems in the teaching and practicing of medicine today. The problems cover such areas as closely examining and touching the reproductive organs (male-female, female-male, male-male, and female-female); looking even at the naked photographs for studying physiology and anatomy; taking pulse, and other vital signs of patients of opposite sex. While the classical decisions were prohibitive in all these cases, majority of the modern Muslim jurists have casuistically accommodated the need to carry out necessary medical training and research.

In the patriarchal family structures, and not necessarily in the *Shari'a*, women were assigned a subordinate role in the household and community. Through certain cultural practices, women's reproductive capacity was controlled. In some parts of the Muslim world, women are victims of traditional practices that are often harmful to their well-being and that of their children. One of the controversial and persistent practices is female circumcision (*khafd* or *khifad*) without which it is believed that girls could not attain the status of womanhood. Islamic views on female circumcision are ambiguous. While there are traditions that can be extrapolated to prohibit the practice, there are some that condone it as a cultural norm. The operation was performed long before the rise of Islam. It is not practiced in many Muslim countries, including Saudi Arabia, Tunisia, Iran and Turkey. There is nothing in the *Qur'an* that justifies female circumcision, especially its most severe form, infibulation. The Prophet opposed the custom found among pre-Islamic Arabs, since he considered it harmful to women's sexual well-being. Yet the official juridical position among majority of *Sunni* jurists is that female circumcision is sanctioned by the *Sunna*. However, the law does not regard it as an obligatory requirement. It is merely a recommended act.

As Islamic jurisprudence became a highly technical process, disputes about method and judicial opinions crystallized into legal schools designated by the names of prominent jursits. The legal school that followed the Iraqi tradition was called "*Hanafi*", after Abu Hanifa (d. 767) the *imam* (teacher) in Iraq. Those who adhered to the rulings of Malik b. Anas (d. 795), in Arabia and elsewhere, were known as "*Malikis.*" Al-Shafi'i founded a legal school in Egypt whose influence spread widely to other regions of the Muslim world. Another school was associated with Ahmad b. Hanbal (d. 855), who compiled a work on *hadith*-reports that became the source for juridical decisions of those who followed him. Shi'ites developed their own legal school, whose leading authority was the Imam Ja'far al-Sadiq (d. 748). Normally, Muslims accepted one of the legal schools prevalent in their region. Most of the Sunnites follow Hanafi or Shafi'i; whereas the Shi'ites follow the Ja'fari school. In the absence of an organized "church" and ordained "clergy" in Islam, determination of valid religious praxis was left to the qualified scholar of religious law. Hence, there emerged a living tradition, with different interpretations of the Qur'anic laws and prophetic traditions, giving rise to different schools of the *Shari'a*.

The scope of *Shari'a*, understood as the norm of the Muslim community as a community, was defined by two essential areas of human life: acts of worship both public and private, connected with the pillars of faith; and acts of public order that insure individual justice. The *Shari'a* reflected Muslim endeavors to ensure that Islam pervaded the whole of life. However, many areas of human existence, including the ethical problems connected with the medical treatment of human ailments received little systematic attention in the classical formulations of the legal thought (Rahman, 1980; Wensinck, 1965; Watt, 1968).

V. Theological and Ethical Tradition

In the first half of the eighth century, the debates about qualified leadership, the existence of injustices in the community, and its appropriate response to redress the situation formed the rudiments of the earliest systematic theology of the group called Mu'tazilites. Before them, some Muslim thinkers had developed theological arguments, including a doctrine of God and human responsibility, in defense of the Islamic revelation and the prophethood of Muhammad when these were challenged by other monotheists. The Mu'tazilites, however, undertook to show that there was nothing repugnant to reason in the Islamic revelation. In defining God's creation and governance of the world, these early Muslim theologians sought to demonstrate the primacy of revelation. At the same time, their theology reflected Hellenic influences. From the ninth century on, translations of the full Greek philosophic and scientific heritage became available in Arabic. The result was the development of a technical vocabulary and a pattern of syntax that enriched theological terminology.

The Ash'arite traditionalists, reacting to Mu'tazilite rationalism, limited speculative theology to a defense of the doctrines given in the *hadith*-reports, which were regarded more reliable than abstract reason in deducing individual doctrines. The Ash'arites emphasized the absolute will and power of God, and denied nature and humankind any decisive role. What humans perceive as causation, they believed, is actually God's habitual behavior. In their response to the Mu'tazilite view about the objective nature of good and evil, and in their effort to maintain the effectiveness of a God, at once omnipotent and omnibenevolent, who could and did intervene in human affairs, they maintained that good and evil are what God decrees them to be. God transcends the order of nature. Hence, the notion of free will is incompatible with the divine transcendence, which determines all actions directly. Ash'arite theological views remained dominant throughout Islamic history, well into modern times, and had profound effect upon scientific and particularly medical theory and practice among the Sunnites. The Shi'ite theological and ethical doctrines were based on Mu'tazilite thesis about the Justice of God and the objective nature of moral values.

At the practical level, medicine, like astrology, involved the training necessary to apply techniques that demonstrated tact and insight in the treatment of patients. Medical practice was based on a tradition of clinical observation, which became the source for encyclopedic works like the *Canon* (*al-Qanun*) of Avicenna (d. 1037). Since dissection of human cadavers was socially impossible because of the prohibition in Islamic law against mutilation of the dead and the requirment of immediate burial, physicians treated their patients partly on the basis of their knowledge of anatomy and partly by relying on their understanding of the rationality and harmony of the cosmos. Diagnosis and prognosis were also based on their insights about psychological and environmental factors. Despite the disapproval of some orthodox Muslims, who rejected Greek medicine as not provided for in the Prophetic medical tradition, many of these philosopher-physicians of society came to be known as the *hakim* (wise) (Elgood, 1951a, 1951b).

VI. Professional Ethics in Islam

Since the *Qur'an* teaches that society as a whole needs to respond to the creation of a just public order, there has been an emphasis on the way an individual needs to be prepared for such a revolution. Acknowledgement of God demands, in the first instance, a personal devotion to moral purity. But personal purity implies a just social behavior: generosity to the weak and curbing the license of the strong. Moreover, it is fully recognized that a person's moral life is usually less a function of his good resolutions than of the level of actual expectations around him. It must be society and not just individuals that should be reformed. The *Qur'an* makes it sufficiently clear that moral path is for everyone, not just for moral heroes, by praising those who urge others to virtue almost as much as those who practice it themselves. The moral life must be lived by a society at large.

Practical piety and reliable character are emphasized in connection with all professions. Although a physician need not be a pious individual in order to be a competent physician (because a physician's work is essentially to take care of his/her patient), nevertheless, piety and good character aid in the general acceptance of the physician's advice and bad character would detract from its value. A physician should be a cultured person, aware of the sensibilities of the people among whom he/she works. In Muslim culture, a physician must work hard to gain the trust of the patient and cultivate professional confidence (*Fiqh al-tabib*, 1993; Rahman, 1989).

Islam lays great emphasis on virtues and obligations in connection with medical profession, because medicine deals with the most valued aspect of existence, namely, preservation of human life. Bad character in a physician is seen as a mortal poison and a sure path to perdition. The sicknesses of heart and the diseases of soul are regarded as a great threat to the normal professional role assumed by a physician. Moreover, the society and the institutions that provide medical care have certain expectations from a person to whom they entrust their physical well-being. Muslim ethicists lay down canons by which virtues become ingrained in the practice of a skillful physician. Techniques of meditation and prayers are suggested for medical professionals to focus their attention to the wholeness of human care, and not simply to their physical condition. In this way, medical professional in a Muslim community is expected to learn not only the origins and causes of sicknesses which cause loss of corporeal life, but he/she also begins to pay attention to the diseases of heart and soul. In this latter diagnosis, Muslim physician goes beyond the role-related technical skill and equips him/herself with a character built on virtuous life to understand the religious/psychological dimensions of the profession. The two most important virtues emphasized in Islamic professional ethics are spiritual and moral consciousness (*taqwa*) and patience (*sabr*). The physician must cultivate these two virtues by leading a balanced and moderate life and by not wasting time and energy indulging in pleasure and amusements.

The question of professional ethics is directly connected to a religious problem of the relationship between action and its impact upon human conscience. To state it briefly, human acts have a direct impact upon the development of conscience which, in Islamic tradition, is regarded as the source of determining the rightness or wrongness of human undertakings. The conscience must be constantly guarded against becoming corrupted. When conscience becomes corrupted as a result of neglecting ethical matters related to the production of daily sustenance, then there is no moral safeguard left to prevent these professionals from engaging into more serious acts that would lead to the destruction of the very fabric of social relations founded upon divinely ingrained sense of justice and fairness. Both intention and reflection must precede all human acts that infringe upon the spiritual and physical well-being of others.

Here it is important to keep in mind that both the patient and physician are required by Islam to observe ethical discipline. Patients should strictly follow their physicians' orders and respect their physicians. Patients are exhorted to regard their physicians better than their best friends. Patient should have direct contact with their doctors and should confide fully in them concerning their sickness. In fact, it is better for people to stay in touch with a physician who can advise them about their health before they actually need treatment (Rosenthal, 1969).

VII. Healthcare Provider: Patient-institution Relationship

When a patient goes to a health care institution, he/she is in desperate need of attention. Islam teaches that fulfilling the needs of the people is in itself an opportunity to recognize the blessings of God on humanity. Hence, it is the duty of healthcare providers to perform their responsibilities with necessary compassion and discernment. The profit motive should not drive the institution to hold back the necessary diagnosis and treatment. In fact, both patient and health providers must observe an ethical discipline founded upon the total wellness of individual (Rispler-Chaim, 1993).

There is much emphasis on free medical services in Muslim culture because of the prevalent poverty in many regions of the world where Muslims are a majority. To refuse to see a patient because she happens to be poor is to forfeit the claim to be human. Institutional responsibility in such cases is enormous because healthcare insurance coverage is not available universally. In the modern Muslim nations health care has become a major part of endeavors to educate population about health hazards and the need to observe daily hygiene as much as keep the home and social environment clean.

VIII. Reproductive Technologies and Related Issues

The ability to bear children is regarded as an important purpose of marriage in Islam. Some Muslim religious thinkers view procreation as the main goal of a marital union. However, normative sources like the *Qur'an* and the *Sunna* do not view sexual relations between spouses merely for the purpose of reproduction (Musallam, 1989). In Muslim culture, children are an important source of a healthy and successful marriage. Since the *Qur'an* does not accord legal validity to reproduction separate from the act of coitus, and since Islamic law does not regard adoption as an option for infertile couples, there has been relatively more sustained interest in reproductive technologies developed by modern medicine. However, a number of techniques infringe upon ethical sensibilities connected with obtaining semen or implantation of spermatozoa into the female reproductive tract (Islam and Family Planning, 1974; Sachedina, 1996b).

(1) Artificial insemination is permissible in Islamic law as long as insemination utilizes the semen of the husband. Semen of a third party or donor insemination is forbidden because, according to Islamic law, the lineage of an off-spring must be properly connected to a male and female joined in a religiously recognized and solemnized marital union. The sanctity of a child's moral and legal personhood is dependant upon his/her untarnished lineage through both parents.

(2) Since artificial insemination involves an element of adulterous implantation in the womb of a surrogate mother, no contract involving such transaction would be legal in the *Shari'a* law. Another problem related to artificial insemination is related to the method of obtaining semen. Masturbation as a method of obtaining semen is rejected

by the law as sinful. Some jurists have argued its permissibility in this case because the purpose is not to derive pleasure. Moreover, they justify their decision based on the principle which states "necessity renders the forbidden permissible." But other methods, such as the use of vibratory stimuli, an alternate possibility of obtaining sperm by using a condom during intercourse or by removing some surgically from the epididymis (the storage depot for spermatozoa), are not a problem.

(3) In general, all legal schools in Islam approve insemination of a wife (*in vivo*) with semen obtained from her husband and artificial insemination (*in vitro*) using the husband's semen. All other forms (e.g., using sperms of a donor or mixing the woman's ovum with semen from a man other than her husband, then transferring the ovum to the uterus of the man's wife) are forbidden. The problem of discarding other fertilized ova will be discussed under abortion (see below).

(4) Surrogate motherhood is also forbidden on the grounds that no other womb than the wife's can be used for the purpose of carrying a fetus to its full term. The main concern for the preservation of properly recognized lineage of the child rules out any ambiguous procedures that may raise doubts about the identity of the child's parents.

Muslim jurists define abortion as the induced ejection of a fetus prematurely with or without a proper justification. The common juristic terminology like *al-isqat* (literally "elimination") suggests the intentional aspect of the miscarriage and not simply discharged fetus with no signs of life (Ebrahim, 1991).

There are no references in the *Qur'an* about abortion. The passages used as documentation to infer prohibitive ruling about abortion refer to the general interdiction about killing (*qatl al-nafs*) and the punishment that accrues to the one who commits intentional homicide: "And slay not the soul God has forbidden, except by right. Whosoever is slain unjustly, We have appointed to his next-of-kin authority; but let him not exceed in slaying; he shall be helped" (Q. 17:33; also 5:32). Even those passages that speak about the embryonic development of a fetus do not spell out the modern day differentiation between a biological animation and a moral and legal existence.

Based on Qur'anic embryology (Q. 23:10-12), some important conclusions have been drawn about the development of embryo to a full human person. First, perceivable human life is possible at the later stage in biological development of the embryo when God says: "thereafter We produced him as another creature." Second, it is possible to make a distinction between biological animation and moral-legal personhood, and, as indicated by the consensus among the Sunni jurists over the interpretation of these verses, to place the latter stage after the first trimester in pregnancy. This consensus is based on the traditions that provide further elaboration of the Qur'anic embryology.

The single most important tradition that has provided religious grounds for legal estimation of fetus inviolability has been reported in both the Sunni and Shi'ite compilations. This tradition describes the embryonic stage when human destiny is recorded by an angel who is sent by God to breathe the spirit either on the fortieth or forty-second night or after 120 days. The jurists have identified this stage as the moment of ensoulment when the fetus attains personhood. The moral-legal implication of the ensoulment is not the subject of these traditions. With the limited knowledge about human embryology, ancient Muslim jurists did not emphasize the distinction between two periods of pregnancy to deduce decisions about the culpability and accruing penalty in the matter of induced abortion. For them deliberate termination of pregnancy at any stage of the embryonic development was sinful. However, after first trimester abortion was absolutely prohibited. Muslim jurists have reported consensus in the matter of complete inviolability of the fetus after 120 days. The differences of opinion in this matter had to wait for the biomedical advancements in modern times when biological data on the embryonic journey to a full human at times contradicted the traditional account of when conceivable life was scientifically discernible.

The opinions of the early Muslim jurists on abortion can be divided in accordance with the first three stages of forty day each, that is the first trimester, in embryonic development:

- *The drop stage*: Majority of the Hanafi, Shafi'i, and Hanbali, and some of the Maliki and Shi'ite jurists allow it. Majority of the Maliki and Shi'ite and some Hanafi, Shafi'i, and Hanbali jurists prohibit it.
- *The clot stage*: Majority of the Hanafi, Shafi'i and some among the Hanbali jurists permit it. All the Maliki, majority of the Hanbali and Shi'ite, some Hanafi and Shafi'i prohibit it.
- *The tissue stage*: Majority of the Hanafi and Shafi'i, and some among the Hanbali jurists permit it. All the Maliki, majority of the Hanbali and Shi'ite, and some Hanafi and Shafi'i jurists prohibit it, because this is the ensoulment stage.

While in agreement about the abortion before the first trimester, the jurists have disagreed about the legal status of the fetus and the rulings inferred from their comprehension of the biological stages. However, on the basis of the penalties prescribed for feticide, there is an agreement that the fetus before ensoulment cannot be accorded a status of a full person. Also, no funeral rites are to be performed for a fetus before the first trimester.

Overall, the law stipulates the fetus' right to life, even when a universally recognized definition of an embryo that specifies personhood is lacking. Accordingly, it requires postponement of a pregnant woman's execution until after she has delivered her baby and made provisions for its care after her death. A majority of the Hanafi, Shafi'i, Hanbali and some Shi'ite scholars rule that abortion may take place during the first trimester if the woman's pregnancy threatens the well-being of an already existing infant. In the case of a pregnancy that threatens a woman's life, a majority of the jurists have given priority to saving the life of the fetus when ensoulment has already occurred.

The phenomenal advancement of biomedical technology in saving the life of a woman faced with a complicated pregnancy, as well as determining the beginning of a life in a fetus, has led to a reconsideration of some classical formulations about abortion. A number of juristic principles, including the "contrariety between two harms" and "protection against distress and constriction" have been evoked to rule the priority of saving the mother's life on whose well-being depends the life of the fetus. Also, in the case of a rape or incest psychological damage suffered by a woman has been duly recognized as a justification for abortion.

Different legal schools hold conflicting opinions as to the appropriate penalty for the act of feticide, but none of the schools punish the crime as homicide. If a man causes a woman to miscarry (or abort) and the fetus is unformed, his crime carries the penalty of *al-ghurra* (monetary compensation); but if the expelled fetus is formed then it is *diya kamila* (full blood money). An additional penalty may be levied, requiring the aggressor to fast for two consecutive months.

IX. Organ and Tissues Donation and Transplantation

In general, Islam encourages all efforts that promote saving human life. The *Qur'an* clearly states: "Whoso gives life to a soul, shall be as if he had given life to humankind altogether" (Q. 5:33). Organ transplantation can save life and hence, with the advanced medical technologies in place, Muslims have been from time to time reminded about the merit of organ/tissue donation. Islamic law prohibits mutilation of the cadaver and, thus, to cremate it. In early 1980s, rulings were issued on the basis of the principle of public interest (*maslaha*) to allow organ transplant from person to person. However, there are cultural factors connected with a strong commitment to intact burial. From the early 1970s, the expansion of organ procurement, especially viable organs from heart-beating cadavers, whose cardiopulmonary function is maintained by machines, introduced the concept of brain death, which generated ambiguities among Muslim jurists. Although musculo-skeletol tissue transplants have increased in the Muslim world, vital organ transplants like heart and kidney have encountered the difficulty of determination of death on the basis of total and irreversible cessation of brain function. The brain death criterion is not universally accepted by Muslim jurists of all legal schools. Since the organ donor must be kept on machines that maintain respiration and heartbeat in order to keep an organ usable for transplantation, the traditional death criterion in the *Shari'a*, which is cessation of breathing, does not apply in the case of brain death. More recently, with the growing education of legal scholars in medical issues connected with brain death, the jurists have permitted the retrieval of organs, as long as medical institutions obtain permission from families. Such permission has not been forthcoming because of the psychological and cultural factors.

Eye banks have existed in the Muslim world for more than four decades, whilc organ banks are relatively new. It was not until November, 1998 that Iran saw its first organ bank, whereas Egypt and other Arab countries have had their system for procurement of tissues and organs in place since the early 1980s. Ethical and legal issues connected with organ transplantation revolve around the procurement, transfer and use of organs and tissues from cadavers. Organ transplantation also raises questions about the appropriateness of viewing human body as property. Egyptian jurists have specifically raised the question about the validity of a living will in which advance directives about the donation of organs are included. They argue that human being cannot claim ownership of his body since it is given to him as a trust. Thus, he cannot make a living will in connection with his cadaver, which should be promptly buried within few hours after death. On the same basis, some jurists identify an intimate relationship between personhood and embodiment and view the cadaver as symbolic of the person. Accordingly, they view the sale of organs as unlawful. This latter opinion is not held unanimously by all, since some Shi'ite jurists regard the sale of organs as permissible as long as it causes no harm to the person or does not lead to the mutilation of the cadaver.

In more recent literature there exists a consensus regarding the right of a living person to donate certain parts of the body with the condition that it would not lead intentionally wounding oneself or forfeiting one's life to save another. However, if it is deemed that by risking one's life one may be able to save his fellow-human from impending death, then one could undertake to donate a part or an organ that is needed. At this point, the discretion is given to the person who can decide after a careful risk-benefit analysis in which the probability of saving the recipient's life is substantially greater than the risk to donor's life or health. It is important to keep in mind that since Islamic tradition emphasizes human relationships as important for individual, if the family opposes the individual's decision to donate, Islamic law favors the family to prevail. In general, the healthcare system is sensitive to the family's wishes, even when the deceased person signed a donor card, and the will can be thwarted after their death (Sachedina, 1988 and 1998).

X. Death and Dying in Islam

Traditionally, Islamic jurisprudence defines death as complete cessation of the heart or respiration. However, a further dimension has been added to this formulation of death in view of the modern medical technology that can intervene to prolong life through the life-support system in the case where all functions of the brain have ceased. This development has given rise to the question whether brain death can be recognized as a valid formulation of death without first defining the criteria of life in Islam. Can innate integration of vegetative functions without cognition in a brain-dead person be used as the necessary and sufficient condition of life? What are the social and moral implications of recognizing brain death as a right criterion for death in Muslim society?

A. Some Conceptual Considerations

Although the Muslim scripture, the *Qur'an*, contains various death themes that add significantly to our insight into the meaning of death, the concept is left undefined and always portrayed in close relationship with the concepts of life, creation, and resurrection. The *Qur'an* is more concerned to determine the nature of death.

> Every person (*nafs*) shall taste of death; and We try you with evil and good for a testing, then unto Us you shall be returned (Q. 21:35-6).

Death is the termination of an individual comprehensive being, capable of believing and disbelieving, and not simply a living organism. Life does not end with death. In the same way that a person does not cease to exist in sleep, so also he does not cease to exist in death. And in the same way that a person comes back to life when waking from sleep, so also will she/he be revived at the great awakening on the Day of Judgement. Hence, Islam views death merely as a stage in human existence. Physical death should not be feared as an evil. One should, however, worry about the agonies of spiritual death caused by living a life of moral corruption. That sinful life is not worth living. Human efforts should be concerned with the revival of human conscience, which will lead to a meaningful life. Does it mean that human body should be simply neglected? No, not at all. It simply means that human death must be viewed as secondary to the spiritual and moral quality of life.

This religious evaluation of death is reflected in Muslim cultural attitudes to life and death. In general, Muslim public does not view, for instance, a persistent vegetative state of an individual as life. Life in Muslim culture has a set of criteria which must be fulfilled in order for the patients, their families, and society in general to regard a person living. These include a person's ability to make decisions and execute them through his own conscious and cognitive competence. In the absence of such competence, close family members or religious and lay leaders in the community assume the guardianship to protect the person's rights. The principle of public good (*maslaha*) for society in Islam allows the community leaders to act as surrogate decision-makers in cases when the person due to mental or any related incompetency is unable to assume that responsibility.

Significantly, in the case of a patient in the vegetative state, ethical deliberations in Islam are not only concerned with determining the value of the patient's life. The principle of public good demands that an individual's life must be weighed in the scale of general well-being of those who are horizontally related to the patient. End of life decisions require to take into consideration an individual's interpersonal relationship with his own family and society in general. If active medical intervention in the case of a severely brain-damaged patient leads to further suffering of the patient and those related to him in society, then the ethical judgement cannot ignore the ensuing general harm, including the rising cost of prolonging such life for the entire society.

It is for this reason that Muslim jurists have adopted the view that it is permissible for the patient in an irreversible vegetative state, either through a prior living will or his immediate family or supreme legal authority (*hakim al-shar'*), to refuse any treatment that simply prolongs the patient's miserable condition. The point is explicitly made clear that, in the eyes of Muslim public, it is pointless and even degrading to intervene medically in the nature's course towards an imminent death. On the basis of the religious and moral duty of rejection of harm (*'usr wa haraj*), if it is reasonably determined by at least three consultant physicians that pursuing a particular course of treatment is proportionally more harmful than allowing the nature to take its course, then it is obligatory to stop the treatment.

This conceptual and cultural understanding of death in Islam is important to keep in mind as we consider the legal and ethical deliberations that were undertaken by Muslim legalists in providing the criteria to determine death. Their decisions were not deduced solely on the basis of what we would call normative sources like the *Qur'an* and the *Tradition*, the *Sunna*; they also took into account cultural understanding of the nature of life and death in the community. In Muslim culture, until recently when modern medical technology admitted the distinction between cessation of cerebral function and cardiorespiratory function, the pronouncement of death was based upon the criteria provided by the vitality of mutually dependent organic system of human body. The terms "cerebral death" and "brain death" are neologisms in Muslim societies, which continue to see death as the cessation of vital functions in a single organ system rather than a part of the organ. Having said this, the question arises whether the Islamic legal tradition provides any criteria to determine when a person can be regarded as dead.

B. The Traditional Legal Criteria

Until recently, determination of death in Muslim culture was not enigmatic at all. In general, Islamic law has depended upon the opinions of scientific experts and professionals, who have used the pragmatic but traditional criteria for death routinely observed in patients. According to the traditional criterion, the life ends with the permanent cessation of respiration and of circulation. In other words, Muslim jurists regarded complete cessation of heartbeat as a sufficient criterion to declare a person legally dead. The problem arose when modern medical technology acquired the ability to keep the signs of life through respiratory support in a brainstem-dead patient. The patients were regarded alive in accord with the traditional definition of death.

There are two interrelated reasons that have prompted Muslim jurists to reconsider the stance on brain death criteria in the case of patients with irreversible brain damage while the cardiovascular system continues to function by means of new techniques of intensive care:

(1) Can recognition of brain death lead to the unethical and illegal retrieval of organs for transplantation in such patients whose cardiorespiratory physiology can be kept functional for successful retrieval? In many poor countries in the Third World, there is an irresistible temptation to make money from the sale of these organs.

(2) Can the government policy authorize the health care providers to withdraw treatment when organ viability can be maintained by active medical intervention? Until recently, health policies in the Muslim countries generally reflected insensitivity to the public's moral and cultural sensitivities connected with death.

The following decision was made as a government policy in Saudi Arabia under the rubric of *Religious Aspect of Organ Transplant* (The Purport of the Senior Ulama Commission's Decision No: 99 dated 6-11-1402 [AH]/25-08-1982):

> The board unanimously resolved the permissibility to remove an organ, or a part thereof from a Muslim or a non-Muslim (*dhimmi*) living person and graft it onto him, should the need arise, should there be no risk in the removal and should the transplantation seem likely successful.

According to two leading medical doctors Ali al-Bar and Nabil Nizamuddin, the latter being the liver transplant surgeon in King Fahad National Guard Hospital in Riyadh, the above policy statement requires the following elaboration:

> Should the diagnosis of brain death be established unequivocally, the physician in charge may keep the corpse ventilated for the purpose of pre-arranged organ donation until receiving the consent of the heirs, or an order from the *Qadi*, the magistrate, in the case of an unknown corpse. The ventilated corpse is considered dead from the time of declaration of brain death and not from the time of turning off the ventilator.

The last statement is contradicted by the Council of Islamic Jurisprudence (*majma' al-fiqh al-islami*), which includes jurists from all schools of thought in Islam and which meets regularly to review some of these new rulings. Their ruling reads as follows:

> It is permissible to switch off the life support system with total and irreversible loss of function of the whole brain in a patient if three attending specialist physicians render their opinion unequivocally that irreversible cessation of brain functions has occurred. This is so even when the essential functions of the heart and the lungs are externally supported by life support system. However, legal death cannot be pronounced except when the vital functions have ceased after the external support system has been switched off (*al-qarar al-thani*, p. 21).

In none of the rulings examined thus far has any Muslim jurists tried to define or determine the criteria for accepting the validity of brain death from Islamic legal perspective. They have depended on the consultant physicians, who are more interested in getting the approval for retrieving organs, to provide their expert opinion. Hence, the debate in North America concerning the acceptance of "higher brain formulations of death" and the controversial aspects of providing medical care of patients with advanced forms of dementia and PVS is absent in the juridical literature dealing with the definition of death.

In its third session held in Amman, Jordan, on October 16, 1986, the Council of Islamic Jurisprudence once again took up and discussed the life supportive system in the ICU. After extensive and exhaustive explanation given by physicians specializing in that field of medicine, they decided the following:

> The person is considered legally dead, and all the guidelines provided by the *Shari'a* to determine death are applicable when following signs are confirmed:
> (a) When complete cessation of the heart or respiration occurs, and the expert physicians ascertain that the cessation is irreversible.
> (b) When complete cessation of all functions of the brain occurs, and the expert physicians ascertain that the cessation is irreversible and the brain is in the state of degeneration.

In this condition it is permissible to discontinue the life supportive system from the patient even when some of the patient's organs like the heart are kept functional by artificial means.

The document then proceeds to list the procedure that must be followed as part of the *Brain Death Documentation*:

> Brain death is the irreversible cessation of all spontaneous brain activity including the brain stem. Before any supportive means is discontinued, the family members must be counseled. This should be documented in the patient's chart.

In a question that was submitted by the Ministry of Health in Tehran to one of their leading jurists, Ayatollah Tabrizi, he was asked about the definition of death in Islamic law – whether it is the cessation of brain function or the function of heart. His response reveals the early stages of debate on brain death in jurisprudence. He says that for that distinction, one must refer to a physician. He says:

> It is necessary to refer to the medical specialist in order to decide whether the first or the second conforms to the definition of death. Some experts are of the opinion that if the brain waves show the cessation for more than two and a half minutes, then death is definite and there is no way that life could return.

He then proceeds to define death as it is accepted in the tradition:

> Death is the passing away of the soul from the body, as some commentators have indicated in their explanation of the verse from the *Qur'an*: "Muhammad is not but a messenger; before him also there were messengers." Death is, then, passing away of the soul and cancellation of life from body. Contrast this with murder. Murder is death when the cause is related to premeditation or something like that. Hence, death is distinct from murder. However, when compared with it, death is natural, whereas murder is just the contrary.

In other words, this jurist hesitates to regard irreversible cessation of brain function as a valid form of death. However, the government appointed Council of Islamic Jurisprudence in Iran, under the section regarding Rulings Concerning Organ Transplantation, writes:

> The criterion for death is that normal pulse and the heart by means of which a person continues to live has come to a complete halt. When a person reaches this stage he is regarded as dead. Reviving the pulse in his heart through an electronic device does not constitute life for him. However, if by means of a ventilator or other mechanical device the heart begins to function or by means of an artificial heart a person's life is restored, then the person is regarded as being alive. Hence,
>
> (a) As long as he is not dead, if he himself gives the permission to remove an organ, with the conditions stated above, then it is permissible to remove that organ for transplantation.
>
> (b) After he dies, even when the heart is kept alive by some electronic device, it is permissible to remove his organs for transplant, provided he has made a will to that effect. Or, there is no problem in removing his organs under the two above-mentioned circumstances.

The redefinition or expansion of the traditional criteria of death is virtually dominated by two factors: retrieval of organs and termination of medical treatment. There is little conceptual or philosophical discussion regarding the confusion over the higher brain conceptions and its implications for continuation of treatment. The true state of patients with irreversible brain damage whose other organ systems continued to function remains non-comprehensible among various sectors of Muslim society. In the absence of any public debate geared towards educating the society that has accepted the brain death criterion for practical reasons without questioning its validity in certain controversial cases, it is unlikely that any well considered definition and a set of criteria for determining brain death will emerge among Muslim jurists.

However, if the brain death criterion is rejected as a valid ground in pronouncing death, it raises the critical issue of justice in distribution of meager resources for health care. What is the responsibility of the health care providers to keep the brain dead person alive with expensive intensive care technology? Here the jurists have resorted to practical principles like rejection of harm and proportionality to provide sanctions for turning off the life-sustaining equipment. In the final analysis, it is pragmatic considerations rather than any philosophical or theological evaluation of the obligation that have determined the course of action. And, like any other ethical judgement that takes into consideration the contextual aspects of a given case at hand, the judicial decision in this and many other matters related to the interaction of traditional values and modern biomedicine, is at the most temporary and open to revision as underlying confusion about brain death becomes clearer to not just the medical community but also Muslim jurists, theologians, and politicians.

XI. Access to Healthcare

Islam is concerned with searching for a just solution to deal with problems that face humanity. And, although Islamic theology treats human suffering as part of the divinely ordained spiritual-moral growth, it treats public health as a shared responsibility between individual and the community. Islamic law, in general, does not use the language of rights in any of its prescriptive directives for the betterment of human society. Its notion of an entitlement is, as a rule, subsumed under its notion of religiously and morally defined duty. A broad range of considerations is recommended in achieving a certain level of the quality of life. Health care needs are treated with everything else a society invests in achieving that end. Dietary laws, prescriptions about habits of eating, drinking, sleeping, physical and moral education: all, according to the *Shari'a*, contribute directly to the development of healthy lifestyles. Taking care of one's health is both an individual as well as a collective obligation. Individually, it requires all men and women to undertake preventive measures to preserve health. Collectively, it puts the responsibility on the community to provide preventive medicine, supportive care, and undertake medical research sufficiently to improve curative medicine (Sachedina, 1999).

There is some tension in the Islamic communitarian ethics between an individual's claim to health care and the well-being of the community as a whole. In Muslim culture, a preoccupation with group rights leads to insensitivity to the needs of individuals. It also leads to an imbalance in source allocation, which are meagre. In many Muslim countries, there is an increasing emphasis on the community's ethical obligation to provide all with equitable access to health care. The community must ensure that all of its members can obtain such care, because health care is so important in relieving suffering, preventing premature death, and strengthening relationships of caring. Since women have been traditionally marginalized in the allocation of health care resources, emphasis on justice-based allocation has led to their preferential treatment with the rest of disadvantaged persons like poor and elderly in the community.

Another problem connected with communitarian ethics in the Muslim world is related to collectively formulating uniform attitudes to societal diseases. The legal tradition and practices in Muslim community are tightly regulated when communicable or non-communicable alcohol, drug, or sex related diseases involve societal interests of the larger community. This causes problems of distribution in publicly administered health care resources, which in many parts of the Muslim world, are limited. When it come to allocation of these resources, the public attitude is informed by religious sensitivities connected with the consequences of willful disobedience of the moral teachings of Islam. Hence, they treat those afflicted diseases like AIDS as undeserving of a share of these limited resources.

Overall, Islamic teachings approach the health care needs of all by prescribing measures within one's control to avoid risky behavior (smoking or overeating) that results in illness. This strategy to deal with improving the health status of the people is secured through family norms and voluntary efforts geared towards sanitation, prevention, and maintenance of religiously prescribed standards. The key to a healthy environment, as the *Qur'an* puts it, is a godfearing individual brought up in a family that is aware of its obligations to God and fellow humans.

Bibliography

Assaad, M.B. (1979). *Female circumcision in Egypt: Current research and social implications.* Cairo: American University, Social Research Centre.

Bakar, O. (1986). Islam and Bioethics. *The Greek Orthodox Theological Review*, *31(1)*, 157-179.

Burgel, J.C. (1973). Psychosomatic Methods of Cures in the Islamic Middle Ages. *Humaniora Islamica*, *1*, 157-172.

Burgel, J.C. (1926). Secular and Religious Features of Medieval Arabic Medicine. *Asian medical systems: A comparative study*. In: C.L. Donald & E.H. Campbell (Eds.), *Arabian medicine and its influence on the middle ages*, 2 vols. Trubner's Oriental Series. London: K. Paul, Trench, Trubner & Co.

Ebrahim, A.F.M. (1991). *Abortion, birth control and surrogate parenting: An islamic perspective*. Indianpolis: American Trust Publication.

Elgood, C. (1951). *A medical history of persia and the eastern caliphate, from the earliest times until the year (1951)*. Cambridge: University Press.

Elgood, C. (1951). *Tibb-ul-Nabbi or medicine of the Prophet*, "Being a Translation of Two Works of the Same Name. I. The Tibb-ul-Nabbi of al-Suyuti. II. The Tibb-ul-Nabbi of Mahmud bin Mohamed al-Chagayni: Together with Introduction, Notes and a Glossary," *Osiris* 14: 33-192.

Fiqh al-tabib [Islamic Laws for Physicians] (1993). Compiled by Drs. Mustafa Najafi, Mas'ud Salihi and Mas'ud Firdawsi, International Congress on Medical Ethics, Tehran, July 14-16.

Giorgis, B.W. (1981). *Female circumcision in Africa*. United Nations Research Series: Addis Ababa.

Hodgson, M.G.S. (1974). *Venture of Islam: Conscience and history in a world civilization*. Vol. I. Chicago: University of Chicago Press.

Islam and Family Planning (1974). 2 Volumes. Proceedings of the International Islamic Conference, 1971 in Rabat, Morocco. Beirut: The International Planned Parenthood Federation, Middle East and North Africa Region.

Islamic Medical Wisdom: The Tibb al-A'imma (1991). B. Ispahany (Trans.); A.J. Newman (Ed.). London: The Muhammadi Trust.

Masoom, S.H.F. (1992). *Collection of articles from seminar on Islam's views in medicine*. Mashhad: Ferdowsi University Press (Persian).

Musallam, B.F. (1989). *Sex and society in Islam*. Cambridge: Cambridge University Press.

Plessner, M. (1974). The Natural Sciences and Medicine. In: J. Schacht & C.E. Bowsorth (Eds.), *The legacy of Islam* (2nd ed.). Oxford: Clarendon Press.

Rahman, F. (1980). *Major themes of the Qur'an*. Minneapolis: Bibliotheca Islamica.

Rahman, F. (1989). *Health and medicine in the Islamic tradition*. New York: Crossroad.

Rispler-Chaim, V. (1993). *Islamic medical ethics in the twentieth century*. Leiden: E.J. Brill.

Rosenthal, F. (1969). The defence of medicine in the medieval Muslim world. *Bulletin of the History of Medicine*, 43, 519-532.

Sachedina, A.A. (1988). Islamic views on organ transplantation. *Transplantation Proceedings*, XX No. 1, Suppl. 1, 1084-1088.

Sachedina, A.A. (1998). Human clones: An Islamic view. In: G. McGee (Ed.), *The Human Cloning Debate*. Berkeley: Berkeley Hills Books.

Sachedina, A.A. (1999). Can God inflict unrequited pain on His creatures? Muslim Perspectives on Health and Suffering. In: J.R. Hinnells & Roy Porter (Eds.), *Religion, health and suffering*. London: Kegan Paul International.

Sachedina, A.A. (1996a). Islam. In: W.T. Reich (Ed.), *Encyclopedia of bioethics*. New York: Macmillan.

Sachedina, A.A. (1996b). Eugenics in Islamic law. In: W.T. Reich (Ed.), *Encyclopedia of bioethics*. New York: Macmillan.

Sachedina, A.A. (1996c). Medical ethics, History, Iran. In: W.T. Reich (Ed.), *Encyclopedia of bioethics*. New York: Macmillan.

Watt, W.M. (1968). *Muhammad at Mecca*. Oxford: Clarendon Press.

Wensinck, A.J. (1965). *The Muslim Creed: Its genesis and historical development*. London: Frank Cass & Co. Ltd.

Buddhism and Bioethics

Damien Keown

I. Introduction

What the West knows as "Buddhism" is a body of religious teachings attributed to an historical individual who lived in North East India in the fifth century B.C. Following a profound spiritual transformation achieved at the age of thirty-five he became known by the honorific title of "*Buddha*" ("enlightened one"). The Buddha claimed no divine provenance or authority for his teachings and understood them as a form of natural philosophy. For this reason the word for the teachings, *Dharma*, also refers to the immutable laws of both the natural and moral orders in which they are thought to be grounded. The religious life in Buddhism consists in living in accordance with *Dharma*, and it is believed that anyone who follows Buddhist teachings can replicate the spiritual transformation achieved by the founder.

In terms of ethical typology, recent scholarly discussion suggests that Buddhism is best understood as a teleological virtue ethic. This means that it postulates a certain goal or end (*telos*) as the fulfillment of human potential and maintains that this goal is to be realized through the cultivation of particular virtues. This kind of ethical system is familiar in the West and is mainly associated with Aristotle and his concept of human flourishing or *eudaimonia*. In Buddhism, the goal of human perfection is known as *nirvana* and is attained through a process of moral and intellectual self-transformation that comes about through following the teachings described below.

Buddhist teachings are encapsulated in the form of four basic propositions known as the Four Noble Truths. These maintain: (i) that life as we now know it is imperfect and unsatisfactory, (ii) that the causes of this unsatisfactoriness are craving and ignorance, (iii) that there exists a state of perfection free from all deficiencies, and (iv) that the way to perfection is by following the Eightfold Path. The Eightfold Path is a program for right living consisting of:

(1) Right understanding
(2) Right resolve
(3) Right speech
(4) Right action
(5) Right livelihood
(6) Right effort
(7) Right mindfulness
(8) Right meditation

These eight factors are grouped into three categories: 1-2, wisdom, 3-5, moral cultivation, and 7-8, meditation. As far as moral cultivation is concerned, the Buddha laid down certain precepts, the most well known of which are the Five Precepts for laymen. The Five Precepts forbid:
(1) Taking life
(2) Stealing
(3) Sexual misconduct
(4) Lying
(5) Taking intoxicants

Buddhism is distinctive as a religion in lacking a belief in a Supreme Being or creator god, as well as denying the existence of a personal soul. In Buddhist thought, the world has evolved simply as the result of natural processes: it had no beginning and will have no end. The human person is understood naturalistically as a complex of material and psychic elements that are constantly in flux. Individuals have free will and their destiny is a function of their moral choices. This is known as the doctrine of *karma*. *Karma* is an important concept in Buddhist ethics and may be defined as a principle of moral retribution, which holds that one inevitably suffers the good or bad consequences of one's moral deeds. *Karma* is linked to a belief in rebirth such that good and bad moral deeds in one life lead to rebirth in a better or worse condition in the subsequent life. There are six possible realms of rebirth, and, in terms of this teaching, a human being who is wicked can be reborn in a lower state, for example as an animal, while one who is virtuous may be reborn in a heavenly paradise. The belief in rebirth has important implications for some issues in bioethics, such as the question when life begins.

The Buddha appointed no successor, and many different schools arose after his death. Buddhism spread widely and influenced every Asian civilization, but it has no head or central authority. The three most important forms of Buddhism encountered today are Theravada (the oldest surviving school of Buddhism), Tibetan Buddhism, and far-Eastern Buddhism (including Pure Land, Zen and other sects). The historical spheres of influence of these have been as follows. Theravada Buddhism has been and remains prominent in South East Asia, notably in Sri Lanka, Thailand, and Burma. Tibetan Buddhism influenced much of medieval central Asia but in modern times has been suppressed following the Chinese invasion of the country in 1959. Buddhism, along with other religions, has suffered a similar fate in the People's Republic of China. Prior to the advent of communism, Buddhism had a history of almost two thousand years in China, and has been present for some 1500 years in Japan and Korea. In modern times Buddhism has also traveled to the West and today there are approximately five million Buddhists in the USA and around one million in Europe. The total number of Buddhists worldwide is approximately 500 million.

Since Buddhism is an amorphous movement with no clear hierarchy or locus of authority, it is difficult to make authoritative statements of the kind "The Buddhist view on issue x is ..." without qualification. Lay Buddhists typically turn to their clergy for religious and moral guidance, and these in turn base their opinions mainly on canonical scriptures, the earliest of which were committed to writing around 75 B.C. Despite the variety of Buddhist schools and sects, however, it does make sense to speak of a "Buddhist view" at least as far as our present purposes are concerned. There is a good deal of consistency amongst the major schools in the field of ethics, both in terms of the dominant pattern of reasoning employed and in the conclusions reached on specific issues. It therefore seems fair to speak of a "mainstream tradition," a term which here denotes the common moral core which can be extracted from the different movements, schools and sects.

Apart from the problem of establishing a locus of authority, a further difficulty arises from the diversity of cultures involved. Some scholars regard cross-cultural ethics as a methodological minefield and contend there are fundamental epistemological problems in understanding alien cultures and deciphering their moral language. Awareness of these problems has been heightened by recognition of the increasing diversity and pluralism in the moral discourse of the West itself. Nevertheless, this concern is balanced by a countervailing trend toward globalism found in beliefs such as universal human rights, and a position of extreme relativism is nowadays difficult to maintain. While cultures influence the evolution of ethical beliefs, many think that the beliefs themselves cannot be immune from scrutiny simply because they are the product of a particular culture. Pellegrino rightly points out that ethics is not grounded by culture:

> The ethical system of any culture is morally defensible because it is grounded in truths that transcend that culture; it is not morally defensible simply because it is a product of a particular culture. Respect for culture and ethics other than our own is the beginning of any intercultural dialogue, not its ending (Pellegrino, Mazzarella, & Corsi, 1992, p. 18).

There are sufficient common denominators between Buddhist and Western thought to permit a fruitful intercultural dialogue. The ethics of medicine is an important bridgehead, and the fact that disease is a cultural universal means that the ethics of medicine has a vital contribution to make to the dialogue. As Pellegrino puts it:

> As the biosphere expands to embrace the whole globe, every nation has a stake in every other nation's health. For these reasons, the practical and conceptual questions of transcultural biomedical ethics are more sharply defined than in some other domains of knowledge (1992, p. 14).

II. History

The study of Buddhist ethics is a recent development brought about by the arrival of Buddhism in the West and largely in response to the demands of Westerners for clarification of where Buddhism stands on a range of contemporary moral issues.

Although Buddhism is widely respected for its humane and benevolent moral values, there is an apparent absence in traditional Buddhist thought of a branch of learning devoted to reflection on ethical issues. Accordingly, very few issues in bioethics have received attention from Buddhist teachers or scholars. There is silence on many questions, and it is difficult to find position papers or pronouncements on controversial matters. Some commentators suggest that there are cultural reasons for this, and that the desire for clear and categorical statements in ethics is a legacy of the distinctive Western religious practice of formulating definitive credal statements on matters of doctrine. This practice is not common in Asian traditions, which tend to see it as divisive and prefer to seek consensus rather than draw boundaries.

Traditional societies, furthermore, do not appear to distinguish between ethics, law and politics in the way the West does. Societies in Asia tend to be much more integrated and homogenous than in the West, and, in the former, duties and obligations at all levels of society are ultimately derived from religious beliefs and customs. Thus what an individual should do, what the law should enforce, and how rulers and states should behave are essentially deductive questions which can be answered by reference to shared religious values and principles. Members of society, moreover, are identified primarily by their social role, and the smooth running of society depends upon them playing their preordained part. The Indian caste system is an example of this. In such a context, a system of ethics concerned with individual responsibility and personal choice is largely redundant since the course of one's life is determined in virtually every detail from birth. Western culture, on the other hand, gives primacy to the autonomous individual, and it may be that the discipline of ethics has evolved in tandem with this distinctive notion of the independent self-directed moral agent who embarks on a self-directed quest for the good.

Another reason for the lacuna in Buddhist ethics would seem to be the lack of precedent set by the tradition itself. Buddhism originated as a movement whose purpose was to renounce worldly life, not to become enmeshed in its problems. Accordingly, there never developed in Buddhism a science of religious law of the kind found in Hinduism, Judaism, Islam, and Christianity. In each of these traditions, jurists and commentators have established codes and digests of laws in a systematic attempt to resolve conflicts between daily life and the demands of sacred law.

A further historical consideration is that much of the Buddhist world has been untouched by modernism. One of the major centers of Buddhist learning, Tibet, was to all intents and purposes a medieval feudal state as recently as half a century ago. Elsewhere in Buddhist Asia, there was nothing to compare with the revolutionary developments such as the Enlightenment and the rise of science that swept away medievalism in Europe. Even in those Asian countries that have seen rapid modernization, such as Japan, it remains to be seen whether the arranged marriage between East and West will be a fruitful union.

The study of Buddhist bioethics has only evolved within the last decade and the literature available is extremely limited.[1] Although Buddhism has only a short history of involvement in bioethics, however, it has a much longer history of involvement in the practice of medicine. R.L. Soni has written, "It is indeed a matter of supreme interest that the noble profession of medicine and the corpus of thought known as Buddhism are both concerned in their own way in the alleviation, control and ultimately the removal of human sufferings" (Soni, 1976, p. 137). In a similar vein, the *Dictionary of Medical Ethics* points out that "The principles governing Buddhism and the practice of medicine have much in common" (Duncan, Dunstan, & Welbourn, 1981).

The Buddhist monastic Order has a claim to be the world's oldest and most widespread continuous social institution, and for over two thousand years it has had a close involvement with the treatment of the sick. Several centuries before Christ, Buddhist monks were developing treatments for many kinds of medical conditions, and, according to the latest research, Buddhism can claim much of the credit for the development of traditional Indian medicine (Zysk, 1991, p. 4).

Kenneth Zysk has recently described the paradigm shift which occurred in Indian medicine in the period between 800 to 100 B.C. involving a change from the older magico-religious healing techniques to "an entirely new empirico-rational approach to disease and its cure" (Zysk, 1991, p. 117). The Buddha raised a dissenting voice to the contemporary religious orthodoxy that went by the name of "Brahmanism," and his followers were not hindered by the restrictions on medical research that arose from orthodox beliefs concerning the impurity of death and disease.

According to Zysk, the early Buddhist monasteries of India were the places where the most significant developments in Indian medicine took place.

> Like the Christian monasteries and nunneries of the European Middle Ages, communities of Buddhist monks and nuns played a significant role in the institutionalization of medicine ... The codification of medical practices within the monastic rules accomplished perhaps the first systematization of Indian medical knowledge and probably provided the model for later handbooks of medical practice; the monk-healers' extension of medical care to the populace and the appearance of specialized monastic structures serving as hospices and infirmaries ... ensured ongoing support of the monasteries by the laity; and the integration of medicine into the curricula of major monastic universities made it a scholastic discipline. In India and elsewhere in Asia, Buddhism throughout its history maintained a close relationship with the healing arts, held healers in high esteem, and perhaps best exemplified the efficacious blending of medicine and religion (Zysk, 1991, p. 6).

At the same time, medical expertise was required as a means to securing the healthy physical constitution necessary to withstand the rigors of the monastic life. Without good health, as Birnbaum points out, the practice of the religious life would have been impossible.

> It is not surprising that medicine bears such significance, for surely great strains were placed upon the physical well being of monks due to their austere life and strenuous meditative practices. Since illness and its indisposition tend to weaken the mind, often causing it to lose its focus on its function as a liberating faculty, the prevention and proper treatment of illness held (and continues to hold) a great importance for the Buddhist monk (Birnbaum, 1979, p. 3).

The Buddha pointed out that since monks had severed all other social ties it was incumbent on them to care for one another:

> You, O monks, have neither a father nor a mother who could nurse you. If, O monks, you do not nurse one another, who, then, will nurse you? Whoever, O monks, would nurse me, he should nurse the sick (Zysk, 1991, p. 41).

With the passage of time restrictions on treating the laity were eased. The great Buddhist monarch Asoka claims, in an edict around 258 B.C., to have instituted an early form of state health-care provision:

> Everywhere in the dominions of King (i.e., Asoka) ... provision has been made for two kinds of medical treatment, treatment for men and for animals. Medicinal herbs, suitable for men and animals, have been imported and planted wherever they were not previously available. Also, where roots and fruits were lacking, they have been imported and planted (Rock Edict II, 1978, p. 64).

Asoka's interest in medicine may have been stimulated by his conversion to Buddhism, and Buddhist monks may well have had some role to play in his "national health service" if, indeed, it involved anything more than the planting of herbs and the like. What is certain, however, is that his royal endorsement of medical provision would have provided a further stimulus to medicine in the monasteries. As Buddhism spread, moreover, the goodwill generated by the provision of medical care would doubtless have encouraged monks to develop their skills in this area. Today it is not uncommon to find monks qualified in traditional medicine, Western medicine, or both.

Given the close connection between medicine and monasticism, it will come as no surprise to find that the Buddhist attitude to the ethics of the care of patients is deeply influenced by its religious beliefs. What is to be done and not to be done by the physician will be determined by the same moral principles which determine what is to be done and not to be done by a monk, since the physician is a monk first and a physician second. Thus, as we might expect, medical ethics in Buddhism involves essentially the application of the wider principles of religious ethics to problems in a more specialized field.

The ancient monastic texts reveal that the Buddha resolved problematic matters on a case-by-case basis as new situations arose. The records of these case histories include medical issues and represent the earliest codification of medical knowledge in India (Zysk, 1991, p. 71). As may be expected, the treatments described are not those of modern medicine, nor are the problems they raise identical in all respects. Given the primitive technology, for example, certain questions that have arisen today could scarcely be imagined. Nevertheless, we are not entirely bereft of guidance in the ancient sources, and although the circumstances today may be new, the moral issues that arise often turn out to be similar in principle.

III. Topics

A. *Bioethics in General*

It should be clear from the foregoing that there are few, if any, important institutions concerned with Buddhist ethics. The establishment of ethics centers, a common phenomenon in the West, has not caught on in Buddhist countries for reasons mentioned in the preceding section. The chief characteristic of Buddhist institutions in general is that they are local and autonomous rather than global and hierarchical. There is no precedent or mechanism for producing statements or declarations that command universal assent among Buddhists. Most collaborative activity is at a national or regional level, and although international assemblies occasionally take place these are rare. Even then, it is rarer still for bioethical issues to feature on the agenda, although in more Westernized Buddhist communities there is some evidence that this is beginning to change. To date, however, there has not been a single conference devoted to Buddhist bioethics, nor are there any research centers, university departments or university chairs dedicated to Buddhist ethics. In Bangkok, the Center of Human Resources Development carries out some research on Buddhist bioethics under the directorship of Pinit Ratanakul, a Yale-educated Thai bioethicist, and more such institutions are urgently required.

In terms of the personalities involved in Buddhist bioethics, these consist mainly of Western and Western-educated academics interested in the study of Buddhism or comparative religious ethics. The names of those most active in this field will be found in the bibliography.

Buddhist monks, who are the traditional source of authority on Buddhist teachings for most lay Buddhists, have been largely silent on bioethics (a notable exception is the Thai monk the Venerable Mettanando, who is also an M.D.). The reason for this silence seems to be that monks are regarded as aloof from the concerns of worldly life and family affairs, and although they may consult them on religious and spiritual matters, most lay Buddhists feel embarrassed to raise practical questions, particularly of a personal nature. For example, women who are considering an abortion almost never consult monks. Many monks, too, feel that these questions are not proper for one who has renounced the world and is pursuing the spiritual life. This attitude is slowly changing as more Westerners join the Order as monks and nuns.

At the present time, it is premature to speak of a dominant bioethical theory in Buddhism. Too little research has been carried out for there to be a consensus among scholars. In terms of Buddhist ethics in general, an earlier generation of scholars inclined to a utilitarian reading of Buddhism. In this they were influenced by an understanding of the doctrine of *karma* in terms of which acts were right simply because they led to the experience of pleasure in the future (such as a good rebirth). This understanding is now less common, partly because *karma* is too complex to be analyzed in such simple terms, but also because of the declining popularity of utilitarianism as an ethical theory. Linked to the renascence of virtue ethics, more recent studies have characterized Buddhist ethics as Aristotelian in form (Keown, 1992; Whitehill, 2000), and it is this theoretical model that is most commonly applied to bioethical issues.

In terms of basic values, one aspect of Buddhist ethics that strikes all commentators is its profound respect for life. The Buddhist respect for life is enshrined in the principle of non-injury or non-harming. Non-injury, and the respect for life it presupposes, lies at the very heart of Buddhist teachings, and this principle plays a fundamental role in Buddhist bioethics. The fact that the imperative to respect life is enshrined in the first of the Five Precepts listed above leads us to conclude that Buddhism shares the respect for life that is fundamental to the moral and legal traditions of the West. This belief in the "sanctity of life"[2] should not be understood as a commitment to "vitalism" (the belief that life must be preserved at all costs) but as the notion that intentional killing always represents a failure to respect the inalienable dignity of living creatures. In the context of bioethics, "life" means human life, but some, particularly far-Eastern, schools of Buddhism come close to adopting a Schweitzerian "reverence for life" whereby plants, micro-organisms, and even natural phenomena are given moral status. Indo-Tibetan schools, on the other hand, tend to see the relationship between plant, animal and human life as hierarchical rather than equalitarian. Human life occupies a place at the top of the hierarchy and is regarded as the most auspicious of all rebirths.

B. Professionalism

There is no one Buddhist perspective on the question of the nature of the ideal relationship among health care professionals. Attitudes and practices vary widely. In Asian countries in general, however, there is a stronger emphasis on respect for authority than is found in the West, and subordinates are less likely to challenge the views and opinions of senior members of the profession. In the earliest times, monks provided medical and nursing treatment, and their conduct was regulated by a monastic code made up of some 250 rules. The rules emphasize non-harming, truthfulness, non-self-aggrandizement, respect, modesty and decorum, and, although these values are intended for those in monastic orders, they may also be thought appropriate to the members of any professional body, including physicians and nurses. Members are encouraged to confess transgressions so as to unburden their conscience and be free to move ahead without remorse. When transgressions occur, the monastic code lays down mechanisms for resolving breaches of the rules including sanctions ranging from a reprimand to temporary or permanent expulsion from the group, in a manner similar to the way doctors may be disbarred from practicing by their professional bodies.

Important Buddhist virtues that should inform the practice of any profession include generosity (with one's time and resources), sobriety, self-restraint, and compassion. A classical formulation of four important virtues includes generosity, kindly speech, helpful action and impartiality.[3] Informed by these virtues, the medical professional should act at all times in a manner consistent with his or her conscience. In the West, conscience is understood as "a mode of consciousness and thought about one's own acts (or proposed actions) by which we judge whether they are blameworthy or praiseworthy according to our own standards" (Ratanakul, 1986, p. 196). In Buddhism, conscience is analyzed into a small cluster of qualities in which the two most important are *hiri* or "self-respect," and *ottappa* or "regard for consequences." These are described as two "bright states which guard the world" and may be seen as concerned with the internal and external dimensions of conscience. *Hiri* causes one to avoid any action that is unworthy of one and causes one's moral integrity to be weakened. *Ottappa* is the concern for the blame or reproach (whether private or public), embarrassment before one's peers, legal sanctions, and also the karmic results of an action.[4] Another quality of great importance in one's personal and professional life is heedfulness. This is described as the basis of all the virtues and is said to be composed of energy and mindfulness. Mindfulness is alert presence of mind that enables one to be focused on the action in hand as well as aware of one's inner mental states, including intentions and motives. Buddhism recommends the practice of meditation as a means of cultivating all the above qualities.

As regards the doctor-patient relationship, Buddhism would analyze this primarily in terms of duties. The language of rights is a peculiarly Western way of stating the requirements of justice, and traditional societies emphasize more the responsibility of the individual towards the collective rather than vice versa. Both doctors and patients therefore may be said to have duties towards one another. There is no Buddhist equivalent of the Hippocratic oath which lays down the duties of physicians, nor a Buddhist version of the Patient Bill of Rights of the American Hospital Association that lays down the standards of services and care patients can expect. Early Buddhist commentaries occasionally digress to discuss the practice of medicine by monks, but the concern is mainly with the protocol for determining which members of society should be treated in the monastery. One ancient text, however, states: "Medicine must be given to those who desire it, and for those who do not know how to prepare it, it must be prepared and administered." In general terms it may be said that the Buddhist health care professional has a duty to enhance the well-being of the patient (the duty of beneficence) and not to cause any harm or injury (the duty of non-maleficence). Since it is generally held that duties and rights are to some degree correlative, we can extrapolate from the duties incumbent on the health care professional to establish a list of the basic rights of patients. For example, when a hospital agrees to treat someone as a patient, the doctors and nurses who care for that patient assume certain obligations towards him. Because of this we may say that the patient has certain rights, most generally the right to a professional standard of medical care, but also related rights such as a right to privacy. Seven major rights are outlined in the Patient Bill of Rights: (1) the right to considerate and respectful care, (2) the right to information, (3) the right to refuse treatment, (4) the right to privacy, (5) the right to confidentiality, (6) the right to know of research and experimentation being done, and (7) the right to receive continuity of care (Ratanakul, 1986, p. 129). All of these would seem appropriate in a Buddhist context. Respect for the autonomy of the patient is particularly important given the unequal nature of the physician-patient relationship. As a result of illness, one party of the relationship is inherently more vulnerable. This inequality is exacerbated by the fact that one of the parties is a specialist and has much greater knowledge and experience than the other in the treatment of the condition. In order to redress this inequality, patients must be treated as active partners in health care decisions and kept fully informed of the available treatments and prognosis.

Of particular importance in this connection is the issue of truth-telling. The traditional stance of "doctor knows best" has often meant that patients have been left in the dark about the true nature of their condition. This medical paternalism has been much criticized in recent decades, and greater emphasis is now placed on the duty of veracity. This is in accordance with Buddhist moral principles that regard lying as wrong, even when there is a benevolent motivation such as to shield the patient from unpleasant facts. The Buddhist principle of "right speech" emphasizes that one should always be truthful while leaving scope for diplomacy and tact in speaking the truth at the right time and in the right way. A blunt statement of fact may not be always the best way to break bad news: it may have a demoralizing effect on patients and give the impression that the physician is anxious to wash his hands of the case. It must also be born in mind that in some cultures speaking forthrightly is regarded as rudeness. Good physicians will therefore seek to establish rapport with patients and communicate with sensitivity. The only exceptions to the duty of veracity are rare cases where there is a reasonable presumption that the patient may overreact and suffer physical or psychological injury, or where placebos are used.

Good communication is also important in ensuring that patients understand clearly the medical issues involved in their treatment and are in a position to give informed consent prior to the start of any procedure. For there to be valid consent the patient must understand the information given, the reasons for the treatment, the available alternative treatments (if any), and be able to foresee the consequences of his or her decision. The consent must be completely voluntary, that is to say given freely without any coercion or deception. In this and in many other respects the obligations upon the Buddhist health care professional do not differ greatly from professional norms of conduct throughout the world. Codes of conduct laid down by professional bodies internationally often coincide, and although there are some cultural idiosyncrasies the similarities in the doctor-patient relationship across the world outweigh the differences, particularly where practitioners have been trained in the methods of modern scientific medicine.

C. Reproduction

A distinctive feature of Buddhist thought is that it does not postulate an initial starting point to the series of lives lived by an individual. Instead, it regards the cyclic course of human existence as potentially eternal: it had no beginning and there is no certainty it will ever have an end. All conception is thus re-conception, and the belief that each individual exists prior to conception provides a distinctive perspective on the question of when life begins.

Although the basic Buddhist position on how and when individual life begins was formulated over two thousand years ago, the conclusions reached are in many respects remarkably modern. Buddhism has always seen conception as an event marking the start of a gradual process of development up to birth and beyond, through childhood into maturity. In adopting this view, Buddhist thinking was very much ahead of the West, which, until the modern era, was hampered by Aristotelian theories of three stages of ensoulment in the embryo. By contrast, and in keeping with traditional Indian medical thought, the Buddha explained conception as a natural process that occurs when three specific conditions are fulfilled. In this understanding, (i) intercourse must take place, (ii) during the woman's fertile period, and (iii) there must be available the spirit (*gandhabba*) of a deceased person seeking rebirth. When these conditions are present a new life comes into being. Interpreting these requirements in the light of modern science most Buddhists regard fertilization as the point at which individual human life commences and believe that the embryo is entitled to moral respect from that time onwards. Abortion is therefore seen as morally in the same category as the intentional killing of an adult. The only exception is likely to be when the procedure is necessary to save the life of the mother, although there is no explicit Buddhist teaching on this point, and there appear to be no examples in Buddhist canonical literature of abortion performed for therapeutic reasons.

Despite the condemnation of abortion in the ancient texts, the sources disclose that, as medical practitioners, monks occasionally became illegally involved in such matters. The motives for an abortion include concealing extramarital affairs, preventing inheritances, and domestic rivalry between co-wives. The methods used to procure abortions included ointments, potions and charms, pressing or crushing the womb and scorching or heating it.

The contemporary legal position varies from country to country. The more conservative Buddhist countries of South East Asia such as Thailand and Sri Lanka have laws prohibiting abortion except when necessary to save the life of the mother. Nevertheless, illegal abortions are common. Somewhat surprising for a country in which Buddhism is the state religion, abortions in Thailand are running at some 50% higher than the number in the USA for the equivalent number of citizens. Married women, who appear to use it as a means of birth control, account for 85% or more of abortions. Recent studies refer to an estimated 300,000 abortions per year, the majority of which are illegal (Florida, 1999, p. 23). Opinion polls in Thailand also reveal a paradox: while most Thais regard abortion as immoral, a majority also believes the legal grounds for obtaining it should be relaxed (Florida, 1999, p. 24).

In East Asian countries, attitudes are more liberal. The rate of abortion in Japan has been very high in recent years, perhaps peaking at over a million (some would put the figure much higher) before decreasing in the last few years as the contraceptive pill has become more easily available. Central to the contemporary Japanese experience is the phenomenon of *mizuko kuyo*, a memorial service held for aborted children. This service involves erecting a small statue to commemorate the lost child and includes an apology to the spirit of the aborted fetus. William LaFleur has explored the complex symbolism and cultural history of the practice (LaFleur, 1992; Hardacre, 1997).

Korea provides an interesting comparison with Japan. Both countries have a very high rate of abortion, but in Japan, it is legal (since 1948), whereas in Korea, it is not. Annual figures of between one and two million are quoted for Korea, a country with a population of around 46 million. Over a quarter of the population are Buddhists, which makes them the majority religious group. Statistics quoted by Tedesco (1999, p. 133) reveal that Buddhists are slightly more likely to have abortions than other segments of the population. In 1985, an anti-abortion movement began to gain ground following the publication of a book by the Venerable Myogak, a Buddhist monk of the Chogye order. His book, entitled *My Dear Baby, Please Forgive Me!* became popular, and readers began to demand rites and services for aborted children similar to the Japanese *mizuko kuyo* service, although distinctively Korean in form.

Some Western Buddhists take a more liberal stance on the abortion question. James Hughes suggests that "clear and defensible distinctions can be made between fetuses and other human life" and finds the moral logic of utilitarianism persuasive in the context of abortion, although tempered by the requirements of a virtue ethic, which takes into account the mindset of the actors. Abortion may therefore be allowable where the intention is compassionate and the act achieves the best outcome for all concerned. One American Zen Buddhist group, the Diamond Sangha, has produced a liturgy that can be performed following an abortion or miscarriage (Hughes, 1999).

The above diversity of opinion is reflected in other reproductive issues such as embryo research. In terms of the more conservative majority view, any destructive experimentation on embryos is considered a breach of the first precept against taking human life. Practices such as IVF or techniques that have some therapeutic end (for example, the repair of chromosomal defects before an embryo returned to the womb) are unlikely to be met with any strong Buddhist objection. There are, however, certain aspects of the IVF technique that Buddhism would not approve of. Chief amongst these is the creation of spare embryos by drug-induced superovulation. Leaving aside the problem of the multiple pregnancies that sometimes arise from this practice (when the "excess" fetuses may be deliberately destroyed in the womb), there is the question of the fate of the "spare" embryos that have not been implanted. They are usually either discarded or used for research.

These aspects of the technique are unacceptable to Buddhism. Essentially this is because they involve either the destruction of a living being (a breach of the first precept) or its use as an object for the benefit of others without its consent. Regardless of any benefits, Buddhism could not countenance the use of a human subject as an object of research that is not in its own best interests and to which it has not consented.

Contraception is widely used and approved of in Buddhist countries, especially where the method does not involve the destruction of fertilized embryos. Methods that prevent implantation, such as low-dose estrogen and progesterone- ("mini") pills and the IUD, are less acceptable, although not uncommon. In Japan the high rate of abortion has been attributed to the fact that until very recently health officials refused to license the contraceptive pill due to concern about side effects. Some commentators, however, believe that doctors are unwilling to prescribe the pill because they derive a large income from managing profitable abortion clinics.

D. Death and Dying

Old age and death are two aspects of suffering (*dukkha*) which are constantly referred to in Buddhist sources. Buddhist teachings emphasize the inherent impermanence of phenomena; as the early sources put it, "Whatever has the nature of arising, has the nature of cessation." All forms of organic life have the nature of arising, since they come into being as integrated wholes at a definite moment in time, namely conception. As such they are compounded entities, and, according to Buddhist philosophy, it is the nature of all compounded entities eventually to lose cohesion and disintegrate. There is a sense in which death encapsulates all the unsatisfactoriness (*dukkha*) of the human condition since it reveals starkly the impermanence of individual life and also the attendant pain and suffering of old age. In this sense death is the paradigm problem for Buddhism, since it is emblematic of all the ills to which karmic life is subject.

An important development in the West in recent years has been the formulation of a criterion for defining death in terms of the cessation of all brain functions. In 1968, an *ad hoc* committee of the Harvard Medical School produced a report (Report of the Ad Hoc Committee, 1968) recommending a definition of death in these terms. This definition has since become widely accepted in medical practice and has been incorporated, sometimes with modifications, into the legal definition of death in many countries. One country where this definition has not been accepted and remains the subject of much controversy is Japan. Although the majority of the medical profession is in favor of it, there is widespread popular dissatisfaction among the population at large due to its connection with organ transplantation. There is no Buddhist objection to organ transplantation in itself, and the distaste for it seems to arise from Confucian teachings that see the body as a gift and the plundering of organs, particularly from older members of the family who are soon to become revered ancestors, as a sacrilege. Some concern does exist among Buddhists concerning the criterion of brain stem death, to which organ transplantation from cadavers is closely linked. To declare death on the basis of this criterion seems premature to some, and not in keeping with Buddhist scriptural teachings concerning the point when death occurs. The ancient sources state that death occurs when three things – vitality, heat, and consciousness – leave the body. At the present time it is not clear whether the ancient criteria can be equated with the modern concept of brain stem death, although some authorities, such as the Thai physician-monk Mettanando, see the two as equivalent and believe Buddhism should accept a definition of death based on the loss of the functions of the brain stem (1991). What does seem clear, however, is that since the traditional Buddhist criteria for determining death are biological in nature, Buddhism would reject any definition of death that focused solely on the loss of consciousness or the higher brain functions controlled by the neocortex. It would appear on this basis that patients in the PVS condition cannot be regarded as dead, and Buddhist principles appear to require that such patients should continue to receive at least basic care including nutrition and hydration (Mettanando, 1991; Keown, 1995).

Concerning euthanasia (here understood to mean the intentional killing of a patient by act or omission), it appears that Buddhism would oppose it in all its forms on the grounds that it involves the deliberate taking of life. The Buddha forbade monks to take their own lives or to play a direct or indirect part in assisting or inciting others to commit suicide (Keown, 1996; 1998-1999). Such acts were declared to be wrong even when motivated by compassion, in the light of which it seems that suicide whether assisted by one's physician or by friends or relatives is contrary to Buddhist ethics.

In recent decades there has been understandable concern about patients being kept alive as prisoners of technology; allowing such patients to die rather than prolonging their lives through extraordinary means is sometimes confused with euthanasia. It is important to bear in mind here the difference between euthanasia and the withholding or withdrawal of burdensome and futile treatment. While Buddhism regards life as inviolable, it does not follow that it is something that must be preserved at all costs. Death is a natural part of the cycle of life and must be accepted as such. The recognition that death is not a final end but the doorway to rebirth and new life leads to the abandonment of medical treatment that serves no useful purpose. From the perspective of Buddhist ethics, there is no obligation on doctors to keep patients alive at all costs. In the case of elderly or terminal cases, it is far more important to assist patients in developing the right mental attitude towards death rather than attempting to deny or postpone it. A caring environment, such as is offered by the hospice movement, is the type of response that Buddhism would endorse in these circumstances.

Buddhism regards death as the gateway to new life and teaches that the dying person's state of mind can influence the circumstances of rebirth in the next life. Accordingly, it sees it as desirable to approach death ideally in a clear and mindful state rather than in a drugged or comatose condition. Nonetheless, it has no objection in principle to administering narcotics as part of a program of pain control. The administering of pain-killing drugs to terminally ill patients which may coincidentally hasten their death is not considered to be euthanasia. When patients are in great pain, it may be necessary to administer drugs and other medication while recognizing that this may shorten the patient's life. The doctor's aim here, however, in contrast to euthanasia, is to kill the pain, not the patient. What the physician is typically endeavoring to do is enhance through medical treatment the condition of the patient overall, in this case by freeing them from pain. In contrast to euthanasia, the physician wills the enhancement of life through the elimination of pain, while accepting that his efforts may hasten the advent of death. Death, however, is neither intended nor chosen either as a means or an end.

E. Access to Health Care

There is no general consensus among Buddhists concerning the financial issues arising in connection with access to health care. Arrangements vary from one country to another and depend more on local customs, traditions, and the current political and economic situation than on Buddhist teachings. The majority of Buddhists live in the third world in countries where health care resources are limited or even non-existent. For the poor, treatment is available in government hospitals and clinics or from charitable foundations. The middle classes typically turn to private medicine for their needs. In this respect, there is frequently a two-tier system in operation. Many governments put what resources they have into family planning programs in order to limit population, or to deal with the prevention of epidemics and diseases such as AIDS. No clear "right" to health care can be established from Buddhist teachings, although it could be said that the state has a general duty to care for the well-being of its citizens, within which ambit the provision of at least basic health care should surely fall.

F. Ethics Consultation and Committees

This is an area where the West has evolved far beyond anything found in Buddhist countries. Over the last two or three decades, the concept of patient autonomy has become increasingly important in Western bioethics as part of a more general program of consumer rights. Medical paternalism is now out of fashion, and patients no longer accept unquestioningly the opinions of their physicians. Against the background of this increasing conflict between physician and patient, ethics committees have evolved in order to monitor doctors' decisions in gray areas and arbitrate in cases of conflict between physician and patient. Buddhism itself allocates no specific role to ethics committees, and where these are found in Buddhist countries it is typically the result of imitating the West.

In general terms, the Buddha seems to have thought that it was good practice to meet regularly to discuss issues of common concern. He states that a community that conducts its business in this way can be expected to prosper rather than decline. This, in fact, is the basis on which the Buddhist monastic community conducts its business, resolving disagreements by majority vote. The practice of developing good relations through regular meetings and making important decisions after thorough discussion seems to accord with good practice for a Western ethics committee and to be one that Buddhism would accept.

IV. Conclusions

Caution must be exercised when drawing conclusions about Buddhist perspectives on bioethics. Ethics as a philosophical discipline is not found in traditional Buddhist canons of thought, and there is a risk of inadvertently superimposing Western categories on the discussion. Buddhism does not fit easily into Western categories nor does it resemble the Abrahamic family of religions with which the West is most familiar. Some doubt whether it constitutes a "religion" at all in the conventional sense. Further difficulties arise from its fragmentary and culturally diverse nature, making it is unwise to be categorical about what Buddhists in general believe. An often-quoted verse from an early text, however, sets out its basic aspirations:

Not to do any evil
To cultivate what is wholesome
To purify one's mind
This is the teaching of the Buddhas
(*Dhammapada*, verse 183).

Buddhism is renowned for the virtues of benevolence and compassion and its scrupulous respect for living beings, both human and non-human. The doctrine of *karma* and the belief in rebirth make it distinctive from an ethical perspective. Along with other Asian belief-systems, such as Confucianism, it lends itself to classification as a form of virtue ethics and resembles Aristotle's teleological concept of human flourishing (*eudaimonia*) attained through a systematic life-long program of character development.

With respect to applied issues in bioethics, Buddhism generally takes a conservative stance. The centrality accorded to the principle of non-injury (*ahimsa*) means that any procedure involving intentional harm is seen as immoral. Utilitarian arguments to the effect that bad acts may be justified by their good consequences are unlikely to find favor among traditional Buddhists. However, the detailed process of how one should reason to particular moral conclusions requires further precision and clarification. As yet little work has been done in this field, and, as Buddhism continues to spread in the West, there is an urgent need for dialogue with Western bioethicists in order to develop a framework in terms of which Buddhist responses to bioethical issues can be articulated with greater precision.

Notes

1. For a bibliographical survey, see Hughes, James J. and Damien Keown (1995). "Buddhism and Medical Ethics: A Bibliographic Introduction," *Journal of Buddhist Ethics* 2, pp. 105-124. Publications subsequent to the compilation of this bibliography include Harvey, Peter (2000). *An Introduction to Buddhist Ethics: Foundations, Values and Issues*, Cambridge: Cambridge University Press; Keown, Damien (ed.) (1999). *Buddhism and Abortion.* London/Honolulu: Macmillan/University of Hawaii Press; and Keown, Damien, (ed.) (2000), *Contemporary Buddhist Ethics.* London: Curzon Press.
2. For a brief statement of the Buddhist position, see Ratanakul, Pinit (1985), "The Buddhist Concept of Life, Suffering and Death and their Meaning for Health Policy," in *Health Policy, Ethics and Human Values*, Z. Bankowski and J.H. Bryant (eds.), Geneva: CIOMS, pp. 286-295; p. 289 ff.
3. Harvey, Peter (2000, p. 110).
4. Harvey, Peter (2000, p. 11).

Bibliography

Birnbaum, R. (1979). *The healing Buddha.* Boulder: Shambhala.

Duncan, A.S., Dunstan, G.R., & Welbourn, R.B. (1981). *Dictionary of medical ethics.*
London: Darton, Longman and Todd.

Florida, R. (1999). Abortion in Buddhist Thailand. In: D. Keown (Ed.), *Buddhism and abortion* (pp. 11-29). London: Macmillan.

Hardacre, H. (1997). *Marketing the menacing fetus in Japan.* Berkeley: University of California Press.

Harvey, Peter (2000). *An introduction to Buddhist ethics: Foundations, values and issues.* Cambridge: Cambridge University Press.

Hughes, J. & Keown, D. (1995). Buddhism and medical ethics: A bibliographic introduction. *Journal of Buddhist ethics, 2*, 105-124.

Hughes, J. (1999). Buddhism and abortion: A western approach. In: D. Keown (Ed.), *Buddhism and abortion.* London: Macmillan.

Keown, D. (1992). *The nature of Buddhist ethics.* London: Macmillan.

Keown, D. (1995). *Buddhism and bioethics.* London: Macmillan.

Keown, D. (1996). Buddhism and suicide: The case of Channa. *Journal of Buddhist ethics*, *3*, 8-31.

Keown, D. (1998-99). Suicide, assisted suicide and euthanasia: A Buddhist perspective. *Journal of law and religion*, *2*, 385-405.

Keown, D. (Ed.) (1999). *Buddhism and abortion.* London/Honolulu: Macmillan/University of Hawaii Press.

Keown, D. (Ed.) (2000). *Contemporary Buddhist ethics.* London: Curzon Press.

LaFleur, W.A. (1992). *Liquid life: Abortion and Buddhism in Japan.* Princeton: Princeton University Press.

Mettanando, B. (1991). Buddhist ethics in the practice of medicine. In: C. Wei-hsun Fu & S.A. Wawrytko (Eds.), *Buddhist ethics and modern society: An international symposium* (pp. 195-213). New York, etc: Greenwood Press.

Pellegrino, E., Mazzarella, P., & Corsi, P. (Eds.) (1992). *Transcultural dimensions in medical ethics* (18). Frederick, MD: University Publishing Group.

Ratanakul, P. (1986). *Bioethics, an introduction to the ethics of medicine and life sciences.* Bangkok: Mahidol University.

Report of the Ad Hoc Committee of the Harvard Medical School to Examine the Definition of Brain Death. (1968). A definition of irreversible coma. *Journal of the American Medical Association*, *205*, 337-340.

Rock Edict II (1978). *The Edicts of Asoka*, Midway Reprint (Ed.), Trans. N.A. Nikam & R. McKeon (p. 64). Chicago & London: The University of Chicago Press.

Soni, R.L. (1976). Buddhism in relation to the profession of medicine. In: D.W. Millard (Ed.), *Religion and medicine* (Vol. 3, pp. 135-151). London: SCM Press.

Tedesco, F. (1999). Abortion in Korea. In: D. Keown (Ed.), *Buddhism and abortion* (pp. 121-155). London: Macmillan.

Whitehill, J. (2000). Buddhism and the virtues. In: D. Keown (Ed.), *Contemporary Buddhist ethics* (pp. 17-36). London: Curzon Press.

Zysk, K.G. (1991). *Asceticism and healing in ancient India: Medicine in the Buddhist monastery.* Oxford: Oxford University Press.

Hindu Bioethics

Cromwell Crawford

I. Introduction: Historical Perspective on Hindu Medicine, Religion, and Ethics

Three features of Hindu bioethics set it apart from other approaches to bioethics, both religious and secular: (1) its connection to a particular form of medicine, *Ayurveda*; (2) its philosophic grounding; and (3) its ethical orientation. While Hinduism shares with most faith traditions a positive attitude toward medicine and the healing arts, Hinduism is distinctive because it has its own system of medicine known as *Ayurveda*, based on medical manuals that comment directly on health issues. Hinduism includes diverse philosophical schools of thought, such as *Samkhya*, *Yoga*, *Nyaya*, *Vaisesika*, and *Vedanta*, that are attuned to matters of medical inquiry and are suited to the demands of our pluralistic age. The contextual structure of the Hindu approach to ethics gives it the flexibility and adaptability necessary for thinking about bioethical dilemmas.

A unique feature of Hinduism is that a full-fledged system of medicine evolved within its complex ethos. Although the details of its historical developments are unknown, it is fair to assume that during the protohistoric Harappa culture, which existed around 2000 B.C.E. and collapsed around 1500 B.C.E., a rudimentary system of medicine was practised in the northwestern region of India. Archaeological excavations at the two main capitals of Harappa and Mohenjo-daro give evidence of a technically advanced society which built its houses, streets, and public facilities with knowledge of the principles of good hygiene and sanitation. Water was valued for its purifying and therapeutic qualities. Terra cotta figurines and images on seals suggest powerful feelings for and bonds to Mother Earth and her bounty of plants and animals. The figure of a horned deity, ritualistically seated in a yogic position, typifies an ancient medicine man.

Data covering the end of the second millennium B.C.E. are drawn from the *Rg Veda*, the earliest literature of India, which gives us clearer glimpses of the state of medicine in the early Vedic period. More important than the *Rg Veda* for knowledge of ancient Indian medical lore are the hymns of the *Atharva*, which should be read with the *Kausikasutra*. Vedic medicine was predominantly magico-religious, but combined sorcery and witchcraft with certain empirical facets of healing. These procedures include surgery, methods for stopping hemorrhage, bone-setting, hydrotherapy, and extensive use of plants and herbs. The power of suggestion and visualization were at the root of many of the healing rituals (Zimmer, 1948, pp. 9ff.).

During the millennium preceding the Christian era, developments took place that precipitated a paradigm shift from the earlier magico-religious tradition to the new empirico-rational medicine of *Ayurveda*. In his *Asceticism and Healing in Ancient India* (1991), Kenneth G. Zysk traces the contribution made by Buddhism to Indian medicine through (a) its institutionalization in monasteries, which led to new models for medical manuals; (b) through the emergence of monk-healers; and (c) the establishment of monastic hospices and infirmaries. During the Gupta period, Zysk states, "Hinduism assimilated the ascetic medical repository into its socioreligious and intellectual tradition," thus making it an orthodox Hindu science (p. 118).

Ayurveda is "the science of living to a ripe age." The term is semantically significant. Basham notes: "its first component (*ayur*) implies that the ancient Indian doctor was concerned not only with curing disease but also with promoting positive health and longevity, while the second (*veda*) has religious overtones, being the term used for the most sacred texts of Hinduism" (Basham, 1976, p. 18).

Ayurveda is divided into eight branches: (1) Internal Medicine (*Kayacikitsa*), (2) Surgery (*Salyapahartrka*), (3) Diseases of the Supra-clavicular area (*Salakya*), (4) Pediatrics, including Obstetrics/Gynecology (*Kaumarabhrtya*), (5) Toxicology (*Visagaravairodhikaprasamana*), (6) Psychiatry (*Bhutavidya*), (7) Rejuvenation (*Rasayana)*, and (8) Knowledge for increase of virility (*Vajikarana*, *Caraka-Samhita*, 1996-1997, vol. 1, p. 242).

The most authoritative texts on *Ayurveda* are certain extant collections known as The Great Trio (*Brhat-Trayi*). They are (i) the *Caraka Samhita* (100 A.D.), (ii) the *Susruta Samhita* (3-4 A.D.), and (iii) *Vagbhata's Astangahrdayam* (mid-7 A.D.). The range of topics covered in the medical manuals of *Ayurveda* read almost like modern medical texts, despite their antiquity. The texts are impressive for their concern for the moral dimensions of medicine. This orientation informs the attempt to construct a distinctive system of Hindu bioethics.

The symbiosis between medicine and morals in *Ayurveda* follows from common assumptions that underlie both disciplines. Here we highlight some of the salient features of Indian medicine, which provide the bases for ethical analysis.

(1) *Ayurveda* replaced the supernatural therapy (*daiva-vyapasraya*) of the Vedic phase with rational therapy (*yukti-vyapasraya*) to make medicine logical and scientific.
(2) *Ayurveda* is holistic. It views the person as an integrated whole and not just an aggregate of several body parts which are the domain of specialists.
(3) *Ayurveda* sees the person as grounded in nature, a microcosm within the macrocosm. Diet, climate, soil, season, time, and place all influence health and well-being.
(4) Health and healing are regarded as acts of nature. In medico-ethical terms, the natural is the good.
(5) Health is a positive state, and not just the absence of disease.
(6) Health is multi-dimensional; the physical, mental, social and spiritual are all relevant.
(7) *Ayurveda* apprehends the person as an individual, having a unique constitutional type and an unmatched set of life experiences.
(8) *Ayurveda* gives prominence to the notion of balance. It promotes an ethics of moderation in matters of sex and abstinence, food and drink, work and play, sleeping and awaking, faith and common sense.
(9) Medicine is essentially preventive and promotive, and caring is more important than curing.

(10) Longevity is measured not in number of days, but quality of time.
(11) Death is an inevitable part of the natural process of living and is therefore not an evil or the object of divine punishment. Death is the opposite of birth, not of life.
(12) Health and disease, happiness and suffering, and life and death are the consequences of an individual's *karma*, thus great emphasis is given to human responsibility.
(13) Health is more than what the doctor does; it is a total life-style that carries one from the cradle to the grave.
(14) Health is not the ultimate good but the penultimate good.

The moral structure of Indian medicine makes it eminently suited to deal with the dilemmas which arise in modern medical practice.

Next, we explore how the integration of the religio-philosophic speculations of Ayurveda along with other schools of Indian philosophy give it a distinctive shape. *Ayurveda* is a compendium of science and philosophy. As a science, its purpose is to ensure health of body and mind, but as a philosophy its goals go beyond the preservation of health and the curing of disease. The present resurgence of *Ayurveda* in the West is as much due to its philosophy as its science, because it appeals to the need for a more humanistic approach to medicine.

The eminent philosopher Surendranath Dasgupta has suggested that the philosophical considerations raised with Hindu medicine ought to be included in the history of Indian philosophy. Any objection to this claim loses its force when, he says, we recall that "medicine was the most important of all the physical sciences which were cultivated in ancient India, was directly and intimately connected with the *Samkhya* and *Vaisesika* physics and was probably the origin of the logical speculations subsequently codified in the *Nyaya-sutras*" (Dasgupta, 1986, vol. 2, p. 273). The medical literature embodies a vision of life supported by ethical instructions not present in general philosophical literature. The manuals "throw a flood of lights on the scholastic methods of Indian thinkers" (p. 273). Moreover, scholars in touch with "the importance of Hatha Yoga or Tantra physiology or anatomy in relation to some of the Yoga practices of these schools will no doubt be interested to know for purposes of comparison or contrast the speculations of the medical schools on kindred points of interest" (p. 273). Dasgupta concludes his case for the inclusion of the medical literature in his *History of Indian Philosophy* by arguing that even "a student of pure philosophy" will find intriguing the medical speculations regarding "embryology, heredity and other points of general enquiry" (p. 273).

Dasgupta's remarks highlight the fact that the development of medicine in India has gone hand in hand with the development of philosophy. The reason for this is that Indian philosophy is more than intellectual curiosity. It is the quest for the elimination of moral and physical suffering, which characterizes all of human existence. The goal of philosophy is to liberate the human consciousness and bring it to its natural level of being. Indian philosophy is a way of life and not merely a way of thinking, such that health is an important companion to philosophy. Sound health is a condition of the philosophical end of liberation. The most characteristic path prescribed for reaching liberation has been a cultivation of the spirit of renunciation. The progressive practice of renunciation produces peace of mind and transforms behavior. A spirit of renunciation gradually produces empathy for all sentient beings, as embodied in the principle of *ahimsa*, which enjoins that we do no harm.

Indian medicine is unique because of the integration of the religious or spiritual and the scientific. Hindu bioethics is unique because of the contextual structure of Hindu ethics. A survey of clinical bioethics cases reveals that dilemmas lie at the root of bioethics, and Hindu ethics is a moral system that acknowledges the existence of genuine moral dilemmas. We encounter a dilemma when values to which we are equally committed are brought into conflict, so that to honor one value requires that we violate the other. Western ethicists admit that moral dilemmas are the Achilles heel of most problems encountered in bioethics. Beauchamp (1978) cites the case of Socrates who was sentenced to die in preson. Crito offers him an escape route along with many good reasons to justify breaking the law. Socrates counters with equally strong reasons to support his commitment to respect the law and allow himself to be put to death. The illustration serves to highlight the central difficulty in bioethics cases:

> The reasons on each side are weighty ones, and neither is in any obvious way the right set of reasons. If we act on either set of reasons, our actions will be desirable in some respects but undesirable in other respects. And yet we think that ideally we ought to act on all of these reasons, for each is, considered by itself, a good reason (Beauchamp, 1978, p. 2).

The Hindu position is to be distinguished both from the religious fundamentalist position that views dilemmas in the light of revelation, and the secular rationalist position that views dilemmas as resolvable through the use of reason. Both the religious fundamentalist and the secular rationalist hold that there are no genuine dilemmas, for cases that appear to present dilemmas can be resolved either by greater faith (religious fundamentalism) or more knowledge (secular rationalism).

Hinduism does not deny the existence of dilemmas. Its scriptures address the tension of irreconcilable alternatives. The best examples are found in epics such as the *Mahabharata* and the *Ramayana*. These ancient works embody the difficulties and dilemmas that arise in society. The *Bhagavad Gita* opens with a moral dilemma faced by Arjuna, a lonesome warrior who must either kill or be killed by his own kinsmen. Bimal K. Matilal in his *Moral Dilemmas in the Mahabharata* (1989), transports us to another episode in the life of Arjuna in which he confronts the difficult claims of promise-keeping versus fratricide. When he chooses to kill his brother, his Krsna (alter ego) asks why he chose fraticide over promise-keeping. Arjuna explains that "he was obliged to commit fratricide in order to fulfil his obligation to keep his promise" (1989, p. 8). Arjuna understood the duty of promise-keeping as inviolable. Matilal observes that the scenario resonates with Kantian ethics, which gives highest priority to truth-telling. According to Matilal:

> promise-keeping or even truth-telling cannot be an unconditional obligation when it is in conflict with the avoidance of grossly unjust and criminal acts such as patricide or fratricide. Saving an innocent life is also a strong obligation; saving his elder brother would naturally be an equally strong obligation, if not stronger. Hence, in fact, according to Krsna, two almost equally strong obligations or duties are in conflict here (1989, p. 10).

In all such conflicts, the dharmic action is to be guided by the demands of the situation. There is no question about the need to maintain the consistency of an ethical system, but sometimes the infraction of virtues such as promise-keeping is permitted to achieve noble ends. This does not reduce ethics to opportunism, but it also does not hold ethics hostage to absolutism. The point is illustrated by Krsna's story about Kausika, a hermit who had taken a vow always to speak the truth. One day, while seated at a crossroad, a band of fleeing travelers begged the holy man not to divulge their escape route to the bandits who were pursuing them and who intended to kill them. Kausika did not reply. When the bandits arrived at the scene, knowing fully well that the hermit could not tell a lie, they asked about the travelers, and Kausika told them the truth. The travelers were caught and killed. Though Kausika had practiced virtue in order to reach heaven, he failed to achieve his goal, because, in this instance, truth-telling was a violent act which emptied his store of merit. Clearly the demand of the situation was the overriding duty to save lives, even though he would have to lie to effect this. But Kausika was an absolutist. He could not see that truth telling was not an unconditional obligation (1989, p. 10). The *Mahabharata* recounts numerous other instances that illustrate the relativity of moral conduct in the context of "duties in distress." A *Brahmana* in distress is allowed to perform sacrifice even for an unworthy person and may eat prohibited food. A *Ksatriya*, unable to subsist by his caste duties when his own avocation is destroyed, is allowed to engage in the duties of a *Vaisya*, agriculture and cattle-rearing. The *Santiparvan* declares it is not sinful to drink alcohol for medical purposes, to accede to a preceptor's wish to cohabit with his wife for the purpose of raising progeny, to steal in times of emergency, to tell lies to robbers, and so on (1989). Similar exceptions are permitted by Manu, the greatest exponent of orthodox morality. Personal survival is of such great importance that it is justifiable for a hungry person to steal food when all other measures fail (Manu, 1992, vol. 11, pp. 11-21). Following Manu, other *Dharmasastra* writers permit perjury to save life as an act of *dharma*.

The dharmic justification of lying and other such acts in situations of moral conflict notwithstanding, Hindu ethics strictly enjoins individuals to maintain their integrity in keeping with the *purusarthas* or values of life. These values are integrated and progressive, culminating in the *summum bonum* of liberation.

The internal flexibility of Hindu ethics gives it a certain advantage over authoritarian and relativistic positions on issues of life and death. Authoritarianism surfaces to different degrees in the moral stances of religious groups such as the Roman Catholic Church, Protestant fundamentalists, and Mormons. These groups base their truth claims on holy books in which they find objectively valid norms of conduct. Certain Protestant fundamentalist groups in particular see human reason as flawed and they rely on revelation for the whole truth. This leads them to see moral issues in absolute terms, allowing for few exceptions, if any. At the opposite end of the spectrum is the position of relativism. Relativists argue that value judgments and ethical norms are reducible to matters of subjective preference. Questions of life and death are considered private issues to be answered by individuals. They, too, minimize the capacity of reason. With hedonic overtones, relativists make the individual's own experience of happiness the standard of value.

Hindu ethics is distinguished from both extremes by the importance it gives to rational authority, although this may seem questionable because of the role played by revelation within the Hindu system. However, Hinduism's recognition of revelation as a conduit of knowledge does not depreciate the role of reason. The Hindu *sastras* make liberal use of reason to support their positions. The validity of reason is questioned only in mystical matters that lie beyond its purview. Thus the use of revelation does not reject reason, for there is continuity between the two. Whereas in Western thought revelation is an external mode of testimony, in the Hindu tradition, revelation is an internal activity, similar to intuition.

As Hirayanna observes, what is revealed begins "as an external opinion inasmuch as we appropriate it from a guru. But we do not merely acquiesce in it. We are under an obligation to intuit it and make it our own, when it will cease to be internal and become inwardly as clear to us as it is to our teacher" (1952, p. 14).

Through reason and intuition, Hinduism finds the source of ethics in the nature of the whole person. It agrees with the relativists that the attempt to find absolute values is illusory and pretentious, because social morality is inevitably the construct of subjective and historical forces. But this admission of subjectivity by Hinduism is not equivalent to saying that all of our choices between life and death are merely the products of subjective preferences. To the contrary, we can arrive at objectively valid norms through our knowledge of deep-seated human capacities for life, love, freedom, and integrity. Our cultural formulations of these psychic strivings will always be relative, and will be refined over time in the light of human experience. This view acknowledges that objectivity is not absolute or unconditional. The notion of absolutism is alien to Hindu ethics, because it is a concept incompatible with the Hindu mind, which never sees ethics as removed from an understanding of human nature and human history.

This approach to moral reasoning shapes Hindu bioethics. It eschews authoritarianism, creedalism, and emotionalism, favoring rationality instead. However, it is not the rationality of the disembodied mind, but the rationality of the whole person that is valued. The autonomous individual gives due weight to scriptural injunctions and the precedents of persons of probity, but in the final analysis he turns to his own conscience, guided by what he considers to be of ultimate value. Notwithstanding its claim to rationality, Hindu bioethics acknowledges that persons of reason might not always agree on what is good, while holding that they can agree more generally on what is evil. Rational people wish to avoid for themselves and for their loved ones evils such as pain, disease, premature death, and the loss of the ability to pursue the ends one chooses. Therefore, the basic agenda of Hindu bioethics is to prevent evil by advocating principles and proscriptions against behavior that inflicts harm to persons and all sentient creatures. Its fundamental principle is to do no harm – *himsam ma kuru*.

The vehicle that brings Hindu ethics into the new world of bioethics is the notion of *dharma*. This is not a static moral concept with limited relevance for other peoples and places. *Dharma* is a catalyst for change; it preserves order in the midst of change and change in the midst of order, and thereby always promotes progress.

II. Topics

A. Professionalism

The professionalization of the practice of Indian medicine dates back to the *Vedas* where the *bhisaj* were introduced. In Ayurvedic literature, the *bhisaj* is now known as the *Vaidya*. The term is a development of *vidya*, or knowledge, which is related to the word *Veda* and thus has a religious connotation absent in the earlier title, *bhisaj*. The Arabic word for doctor, *hakim*, is similarly related to *hikmat*, meaning knowledge. By contrast, the English word "doctor" (Latin, *docere*) connotes the physician's communication of knowledge, instead of the acquisition of knowledge. Thus from the earliest times, the

Indian doctor was seen as a man of learning. By the time of Caraka, knowledge took on a specialized connotation, as the *vaidyas* were organized into a recognized profession (Basham, 1976, p. 18).

A primary indicator of the professionalization of the *vaidya* is its strict defense of the ethics and practice of the medical profession by shutting out all impostors. There is evidence that there were itinerant quacks and charlatans who offered their "services" much like modern "ambulance chasers" do.

The exclusivity of the medical profession is also evident in the fact that admission to medical studies was open only to the three higher stratas of society. In all cases, the ambitions and aspirations of the practice of medicine are grounded in the belief that there are three values in life worthy of pursuit: virtue, wealth, and enjoyment (*Caraka Samhita*, vol. 11, vs. 3). Some further distinctions are made among the classes. *Sudra* students could be admitted, provided they had "good character and parentage," but they were admitted without the benefit of the recitation of initiation mantras. All candidates were to be motivated by the pursuit of virtue, wealth, and enjoyment. But some differences in purpose or aim were recognized among the different classes of students. Members of the priestly class should study *Ayurveda* "for welfare of living beings," the warrior class "for their protection," and members of various occupations would study for professional reasons.

Medical education was morally structured and began long before a student was admitted to the profession. According to Caraka, the candidate should be:

> Of tender years, born of a good family, possessed of a desire to learn, strength, energy, contentment, character, self-control, a good retentive memory, intellect, courage, purity of mind and body, a simple and clear comprehension, command a clear insight into the things studied ... A man of contrary attributes should not be admitted into (the sacred precincts) of medicine (*Caraka Samhita*, vol. 8, vs. 8).

The doctor's "Oath of Initiation" is at the heart of professional medical ethics in *Ayurveda*. It shares with the Hippocratic Oath the importance of total commitment to the good of the patient, but the Indian code has unique features, most notably the doctrine of *karma*, the obligation to remain celibate, as well as the obligation to abstain from eating meat, bearing arms, causing another's death, and the obligation to withhold medical assistance from those who oppose the social and political order. Some of the central elements of the Oath are:

> ... Thou shalt lead the life of a celibate, grow thy hair and beard, speak only the truth, eat no meat, eat only pure articles of food, be free from envy and carry no arms.
>
> There shall be nothing that thou should not do at my behest except hating the king, causing another's death or committing an act of great unrighteousness or acts leading to calamity.
>
> ...
>
> Thou shalt behave and act without arrogance, with care and attention and with undistracted mind, humility, constant reflection and ungrudging obedience. Acting either at my behest or otherwise, thou shalt conduct thyself for the achievement of thy teacher's purposes alone, to the best of thy abilities.

> ...
>
> Day and night, however thou mayest be engaged, thou shalt endeavor for the relief of patients with all thy heart and soul. Thou shalt not desert or injure thy patient for the sake of thy life or thy living. Thou shalt not commit adultery even in thought. Even so thou shalt not covet others' possessions. Thou shalt be modest in thy attire and appearance. Thou shouldst not be a drunkard or a sinful man nor shouldst thou associate with the abettors of crimes. Thou shouldst speak words that are gentle, pure and righteous, pleasing, worthy, true, wholesome, and moderate. Thy behaviour must be in consideration of time and place and heedful of past experience. Thou shalt act always with a view to the acquisition of knowledge and fullness of equipment.
>
> No persons, who are hated by the king or who are haters of the king or who are hated by the public or who are haters of the public, shall receive treatment. Similarly, those who are extremely abnormal, and of miserable character and conduct, those who have not vindicated their honor, those who are on the point of death, and similarly women who are unattended by their husbands or guardians shall not receive treatment.
>
> No offerings of presents by a woman without the behest of her husband or guardian shall be accepted by thee. While entering the patient's house, thou shalt be accompanied by a man who has permission to enter; and thou shalt be well-clad, bent of head, self-possessed and conduct thyself only after repeated consideration. Thou shalt thus properly make thy entry. Having entered, thy speech, mind, intellect and senses shall be entirely devoted to no other thought than that of being helpful to the patient and of things concerning only him. The peculiar customs of the patient's household shall not be made public. Even knowing that the patient's span of life has come to its close, it shall not be mentioned by thee there, where if so done, it would cause shock to the patient or to others.
>
> Though possessed of knowledge one should not boast very much of one's knowledge. Most people are offended by the boastfulness of even those who are otherwise good and authoritative.
>
> There is no limit at all to the Science of Life, Medicine. So thou shouldst apply thyself to it with diligence. This is how thou shouldst act. Also thou shouldst learn the skill of practice from another without carping. The entire world is the teacher to the intelligent and the foe to the unintelligent. Hence, knowing this well, thou shouldst listen and act according to the words of instruction of even an unfriendly person, when his words are worthy and of a kind as to bring to you fame, long life, strength and prosperity ... ("Oath of Initiation," 1989, pp. 130-132).

The pursuit of these high standards among students without the use of force is the result of the student-mentor relationship, which Murthy describes as "intimate and affectionate, yet rigid and disciplined" (1989, p. 127). Though this relationship may appear paternalistic by contemporary standards, the "moral and noble behavior of the teacher molded the novice into an efficient physician" (Zimmer, 1948, p. 76) and it is through this relationship that the professional ethics of ancient India has survived (Murthy, 1989, p. 128).

The model for medical practice is described as "Four-legged Therapeutics" and it focuses on the ethics of teamwork. Medical success is seen as a joint effort in which four agents, each with its own excellence, participate: physician, drug, attendant, and patient (*Caraka Samhita*, vol. 9, vs. 3). The excellence of the physician lies in four professional qualities of theoretical knowledge, extensive practical experience, dexterity and cleanliness (*Caraka Samhita*, vol. 9, vs. 6). These qualities enable the physician to grasp "the four aspects" – "cause, symptoms, cure and prevention of diseases." His role is therefore indispensable. One who holds the honorable degree of *Vaidy* is assumed to possess exceptional "learning, rationality, specific knowledge, memory, devotion and action," whereby he "showers happiness on the living beings" (*Caraka Samhita*, vol. 9, vs. 21). In addition to possessing the four qualities and four aspects of knowledge, the physician is known by four philosophical attitudes – "friendliness and compassion towards the diseased, attachment to the remediable and indifference to those who are moving towards the end" (*Caraka Samhita*, vol. 9, vs. 26).

The second leg of the quadruplet is the drug. It must have the following four qualities: "abundance, effectiveness, various pharmaceutical forms and normal composition" (*Caraka Samhita*, vol. 9, vs. 7). The third leg is the attendant. The four qualities he must possess are "knowledge of attendance, dexterity, loyalty and cleanliness" (*Caraka Samhita*, vol. 9, vs. 8). The patient is the fourth leg. His four qualities are: "memory, obedience, fearlessness and providing all information about the disorder" (*Caraka Samhita*, vol. 9, vs. 9).

Thus, therapeutics in *Ayurveda* is four-legged and each leg has qualities, which are a blend of noetic and moral values. Medicine is a participatory effort in which professionals, medications, attendants, and patients work together. Participation, not passivity, is the virtue of the Indian patient.

This brings us to a discussion of the physician-patient relationship. The importance of the physician-patient relationship lies in the fact that it is a microcosm of medical ethics as a whole. Currently, the subject is under public and governmental scrutiny because of instances in which physicians have failed to treat patients with due diligence as a result of pressure from their HMOs to limit services in exchange for bonuses.

Robert Veatch considers four models for ethical medicine: (1) The Priestly Model, (2) The Engineering Model, (3) The Collegial Model, and (4) The Contractual Model (1988, p. 89). Elsewhere (1997) I have weighed the merits of each model with reference to Ayurvedic principles; here those principles are used to construct a new model – the Participatory Model.

In the priestly or patriarchal model the physician is viewed as a priest who exercises moral authority in a way that eclipses the freedom and dignity of the patient. In the engineering model, the patient is in full control and the doctor is denied the opportunity to act on his own ethical judgments. In the collegial model the physician and patient are friends; and in the contractual model emphasis is given to the financial and legal aspects of their relationship. The participatory model recognizes valuable elements in each model. The patient's dependence brings forth the need for the physician to act with beneficence, and the patient's sense of responsibility for himself requires that he be able to act autonomously. Neither the doctor nor patient is accorded a role of primacy; both are expected to work as a team, meeting each new situation as it arises.

The centerpiece of the participatory model is Caraka's paradigm of Four-legged Therapeutics in which each leg of the table is necessary to alleviate disorders and foster health. The arrangement clearly is one of complementarity among equals, and without any one part, the system collapses.

The patient contributes to his healing and health by carefully monitoring himself and all developments. He must entertain no negative emotions, maintain faith in his doctor, keep the physician fully informed because the physician depends on the patient for accurate feedback to make a diagnosis and prescribe a treatment, and follow directions. The physician is important not because of his professional status but because of his competence and character. All pretensions of a patriarchal attitude in a physician are warded off by the need for professional modesty.

The doctor-patient relationship also mandates that patients have a right to privacy. The physician must not make public information about the patient or the patient's household. When a physician enters a patient's home, he should attend only to the patient's needs and he should not take inventory of his private and personal matters. He is also forbidden to make known to other parties any of the privileged information he has gained from his house call. Such safeguards were set in place to build trust and confidence in doctors. In the modern setting, the right to privacy prohibits the *vaidya* from disclosing information to employers and insurers.

The doctor-patient relationship is also governed by rules of disclosure. Caraka counsels that the doctor should not disclose the imminence of death to the patient or to family members when he knows that it is likely to shock them. It would be recognized that this injunction is embedded in a cultural context in which the physician and the family are closely united. Where it is predictable that disclosure will make the situation worse, it is prudent not to traumatize the patient or family. Where the news is not expected to produce shock, there is no policy against full disclosure. This may sound like disguised paternalism because beneficence is elevated over patient autonomy. However, the *vaidya* limits disclosure only in light of (1) his intimate knowledge of the patient, based on past responses; (2) his familiarity with the family; (3) his knowledge of the stage of the disease; and (4) the paramount importance of ensuring a peaceful death. Caraka's dictum that doctors may withhold information from the patient if disclosure is likely to negatively affect the patient's mental or physical health applies only in cases in which standard therapies are being pursued. When a patient faces a non-traditional therapy, the *vaidya* must disclose all information to the patient.

Focus on the *vaidya's* relationship with the individual patient should not be taken to imply that the doctor's duties do not also have a social dimension or that the social dimension is unimportant. Traditionally, treatment had to be withheld from persons who had violated the law, those involved in risky behavior, and women separated from their families. The physician, under license by the state, was obliged to observe all of the social sanctions against such persons, presumably for the greater good ("Oath of Initiation", 1989).

B. Reproduction

B.1. In Vitro *Fertilization and Embryo Transfer (IVF-ET)*

Hindu bioethics finds no difficulty with IVF-ET with respect to the harm/benefit ratio. One must consider the possible risks and harms associated with the hormone therapy that precedes IVF-ET and the surgical laparoscopy under general anesthesia through which eggs are retrieved as well as the risks incurred by the extra-corporeal management of the egg, sperm, and embryo; the limited rate of success; and the high emotional and financial costs. These harms, however, must be measured against the wishes and rights of the couple seeking to have a child. In addition to the basic human urge to have biological children, the Hindu religion gives great importance to procreation. The Law Books state: "To be mothers were women created, and to be fathers men; religious rites, therefore are ordained in the Veda to be performed (by the husband) together with the wife" (Manu, 1980, 9.96). Male children are especially prized.

In ordinary cases, Hindu bioethics would want to limit IVF-ET to married couples who were using their own gametes in order to maximize the chance of both physical and emotional success for the child. However, there is a provision in the Hindu tradition for use of donor sperm. One precedent for this exigency is found in an ancient form of sexual union known as *niyoga*. Its purpose was to impregnate the wife of an impotent or dead man so that his family could be preserved and so that he might have sons to offer oblations for the welfare of his soul in the next world. The custom has Vedic origins, possibly going back to the practice whereby the brother-in-law extended his hand to the wife of the deceased on the funeral pyre. In the Law Books, *niyoga* was strictly accepted as a dispassionate duty.

B.2. Contraception

Hindu bioethics holds that there are two meanings of the conjugal act: the *unitive* meaning that brings husband and wife together, and the *procreative* meaning that brings forth new life. The connection between the unitive and procreative is inseparable. However, Hindu bioethics holds that the procreative value of the conjugal act need not be bound up with every individual act of intercourse. Moreover, the basic criterion for the meaning of human actions is the total person and not some isolated aspect of the person. For humans, sexual activity is not merely for procreation and gratification, but for expression. We enrich our lives through our sexuality. Contraceptives help free couples of the anxiety of conceiving an unwanted child with every act of intercourse.

Indians have sought such sexual freedom from earliest times. The *Brihadaranyaka Upanisad* states:

> Now, the woman whom one may desire with the thought, "May she not conceive offspring!" – after inserting the member in her and joining mouth with mouth, he should first inhale, and then exhale, and say: "With power, with semen, I reclaim the semen from you!" Thus she comes to be without seed (*Brihadaranyaka Upanisad*, 1931, p. 169).

The effectiveness of this method may be questioned. However, there is no doubt that the intent to contracept was evident in early Indian society. Ethicist Seshagiri Rao correctly observes, "contraception is generally acceptable to the Hindus and is to be encouraged in the interests of domestic felicity and welfare of society" (1978, p. 1271).

B.3. Abortion

Common themes of the epic and legal literature identify abortion as a heinous sin. They collectively affirm the ancient view that life in the womb is not a tissue of the mother's body, but a separate life bearing the essential marks of humanity from conception. For example, in Yajnavalkya's view, the soul takes form in the moment of conception and is progressively invested with all elements for human development. According to Manu, the process of becoming human begins with conception. At the time of conception, the husband is born again as the fetus in the wife's womb. She is thence known as *jaya*, because "the husband is again born in her" (Manu, 1980, 9.8). The value that cradles this view of the unborn is *ahimsa* (non-violence).

Turning to the medical manuals' account of abortion, we begin with Caraka. The central question for our discussion of abortion and the tradition of the Hindu medical manuals is: does this medical treatise view the unborn as a human person, with full rights to protection, or is it a human being who has not yet achieved personhood, and hence does not have the moral safeguards attached to persons? The notion of personhood is the determining factor. Caraka sees the human individual and the natural world as manifestations of the eternal *Brahman*. The person and nature are constituted of six elements: earth, water, fire, air, ether, and the spirit or self in the person and Brahman in the universe. In addition to the five *mahabhutas* (gross elements) and the *atman* (soul), the individual is invested with intelligence (*buddhi)* and ego (*ahankara*). The ego is independent of the body and is made up of action, the fruit of action, reincarnation, and memory. It can exist without the physical body. Conscious perception is brought about in the individual by the agency of the transcendent spirit (*Purusa*) which integrates the *atman*, mind, senses, and sense objects (*Caraka Samhita*, 1996-1997, p. 400).

On the subject of fetal development, Caraka delineates the factors from which the embryo originates, the definition of the embryo, factors producing the embryo, and the order of its development. Conception occurs when the male sperm cell and the female ovum are united with the spirit which, in association with the mind, "descends into the zygote situated in the uterus" thus forming the embryo. It is important to note that the spirit is an original and necessary constituent of the embryonic existence. In addition to the contributions made by its parents, Caraka asserts that the past *karma* of the individual is carried over into the present embodiment and imparts to the newborn child its special features (*Carakh Samhita*, 1996-1997, p. 415).

Thus the *Caraka Samhita* like the legal and epic literature, demonstrates opposition to abortion as morally evil. It does so on the assumption that spirit is present in matter from the moment of conception and is the causal agent in the progressive development of an embryo. This creative manifestation of the spirit in the micro-cosmos is similar to the process of creation in the macro-cosmos. The moral character of the individual is also given in conception because *karma* is carried over from one life to the next. Together the spiritual and moral constituents of the individual produce a person through a continuous process that is *developmental* but *not disjunctive*. It is therefore impossible and impermissible to differentiate degrees of human existence or potentiality in terms of "ensoulment," "viability," and the presence of "brain-waves." The new life is an intimate, inseparable blending of personal and physical-biological existence. According to Caraka, at no time within embryonic development is there a state of pure matter in which the termination of that life is morally justified.

The *Susruta Samhita* has a different timetable of fetal development. It places the emergence of consciousness in the fourth month of gestation (*Susruta Samhita*, 1996-1997, p. 415). It seems that if conscious experience is the mark of ensoulment, then abortion may be deemed morally permissible inasmuch as the fetus is not yet a person. Julius Lipner rules out this possibility, noting that

> nothing is said here to indicate that in its development the embryo undergoes a quantum leap, passing from one kind of human moral status (human being) to another (human person). On the contrary, in characteristic Hindu fashion, the language here is progressive MANIFESTATION, of a personhood previously only latent rather than origination of personhood *ab initio*. The *Susruta Samhita* confirms this conclusion when, after describing the development of the foetus, it observes in the face of opposing views that the foetus undergoes an all-round (rather than sporadic) development from the very beginning (Lipner, 1989, p. 56).

C. *Death and Dying*

C.1. *Death*

Hindu views of death have evolved over some 2,500 years and are expressed in myths, rituals, religion, and philosophy. We focus on views found in the *Upanisads* (700-500 B.C.E.).

The *Upanisads* distinguish between the essential self and the empirical self. The essential self, which is of the nature of existence-consciousness-bliss (*sat-chit-ananda*), is at the core of each person's being. In reality it is one, but through the power of ignorance and desire for bodily attachment it assumes the character of the empirical self, namely body, mind, and intellect. The empirical self is then erroneously taken for the essential self. As a result, the self or *atman* becomes a prisoner in an ongoing cycle of suffering, death, and rebirth. Freedom from this cycle, *jivanmukti*, is brought about through the experience of enlightenment and is possible in the here and now. The I affirms: "when all the desires the heart harbours are gone, man becomes immortal and reaches Brahman here."

The implications of the Hindu views on death and dying for bioethics are many: Death is not the opposite of life. It is the opposite of birth. As such, it is the end of the body (*dehanta*). It occurs with the dissolution of the subtle body from the physical body. Death and birth are markers on one continuous trajectory of life. Birth does not mark an absolute beginning and death is not a final end. The *atman* is indestructible, and this reduces the sense of helplessness in the face of death. Moreover, *karma* connects a person with the past, present, and future dimensions of his life and gives moral meaning to all events and actions.

Present experiences are seen as the consequences of deeds done in the past, which must be endured. Anything accidental or unexpected, for which there is no apparent explanation, is usually attributed to the unseen hand of *karma*. *Karma* is invoked to answer the "why me?" question patients often ask. However, ordinarily Hindus do not dwell on *karma* and focus on doing the best they can. When things do not turn out as expected, *karma* is invoked to help explain disease and death (Desai, 1989, p. 94). This does not reflect fatalism, however. Hindus recognize that choices made in the present shape the future both in this life and the next.

Perhaps because of the understanding that death is not an absolute end and because of the realization that all must die, only untimely death is profoundly mourned, and quality of life is prized more than the length of time a person lives. Death is preferable to distress and decrepitude.

Death is a social event, not a personal one. The extended family comes together to express its love and grief while the patient is alive and they continue to participate in the event through ritual devotion after the patient dies. Thus a good death is one that takes place at home among family.

Again because Hindus do not understand death to be an absolute end, the method of disposition of the body is important. The dead are cremated because fire purifies and returns us to our original state. Children and those who live holy lives in the forest are considered pure and therefore are not cremated.

C.2. Suicide

The core of Hindu views of suicide is the set of scriptures and traditions that are based on the *Upanisads*. The goal is to attain the highest human value, namely liberation from *samsara*, or the cycle of suffering, death, and rebirth. The moral values that facilitate this goal are those that preserve and promote a quality of life that is commensurate with its rational basis and spiritual aspiration. Within this philosophic framework, Hinduism condemns suicide as evil when it is a direct and deliberate act with the intention to kill oneself for self-regarding motives. Suicide is evil because, subjectively, the act is the product of ignorance and passion. Objectively, the act is evil because it produces karmic consequences that impede the progress of liberation from *samsara*. It is with this understanding that the scriptures vehemently prohibit suicide. At the same time, as Kane (1975) observes, the scriptures make exceptions for recourse to suicide when it is religiously motivated in situations of distress (p. 924). The ideal that distinguishes licit and illicit suicide is the perspective of the enlightened person who has renounced all and lives in the forest.

Manu clearly distinguishes between courses that are ordinary and extraordinary for the *sannyasin* – the individual in the fourth and final stage of life. He points out the normal path to be followed:

> He should sleep on raised ground (*sthandila*), should feel no concern if he suffers from an illness, he should neither welcome death nor should he feel joy for continuing to live, but he should patiently wait the time of death, as a servant waits till the time he is hired expires (Manu, 1980, 6.45).

The instructions of Manu are in accord with the teachings and spirit of the *Upanisads*, which elevate the knowledge of *atman* and *Brahman* to the highest place and ascribe greater value to study and meditation than to performing sacrifices and self-immolation. The only prayer of the sage is to be led from the unreal to the real, from darkness to light, and from death to immortality (Manu, 1980, 6.45).

The bliss of *Brahman* is not just an eschatological possibility, but an empirical reality. The union can be had in the here and now and is known as *jivanmukt* (*Katha Upanishad*, 6.14). And so the *moksa* doctrine supplies the basis for moral optimism that perfection can be realized in the present. It is this possibility and progress toward this ideal that makes the human state so precious.

The premium placed on reason and autonomy as the means to *moksa* clearly contradict later beliefs in the magical and meritorious efficacy of dying in holy places such as *Benares* or *Prayaga*, or of dying in performing daredevil acts such as jumping from cliffs. The fact is that, to the extent the influence of the *Upanisads* prevailed, some of the *Dharmasastras*, such as Gautama, declared their opposition to those who willfully died "by starving themselves to death, by weapons, fire, poison, or water, by hanging themselves, or by jumping (from a precipice)" (Gautama, 1980, vol. 2, p. 250). Likewise, Harita and others condemn penitential deaths that require the murderer of a Brahmin to expiate his guilt by becoming a target in battle.

Once we exclude the number of suicides performed in the name of religion, those that are the result of socio-economic pressures, or those performed for selfish desires, the question still remains as to the legitimacy of suicide in Hinduism. The answer is not always consistent, but given the Upanisadic perspective with which we began this discussion, the following norms emerge.

Though empirical existence is clouded by ignorance and mortality, and is not reflective of ultimate reality, it is also the place of soul-making. This polarity creates tension between making the most of the world while at the same time renouncing it. On the one hand, we must look upon the world as our home and not be anxious, even in cases of dire circumstances, to make a hasty exit. On the other hand, should we reach the point at which, through disability, age, or disease, one's body is no longer capable of keeping pace with one's spirit, then the body may be respectfully left behind. Life on earth must not be allowed to interfere with Life. Our essential existence, as the bearer of *moksa*, must ultimately prevail over empirical existence, the bearer of *samsara*. The whole of Hindu discipline is an exercise in progressive renunciation, and suicide is the supreme act of renunciation. For the spiritually mature, suicide is the death of Death.

Although Hinduism allows for the possible permissibility of suicide, only those who have met their obligations to society, who have been enlightened, who act with knowledge, and who are not driven by pressures from without or passions from within may commit suicide. The ultimate threshold for making suicide licit is when spiritual equanimity before the onset of death is placed in jeopardy.

C.3. *Euthanasia*

There are different forms of euthanasia: passive versus active and voluntary versus involuntary versus non-voluntary. Passive euthanasia is the intentional ending of life by refusing treatment that is beneficial and not burdensome. It is synonymous with passive suicide, which involves the refusal of beneficial treatment with the intent to die. Hindu bioethics condemns passive suicide because it violates the moral obligation we have to do what is beneficial and reasonable toward preserving ourselves. Hindu bioethics considers passive euthanasia a failure of our duty to employ all necessary means to save life. Passive euthanasia should not be confused with the termination of treatment that is no longer beneficial to the patient. Technically, withholding or withdrawing life-sustaining treatment is not a form of euthanasia as long as the intention is not to kill the patient. Consider a patient who is kept alive by mechanical ventilation and other artificial means. His condition gradually deteriorates, and he will eventually die, though there is no certainty as to how and when. With full knowledge that his condition is irreversible, the patient requests that he be removed from his respirator and that, in the event of a cardiac or respiratory arrest, he be allowed to die. Hindu bioethics does not treat this as a case of euthanasia, because the treatment is of no benefit to the patient; instead, it is seriously burdensome. The dying process, rather than the patient's life, is being prolonged. As long as the individual has a good chance to regain health, the Hindu doctor would acknowledge the obligation to preserve life. But where such prospects are non-existent, that obligation diminishes.

Unlike passive euthanasia that involves withholding or withdrawing care with the intent to kill the patient, active euthanasia involves intentionally doing something, such as administering a drug, to kill a patient. Both passive and active euthanasia may be voluntary, involuntary, and non-voluntary.

Involuntary euthanasia involves the taking of an individual's life, supposedly for his own good, but either against his wishes or without the benefit of consultation. Hindu bioethics repudiates involuntary euthanasia, because it violates the respect Hinduism has for personal autonomy and is fraught with ominous side-effects.

Non-voluntary euthanasia also involves the taking of a person's life, supposedly to protect the patient's interests, but under conditions in which the patient is incapable of formulating a preference or being able to communicate it. There are times when patients' lives appear to be more horrible than death, but they are incapable of expressing wishes or decisions, including the desire to be put to death. This category of patients can include severely abnormal babies, the senile, the totally paralyzed, and the comatose. For instance, a husband of a wife with Alzheimer's might seek to end her life out of compassion, but he may be unable to obtain her consent. This would be a case of non-voluntary euthanasia. Hindu bioethics promotes the use of legal instruments, such as the *Patient Self-Determination Act (1991)*, to identify and follow patients' wishes. At the time of hospital admission, patients are asked if they wish to make a living will – a directive to cease life-sustaining measures if there is no chance for recovery. The document gives doctors the legal authority not to connect life-support systems if the patient is terminally ill or, if the patient is already on life-support, the directive gives physicians permission to discontinue treatment. For more powerful legal protection, patients should draw up a durable power of attorney for health care, which names another individual to make one's health care decisions should one become incapacitated.

Voluntary euthanasia involves either withholding or withdrawing care so that a patient dies or administering a drug either with the patient's permission or at the patient's request. In the current debate, Hindu bioethics does not stand firmly on either side of the debate. It does not support the position of those who are opposed to voluntary euthanasia, whether passive or active, on the grounds of the sanctity of life. Nor does it support those who favor it on the grounds of quality of life. Hindu philosophy and the reverence for life that emerges from it favor protecting and preserving life in all circumstances. As such, Hindu bioethics condemns all acts that destroy life. At the same time, Hindu bioethics displays a certain tolerance and flexibility in the context of individual intentions, motives, and circumstances. That suggests that euthanasia may sometimes be permissible. These apparently opposite poles emerged in the discussion of suicide below. There is philosophical support for the right to assisted suicide in terms of the principles of autonomy and rational choice, but this is only a limited right, a religious option permitted in the pursuit of higher, existential goals. The case for euthanasia in the Hindu tradition follows from its acceptance of assisted suicide on religious grounds.

Physician-assisted suicide (PAS) differs from euthanasia in that the patient actually kills himself. The physician supplies the patient with a causative agent, usually a medication, with the understanding that the patient will use it to commit suicide. The most publicized instances of this form of euthanasia are the cases involving Dr. Jack Kevorkian and his "suicide machine."

Hindu bioethics has a prima facie bias on the side of protecting life. Therefore, it is wary of all acts that would destroy life. Requests to terminate life could be a hidden plea for attention, a cry for the relief of pain, or a covert expression of the fear of abandonment. All of these considerations prevent Hindu bioethics from hastily endorsing PAS. Effective pain control and hospice care are available to ease the suffering of the dying, and efforts should be made to implement appropriate pain relief for the suffering.

Earlier we saw that there is some philosophical support in the Hindu tradition for the right to commit suicide grounded in the principles of autonomy and rational choice, and the importance given to quality of life. But this support must be understood within the religious context of Hinduism that sees spiritual alertness as essential for a good death. Pain or stupor must not be allowed to cloud such alertness. Neverthelss, there are cases in which PAS would be accepted on religious grounds. Hindu scriptures discuss various methods by which pious individuals may end their lives – immolation, drowning, poisoning, falling, and fasting. Most of these forms, with the exception of fasting, require the direct participation of another individual acting upon the request of the person who wishes to die. Imagine a friend or family member helping the infirmed to the water's edge, carrying him up to a precipice, lighting a brisk fire for him, or preparing a lethal potion for the patient. Once the preparations are made, the old, handicapped, or otherwise incapacitated person takes the final leap over the edge or into the fire, or drinks the cup of poison. This is an ancient version of assisted suicide as practiced by Hindus.

The discussion of PAS further informs the Hindu perspective on active voluntary euthanasia. On the basis of its ancient practice of assisted suicide, we can make a moral argument for active voluntary euthanasia in Hindu bioethics, because the two practices are essentially the same from a moral point of view. The only difference between assisted suicide and active voluntary euthanasia is that in the case of the latter the decisive deed is performed by another. In terms of intention, attitude, and outcome, both forms of participation are virtually the same. In the modern setting, there appears to be no real difference between a medical professional putting a lethal pill in the mouth of a quadriplegic and the patient performing that final physical act himself, had he the capacity and wish to do so. In principle, assisted suicide as practiced by the ancient Indians and active voluntary euthanasia are only instrumentally different; the consequences are the same.

The fact that the Hindu scriptures teach that peoples' lives follow the course of nature and *karma* might be used as an objection to allowing PAS and voluntary active euthanasia. If the body is terminated before its *karma* is completely consumed, the person misses the opportunity to destroy *karma* in the present life and thus must continue to live out that *karma* in the next life. The response of *Ayurveda* to this interpretation of Hindu scriptures is that the fruits of all ordinary actions can be stopped by means of well-balanced conduct, proper medicines, and so forth. This suggests that our ordinary non-moral actions in health care can change or halt the ordinary course of the fruition of our *karma*. Thus I may have taken ill as a result of my ordinary *karma*, but, if I should take proper care, it is possible to avoid such effects and enjoy good health. Other philosophies hold that the law of *karma* is immutable, that only the fruits of unripe *karma* can be destroyed by true knowledge, and that the fruits of ripe *karma* have to be experienced in any case, even if true knowledge is attained. Caraka's theory does not introduce this immutability to ripe *karmas*: "The effects of all *karmas*, excepting those which are extremely strong, can be modified by an apparently non-moral course of conduct" (Dasgupta, vol. 2, p. 403).

This evidence alleviates the fear that unless a person's *karmas* are allowed to terminate with natural death, they will have to be purged in the next life. In keeping with the ancient tradition which allowed for an enlightened person voluntarily to choose the precise moment of his death, in rare cases it is morally permissible for a spiritually elevated person to achieve that end with the help of a doctor, should he find himself terminally ill and in persistent pain. The individual knows that today his mind can control his body, but tomorrow his body will control his mind. Excruciating suffering may rob him of the equanimity he cherishes for his final moments of life. Euthanasia ensures a merciful death because he can leave this life with consciousness unclouded by the stupor of drugs, and without fear that some unexhausted *karmas* will plunge him back into mortal existence. This is an enlightened act of stupendous faith in the Supreme. Such faith is invested with its own power to wipe clean the slate of life, expressed beatifically in a good death.

C.4. *Death with Dignity*

Caraka provides a careful analysis of the signs of life and death in the *Indriyasthanam*. He makes a division between untimely death, caused by accident or disease prior to the end of the life span, and timely death which comes at the end and which cannot be indefinitely postponed. The role of the doctor is to look for signs indicating that the person has died (*Indriyasthanam*, 12.43-46).

When he observes the signs of death, the physician should not disclose this fact, even if asked, so as not to precipitate the patient's death or add affliction to the family. In the Hindu ethos, the process of dying and death itself are a family affair. The attending physician is sensitive to this situation in his handling of information pertaining to the patient's condition. If a physician declares that he sees signs of death, he may limit the patient's and family's will and tranquility. The physician may calmly call to the bedside "those who need to be present" without explicitly stating that the patient is dying (Desai, 1989, p. 94).

Moreover, when death is imminent, the physician should not continue to treat the patient. The medical manuals classify diseases as "curable" and "incurable," and instruct the physician not to waste resources on treating those diseases that fall into the latter category. Once signs of death are definitively observed, all extraordinary means are prohibited on medical and moral grounds. This decision is bolstered by considerations of professional interest, because "the physician treating an incurable disease certainly suffers from the loss of wealth, learning and reputation and from censure and unpopularity" (*Caraka Samhita*, vol. 1, vs. 7-8).

Commenting on this situation from the perspective of a physician, Desai remarks, "It is difficult to imagine a controversy either between ethicist and physician or between family and physician on an issue like 'Do not resuscitate' orders." He acknowledges that modern technology is not as widely available in India as in the United States, but this factor alone does not sufficiently explain the absence of controversy in India regarding such matters. "The Hindu is generally allowed to die peacefully, for artificially or mechanically sustained life is held to be of little value. Most people prefer to die in their own beds" (Desai, 1989, p. 94).

Desai's remarks suggest that Hindu bioethics may have a role to play toward helping Western medicine reconsider its goals and values, especially in the care of the dying. When a physician takes the Hippocratic Oath upon receiving his medical degree, he commits himself to two fundamental values of medicine: to prolong life and to minimize pain and suffering. It does not take too many years of practice to discover that these benign principles can conflict with each other.

Timothy E. Quill, a leading physician in the "Death and Dignity" movement, speaks from experience:

> Modern medical treatment has a powerful potential to extend life, yet this same intervention sometimes unintentionally contributes to increased pain and suffering prior to death. Medicine's remarkable success in treating some diseases have led many in our society to value the prolongation of life no matter what the personal consequences, while inadvertently minimizing the increase in human suffering that is often a byproduct. Rather than extending meaningful human life, as the Hippocratic Oath intends, medical interventions sometimes result in the prolongation of a painful death. The power and potential of medical technology to produce such diametrically opposed effects should be exercised with the utmost care and restraint (1993, p. 43).

For its part, Hindu bioethics holds to the position that no person may morally hasten his or her own death or the death of another person by direct means. However, the individual is not obliged to resist the natural and inevitable approach of death as though it were the enemy of life. Once ordinary means of treatment have failed, and the person chooses to accept the end and prepares for the last steps of life's journey, the doctor should not prolong the dying process by heroic means. In this context, the mandate of *ahimsa* for the physician goes beyond the old command: "Thou shalt not kill," to a new command: "Thou need not strive intrusively to keep alive" (Clough, Hugh, & Wassmer, 1978, p. 732).

III. The Future of Hindu Bioethics

In his *Cross Cultural Perspectives in Medical Ethics: Readings*, Robert Veatch observes, "The religions of Judaism and Christianity and the secular thought of the political philosophy of liberalism in the Anglo-American West are not the only alternatives to a Hippocratic medical ethic" (Veatch, 1989, p. 96). In fact, the new pluralistic approach to world cultures is introducing us to several religious and philosophical alternatives from outside the Anglo-American West. Just as alternative medicine is becoming recognized and respected and is being incorporated into mainstream medicine, there is a growing admission that the ethical problems we face today have dimensions that are not adequately addressed by the standard responses of Judaism, Christianity, and secular philosophies. From among these new Eastern perspectives, Hindu bioethics stands out. Its strength lies in the fact that it is integrated in an indigenous system of medicine more alive today than at any time in its 2000-year history. It addresses the preventive and health-promoting aspects of medicine, the mind-body connection, connections between the micro-cosmos and macro-cosmos, and it employs only those therapies that assist nature. In addition Hindu bioethics is philosophically pluralistic and ethically contextual, giving it the conceptual flexibility often missing in its Western bioethics but which the complexities of contemporary issues demand. This flexibility originates in the focus of Hindu bioethics on the person as a composite of somatic, psychic, social, and spiritual dimensions.

In their quest to cure illness efficiently, modern physicians have overlooked compassion and understanding. Today, patients are more likely to be treated by teams of experts who use technology to diagnose and treat. While the technical quality of care has improved extensively, there is a growing sense that we are losing the qualities of an earlier generation of doctors, namely listenting carefully and responding empathetically to patients. The time physicians can spend with individual patients is being limited. At times, patients' understandings of their diagnoses and treatment options suffers, or they fail to understand a doctor's instructions.

Hindu bioethics gives great importance to the patient-physician relationship and to understanding the patient as a whole person. It eschews physician-centered conversation in the medical setting in which physicians ask questions that require "yes" or "no" answers. This "yes-no" conversational style derives from a disease-oriented view of health in which the goal is to establish a correlation between the patient's complaint and some organic pathology. The best way to achieve this goal is to let the expert determine what is relevant and what is not. Such medical interrogation is alien to *Ayurveda* because of its positive view of health and its understanding of the patient as an individual having many dimensions.

The participatory role accorded to patients in Hindu bioethics means that they have to bear much of the responsibility for establishing a good rapport with their physicians and promoting health by communicating with their doctors. Here again we see the importance of all participants in health care; obligations cannot be accorded solely to the physician. Health care is a holistic endeavor requiring the participation of patients and physicians alike.

Bibliography

Basham, A.L. (1976). The practice of medicine in ancient and medieval India. In: C. Leslie (Ed.), *Asian medical systems: A comparative study* (pp. 18-43). Berkeley: University of California Press.

Beauchamp, T.L. (1978). Ethical theory. In: T.L. Beauchamp & L. Walters (Eds.), *Contemporary issues in bioethics* (pp. 1-5). Belmont, California: Wadsworth Publishing Company.

Clough, V., Hugh, A., & Wassmer, T. (1968). Ethical and moral issues involved in recent medical advances. *Villanova Law Review, 13*, 759-783.

Crawford, C. (1997). Hindu developments in bioethics. In: B.A. Lustig (Ed.), *Theological developments in bioethics, 5*. Boston: Kluwer Academic Publishers.

Dasgupta, S. (1968). *A history of Indian philosophy*. Cambridge: Cambridge University Press.

Desai, P. (1989). *Health and medicine in the Hindu tradition*. New York: Crossroad.

Hiriyanna, M. (1952). *Popular essays in Indian philosophy*. Mysore: Kavyalaya Publishers.

Hume, R.E. (trans.) (1931). Brihadaranyaka upanisad. In: *The thirteen principal Upanishads* (pp. 73-176). London: Oxford University Press.

Kane, P. (1973). *History of Dharma sastra*. Poona: Bhandarkar Oriental Research Institute.

Kaviratna, A.C. & Sharma, P. (trans) (1996-1997). Caraka samhita. In: *Chaukhamba orientalia*.

Lipner, J. (1989). On abortion and the moral status of the unborn. In: H.G. Coward, J. Lipner, & K.K. Young (Eds.), *Hindu ethics* (pp. 41-69). New York: State University of New York Press.

Manu (1984). *The sacred books of the east*. Muller, F.M. (Ed.). Delhi: Motilal Banarsidass.

Manu (1992). *The laws of Manu*. W. Doniger (trans). New York: Penguin.

Matilal, B. (1989). Moral dilemmas: Insights from Indian epics. In: B.K. Matilal (Ed.), *Moral Dilemmas in the Mahabharata*. New Delhi: Motilal Banarsidass.

Menon, A. & Habermas, H. (trans.) (1989). Oath of initiation, in Caraka Samhita. In: R.M. Veatch (Ed.), *Cross cultural perspectives in medical ethics: Readings* (pp. 130-132). Boston: Jones and Bartlett Publishers.

Quill, T. (1993). *Death and dignity*. New York: W.W. Norton & Company.

Rao, S. (1978). Population ethics: A Hindu perspective. In: W.T. Reich (general Ed.), *Encyclopedia of bioethics* (1271), New York: The Free Press.

Saraswati A. (Ed.) (2001). *Katha upanisad*. San Francisco: Viking Press.

Srikantha Murthy, K. (1989). Professional ethics in ancient India. In: Veatch 1989 (pp. 126-130).

Veatch, R. (1988). Models for ethical medicine in a revolutionary age. In: J.D. Callahan (Ed.), *Ethical issues in professional life* (pp. 89-92), New York: Oxford University Press.

Veatch, R. (1989). *Cross-cultural perspectives in medical ethics: Readings*. Boston: Jones and Bartlett.

Zimmer, H.R. (1948). *Hindu medicine*. Baltimore: The Johns Hopkins Press.

Zysk, K.G. (1991). *Asceticism and healing in ancient India*. New York: Oxford University Press.

Sikh Perspectives on Bioethics[1]

Devinder Singh Chahal

I. Introduction

Religion has been an element of human life since man became aware of himself and his environment. As such, religious traditions and rituals can have significant influence on the human mind. Nevertheless, the scientific age within which we now live challenges the often unscientific and illogical traditions and rituals of various religions.

Sikhism, founded by Guru Nanak during the 15th century, is one of the youngest, most scientific, and most logic-oriented religions of the world. Although it originated before the results of dramatic changes in science, technology, economics, and psychology yet influenced culture, Sikhism rejected the myths found in existing religions. Guru Nanak also challenged most of the religious and social laws the priestly class and ruling parties had developed to control the peoples of south Asia.

In light of the challenges Sikhism poses to ancient traditions and rituals, its approach to bioethics ought to be distinctive. However, very little has been written on bioethics from the Sikh perspective. What has been written generally does not give reference to Sikh religious texts or authorities. For example, Sahni (1993, pp. 25-27) has written on religious faith and modern medicine, and Singh (2000, pp. 16-21) has written on science, religion and bioethics in a Sikh journal without giving any reference to the Sikh religious text or Sikh approach to bioethics. Moreover, I have been unable to find any reference to the Sikh perspective on bioethics from any Sikh religious authorities in India. From Balambal (1997), we can infer that the development of bioethics in Sikhism remains indistinctive because the Indian Constitution groups Buddhism, Jainism, and Sikhism with Hinduism. Whenever bioethical issues arise, they are discussed in terms of Hinduism, Islam, Christianity, Judaism, Zoroastrianism, etc. without reference to the Sikh perspective. This is in part the fault of Skikh religious authorities that have, for the most part, remained silent on issues in bioethics. Abortion of female fetuses and infanticide, *sati* (self-immolation by a wife in the funeral fire or pyre of her husband), and genital mutilation are the exceptions. For the most part, however, the primary concern of Sikh religious authorities has been on the importance of maintaining an external physical identity for the Sikhs.

This chapter may be the first discussion of bioethics from the Sikh perspective in which the views presented are supported by quotations from a religious text, the *Aad Guru Granth Sahib* (*AGGS*).

II. History

"Medical ethics" or "bioethics" traces its roots to several early codes of ethics. The first was the ancient Greek Hippocratic Oath, which required physicians above all to "do no harm." It also referred to professional codes of ethics, such as that written by English physician Thomas Percival in the 18th century, which also provided a foundation for the first code of ethics established in 1846 by the founders of the American Medical Association. The last was the Nuremberg Code for research ethics on human subjects, established during the war crime trials at the close of World War II (1939-1945) in response to the gross abuses in human experimentation in Nazi Germany. The advent of new medical and reproductive technologies after the 1950s further complicated the moral and societal issues of medical research and practice, prompting further discussion of bioethical issues. A few examples of bioethical issues that developed during the evolution of Sikhism during the 15th and 17th centuries are discussed below.

A. The Practice of Sati

Before the advent of Sikhism during the 15th century, the practice of *sati* was very common in India. *Sati* refers to the practice of a wife burning herself in the pyre of her husband in order to meet her husband in the next world. She will remain in heaven as many years as the number of hairs on the body of her husband. This practice is a disgrace to the wife, who might otherwise have many years of life ahead of her, perhaps with another man, and be able to raise her children to be good citizens. The *sati* practice was condemned by the Sikh Gurus during the 15th and 16th centuries in their *Bani* ("sacred words"). They declared that the practice of *sati* to obtain salvation or to meet one's husband in the next world is an unscientific, illogical, and unacceptable practice: "It was a custom for the wife to burn herself in the pyre of her husband. By doing so she cannot meet her husband in the next world, but instead falls in the cycle of rebirths" (*AGGS*, M5, p.185).[2]

The Sikh Gurus initiated a change in the religious thought of the people so that they began to oppose *sati* during the 15th century. *Sati* is worse than euthanasia, which has been discussed so often in the field of bioethics. In euthanasia, the affected person may request to be killed. In the case of *sati*, the widow has no choice; she is forced to burn herself in her husband's pyre by her in-laws and society at large. If she does not burn herself willingly, she is forcibly thrown into the fire. *Sati* is equivalent to murder.

In light of Sikh teachings on *sati*, Raja Ram Mohan Rai, founder of Brahm Samaj asked Lord Bentinck to ban the practice of *sati* in the early 19th century. He banned this practice on December 7, 1829, in the Punjab and then in the adjoining state, Rajputana, in 1847 (Singh, 1981). Now *sati* is banned throughout India.

B. Genital Mutilation

In Sikhism, circumcision (genital mutilation) is banned on the grounds that it in no way helps one to be a good person. For example,

> Make every hour of time as auspicious. Remember the Almighty all the time. Suppressing your ten senses be your rosary. Following the principles of self-discipline be your circumcision.
> [and]

> Apply your body to do good deeds to make it as your faithful wife. And enjoy the Holy delights. Purifying your mind and keeping your body complete (without circumcision) should be your Hadith (Code of Conduct). That will be an honor like a turban on your head (a feather in your cap) (*AGGS*, M5, p. 1084).

III. Nanakian Philosophy and Bioethics

There are no bioethics centers in Punjab, the region of India where the majority of Sikhs live. The FIAMC (Federation Internationale des Associations Medical Catholique) Bio-Medical Ethics Center in Bombay, established in 1981, claims to be secular in nature and it includes representatives of diverse religious beliefs (Hindus, Buddhists, Muslims, Jews, Zoroastrians, Christians, as well as atheists and agnostics). However, there is no Sikh representative, and Sikhs were not involved in their early discussions on euthanasia held during 1982.

The Shiromani Gurdwara Parbandhak Committee (SGPC), the Religious Authority on Sikhism, in Amritsar, has not appointed anyone to develop the Sikh perspective on bioethical issues. There appears to be only one person, Dr. Surjit Kaur Chahal of the Department of Philosophy at University of Pune, Pune, India, who is involved in bioethics and environmental issues in Sikhism. However, she has not yet published on the issue such that the Sikh perspective on bioethics is not represented in the bioethics literature.

The Sikh religious authorities during the 19th and 20th centuries focused on maintaining the physical identity and social ethics of Sikhs. The *Sikh Rehit Maryada* (*SRM*, "Sikh Code of Conduct"), which was formulated during the 1930s by the top scholars in Sikhism, was presented to the Shiromani Gurdwara Parbandhak Committee (SGPC), Amritsar, India, in 1945. The *SRM* is followed by all Sikh religious authorities, institutions, and individuals as a code for religious and ethical behavior. The key teachings include the prohibition of female feticide and infanticide, smoking, the consumption of drugs, and adultery. Physical identity requires uncut hair, and Sikh men must wear a turban, shorts as underwear, an iron bangle on the right hand, and a *kirpan* (sword) for the *Amritdhari* Sikhs (initiated Sikhs). If the hair is to be removed for some reason, such as an operation, the affected *Amritdhari* Sikh can ask the *Punj Pyaras* (Five Initiated Sikhs) for exoneration. Sikhs are also not to eat kosher or *halal* meat, meat prepared by killing the animal by slow bleeding. Therefore, in hospitals, the *Amritdhari* Sikhs should not be served with kosher meat. Although these teachings are important for Sikhs, many other issues, including those raised by medical and scientific advances, must also be addressed. The *SRM* must be revised to apply Sikh religious texts to biotechnological advances.

Progress in biotechnology is proceeding at a rapid pace and it is becoming difficult for almost all religions, including Sikhism, to monitor and respond to new developments. For this reason, as well as the fact that there are no official Sikh teachings on bioethics, we must understand some important features of Sikh religious texts to formulate an understanding of bioethics from the Sikh perspective.

A. Nanakian Philosophy

Guru Nanak promulgated a unique philosophy, which is understood as scientifically and logically sound and as having the potential to be universally acceptable. His philosophy, known as "Nanakian philosophy," is often called *Gurbani* in Punjabi. It was preached and enriched by the nine Sikh Gurus who succeeded him in the House of Nanak or the Nanakian School. Followers of his philosophy are known as *Sikh* ("disciple") in Punjabi and his philosophy is called *Sikhi* in Punjabi. According to the *AGGS*, "*Sikhi* is the teachings of the Guru's philosophy" (*AGGS*, M1, p. 465). The Guru referred to in this definition is *Sabd* ("word") (*AGGS*, M1, p. 943). The word *Sikhi* gave rise to the modern anglicized word "Sikhism."

The Nanakian philosophy was incorporated into a *Granth* ("Holy Book") in 1604 by Guru Arjan, the fifth Guru in succession to the House of Nanak. The *Granth* is now called *Aad Guru Granth Sahib* (*AGGS*). Around 1705-1706, Guru Gobind Singh, the Tenth Guru to the House of Nanak, added the *Bani* of the Ninth Guru, Guru Teg Bahadur. Since then, the *AGGS* has been the only authenticated source of Nanakian philosophy.

Although some Sikh theologians try to maintain significant distance between science and Nanakian philosophy, Nanakian philosophy is scientific and logical in its origin (Chahal, 2000a, 2000b). Because of the close relationship between science and Nanakian Philosophy, good knowledge of science is necessary to understand and interpret Nanakian philosophy. The theologians who try to distinguish and separate the two are unable to interpret Nanakian philosophy appropriately.

B. Central Features of Nanakian Philosophy Regarding Ethical Decision-Making

Nanakian philosophy emphasizes critical thinking and analysis. This is central to understanding its approach to bioethics. The most important characteristic of Sikhism is that one must evaluate each act or choice by asking whether it is good for an individual life or for humanity. If it is, then one should pursue it: "One must evaluate the things/philosophy, if convinced, then adopt/follow it" (*AGGS*, M1, p. 1410). In order to do this, one must use one's intellect to distinguish between good and bad, true and false, right and wrong, etc: "Those who have discriminating intellect can understand things in their real perspective" (*AGGS*, M5, p. 285). To formulate positions on issues in bioethics, therefore, one must use one's discriminating intellect to evaluate practices and uses of technology. Finally, it has been emphasized that it is important to do research to resolve mysteries and obscure phenomena before formulating any ethical code: "The researcher progresses while the other (discursive and aimless) perishes, (Nanak) sacrifices himself on the Guru, the Creator" (*AGGS*, M1, p. 1255). Therefore, to formulate positions on bioethical issues may require further research.

C. Some Concepts in Nanakian Philosophy

Here I discuss some key concepts in Nanakian philosophy that would inform the Sikh understanding of bioethical issues, both those we face today and ones that might arise in the future. These are basic ways of understanding the world that shape the Sikh outlook.

C.1. Concept of Life and God

A clear concept of life and God is necessary before one can make decisions regarding the application or use of biotechnological advances (Chahal, 2002).

Scientists in recent years have mapped the human genome. Humans share many genes with yeast, mold, slime, worms, fruit flies, and lettuce; about 90% of our genome is indistinguishable from that of mice and approximately 98% is the same as chimpanzees'. Thus small differences in our DNA mark us as human rather than anything else. Moreover, a variation of only 0.2% separates individual humans from one another (Munro, 2000). The impact of the human genome map is expected to be enormous. It will help us determine if an individual is prone to develop a particular disease, such as Alzheimer's disease, heart problems, high cholesterol, or addiction to tobacco or alcohol, for example. Gene therapy may help to alter the course of such conditions or diseases. The transfer of human genes to pigs may make it possible to produce organs for transplants into humans (Munro, 2000).

In light of these facts, we now consider elements of Sikh philosophy that can inform decisions regarding appropriate responses to these possibilities.

First, the similarities between our DNA and that of other organisms is compatible with the Sikh view that our roots ultimately lie in the *Jyot*, the Energy or the Almighty: "Hey Mind! Recognize your roots. You are from the primordial Energy (the Jyot – the Almighty)" (*AGGS*, M3, p. 441). The close genetic relationship between humans and microorganisms is compatible with the Nanakian philosophical view that we have evolved from these tiny beings: "After passing through many lives of microorganisms. ... and other lives successively man was evolved" (*AGGS*, M5, p. 176). Second, as the most highly evolved being, Nanakian philosophy holds that man is the commander on earth and that all other forms of life are at his service: "All the other forms of life are at your service. (Therefore) You are the commander on this earth" (*AGGS*, M5, p. 374). As a highly evolved being who is the master of the earth, it is the duty of every human being to maintain good health and to be productive. No human should be allowed to damage another human being.

Third, Sikhs hold that the Almighty has always existed and will always exist: "It (the Almighty) was in existence before the appearance of time and space. And was in existence in the Past. It is in existence in the present and will be in existence forever" (*AGGS*, Jap, p. 1).

Fourth, according to Nanakian philosophy, human life is precious and it is a gift we receive only once; it cannot be attained again and again through rebirth. Thus human life should be preserved at all costs and we must always focus on the future of our one life: "Think about the future, look not in the past. Make the present life a great success because there is no birth again" (*AGGS*, M5, p. 1096).

C.2. The Laws of the Universe

The basic Laws of the Universe govern every action and reaction. Nanakian philosophy makes reference to these laws in various verses. First, the Nanakian account of the origins of the universe, offered in the 15th century, is similar to the "big bang" theory widely held today. According to Guru Nanak: "The universe exploded with one sound (big bang) and started to expand. Thereafter appeared many things" (*AGGS*, M1, p. 3). "Many things" here refers to gases, particles, matter, and laws.

Second, Guru Nanak taught that after the big bang and the creation of the laws of the universe, everything was subject to these laws, with the exception of the Almighty:

> Under the laws of the universe, air always blows; hundreds of thousand rivers flow; the energy performs different works; earth moves; clouds move; and birth and death are under the laws; sun and moon (planets) are moving tens

> of millions of miles; *Sid, Budh, Sur, Naath*; the sky; the soldiers and strongest warriors; all of them appear and disappear under the law. In Fact everything is under the laws of the universe (*AGGS*, M1, p. 464).

Third, Guru Nanak teaches that the key to rejecting egoism is to understand the laws of the universe and the fact that all beings are within the bounds of these laws (*AGGS*, Jap1, p. 1).

In light of this view of the universe, Sikh theologians formulating views on issues in bioethics should recognize that biotechnological advances are developing under the laws of the universe, which are laws of the Almighty. When these laws are applied for the benefit of human welfare, then nothing violates the Will of God.

C.3. Diet

With advancement of genetic engineering, new vegetables and fruits, milk- and meat-producing animals, and eggs have been introduced in the food market. Many religious people are against the use of such genetically-modified foods. As these advances are taking place under the laws of the universe, there is no reason to universally prohibit them from the point of view of Nanakian philosophy.

A more controversial topic among Sikhs today is the permissibility of eating meat. The Sikh code (*SRM*) does not permit the consumption of meat if the animal was slaughtered by bleeding slowly under rituals, i.e., kosher or *halal* meat. However, according to the *Hukmnama* (edict) of Jathedar Sadhu Singh Bhaura of the Akal Takht dated February 15, 1980, it is permissible to eat *jatka*, the flesh of animals slaughtered with one stroke of *kirpan* (sword).

Many people who are against meat-eating hold this position because they think that it is sinful to kill conscious living organisms. They eat plant material because they think that plants are not living organisms who are conscious of being killed. The distinction between the level of conscience of animals and plants is grounded in the belief that every living organism, whether single-celled or multi-cellular, whether plant or animal, is conscious and is aware of the conditions inside of its body as well as in its environment. The fact that they try to protect themselves from the adverse conditions as soon as their lives are threatened supports this claim. Most importantly, Guru Nanak's teachings suggest the universality of conscience among living organisms:

> The Almighty has given same consciousness to all the living beings. No living being is without consciousness. The living beings will follow the way of life according to their level of consciousness. They come into existence (take birth) and go away (die) according to the information written (on their genes) (*AGGS*, M1, p. 24).

Because of the universality of consciousness, it is questionable to permit the consumption of plants and not animals because it is very difficult to distinguish between a plant and an animal in some cases. For example, *Euglena* is an organism, which has chlorophyll and, like plants, can synthesize its own food under certain conditions. However, it depends on ready-made food under other conditions. At those times, it ingests food particles and excretes waste like an animal. *Euglena* is a link between plants and animals.

Guru Nanak explains this phenomenon to convince people that plants and animals share some characteristics that make it impossible to distinguish between them: "Only fools wrangle about eating of meat [because] they don't know what is called a meat (animal), and what is called a *saag* (plant) and eating of which results in committing of a sin" (*AGGS*, M1, p. 1289).

If the plants and animals are indistinguishable, Guru Nanak asks how we are to determine what we may and may not eat. The key is whether or not the food in question promotes health or causes harm. If a particular food, whether plant- or animal-based, whether "natural" or obtained from genetically engineered plants or animals, is harmful to a person's health, disturbs the mind, or causes an allergic reaction in him, then the person is forbidden to eat that food (*AGGS*, M1, p. 16). According to Nanakian philosophy, no food should be declared as universally forbidden, whether plant or animal. Therefore, according to Nanakian philosophy, Sikhs may consume any food that is safe for humans.

C.4. Altruism

Altruism is the most important feature of the Nanakian philosophy, because every human being is considered a child of the Almighty such that we are all brothers and sisters. Therefore, Nanakian philosophy emphasizes that we should perform good deeds, treat everyone equally, and use our education to improve the welfare of humanity. This is what it is to live in service to the Almighty.

Guru Nanak explains that service to the Guru/Almighty is doing good deeds and treating everyone equally: "The service of the Guru is to comprehend his philosophy. Killing your ego and doing good deeds are equal to all your meditation, austerities and reading of Puranas" (*AGGS*, M1, p. 223). Second, we are called to treat everyone equally: "Call everyone high, none appears to be low; everyone has been molded from the same matter; and the same source of light shines in all" (*AGGS*, M1, p. 62). Third, whatever type of education is obtained, it should also be applied for the welfare of humanity (*AGGS*, M1, p. 356).

IV. Topics in Bioethics

A. Reproduction

A.1. Abortion

Abortion is a sensitive issue because it involves social, religious, and economic elements. There also are cases in which the health of the mother is a factor. From the social and religious points of view of Sikhs, for a child to be born out of wedlock or as a result of rape is so serious that either an abortion is performed secretly or the pregnant woman commits suicide. Some mothers have abortions not for social and religious reasons but for economic or family planning reasons.

Recently, with the advancement in science and use of ultrasound, the sex of the fetus can be determined. As a result, the abortion rate of female fetuses in Sikh families in Punjab villages has increased so much that it has threatened natural balance of males and females. Before the availability of such technology, female infanticide was common in some Sikh families, even though such killing is against the codes in the *Sikh Rehit Maryada* (*SRM*) (Sikh Rehit Maryada, 1945).

A.2. In Vitro *Fertilization (IVF)*

Some have argued that IVF is an unnatural means of procreating disconnected from God's design because fertilization occurs outside the womb without the intimacy of a husband and wife. However, a close examination of IVF reveals that it proceeds under the laws of the universe. Despite the location of fertilization and the role of physicians and scientists, it coheres with the Laws of the Almighty. Therefore, IVF is not against the Will of God.

It is now possible not only to fertilize an egg *ex utero* but to examine the developing embryo for defective genes before implanting the embryo in the womb of the mother. Parents may use this information to decide whether or not they will keep the embryo. This is where the issue becomes complicated for Sikhs. There are no specific guidelines on this issue in the Nanakian philosophy. In such cases, we are to use our discriminating intellect (*Babaek Budhi*) in consultation with doctors and scientists to determine an appropriate course of action.

A.3. Birth Control

There is no direct reference to birth control in Nanakian philosophy. Here again one has to use one's discriminating intellect (*Babaek Budhi*) to make choices.

B. Death and Dying

B.1. Euthanasia and Physician-Assisted Suicide

Euthanasia is a complex issue, and decisions regarding euthanasia must take into consideration a patient's health. There are no specific guidelines either in the *SRM* or in Nanakian philosophy on this issue. However, decisions on this matter should be made after careful consideration of the position of doctors, scientists, the patient's family, and the patient, if he is capable of participating in such decisions.

B.2. Hospice Care and Care of the Dying

In Sikhism, hospice care for the destitute, the mentally ill, and the handicapped is thought of as a service to humanity. Puran Singh (1904-1992), often addressed as *Bhagat* (a devotee of the Almighty), began providing hospice care in 1947 to a leper in a one-bed facility at Amritsar after Punjab was divided into Pakistan Punjab and India Punjab. It soon became a 7-bed hospice with only the shade of a tree as cover. Now his hospice is managed by All India Pingalwara Society and is funded partly by the SGPC, and partly by public donations. The center has 450 beds. Destitute members of any religion, including Hinduism, Sikhism, Islam, and Christianity, are welcome there. Khushwant Singh (Singh, 2000) has given Puran Singh the title of "Bearded Mother Teresa of Punjab," comparing his work with that of Mother Teresa in Calcutta. The importance of providing care to the dying is supported by the importance of altruism in Nanakian philosophy.

C. *Access to Health Care*

The objective of the SGPC is to provide health care to everyone in need either for free or at the lowest possible charge. For this purpose, the SGPC fully funds a 700-bed Medical College (Guru Ram Das Medical Educational and Research Hospital, Amritsar) and a Dental College with a Hospital (Guru Ram Das Institute of Dental Sciences, Amritsar). Nanakian philosophy emphasizes equality such that Sikhism accepts no disparity among persons. Thus all are treated equally in these facilities.

One area in which Sikhs were leaders in providing access to health care for those who otherwise would not receive care was in the battlefield. Bhai Kanhaiya became the follower of Guru Gobind Singh, the Tenth Guru, in 1705. He was advised by Guru Gobind Singh to treat the wounded soldiers after battle. They were cared for regardless of whether they belonged to the army of Guru Gobind Singh or to that of the foes (Singh, 1992-1999). Guru Gobind Singh and Bhai Kanhaiya were the first who established the system of treating the wounded soldiers, a practice later adopted by Jean Henri Durant and pursued by the Red Cross. Durant, a Swiss citizen who visited the battlefield after the clash between the Austrian and French armies on June 24, 1859, gathered the people from neighboring villages and organized the care of all the soldiers regardless of their origin. On the recommendation of Durant, on February 9, 1863, the Geneva Society for Public Welfare created a Red Cross Society, now called International Committee of the Red Cross. Durant was awarded a Nobel Peace Prize for this achievement in 1901. However, idea behind the Red Cross, caring for all in need regardless of their alliances, had been practiced by the Sikhs over 150 years prior to Durant's work.

D. *Ethics Consultations and Ethics Committees*

The SGPC at Amritsar is the only Sikh Religious Authority that can play a role in promulgating positions on bioethical issues from the Sikh perspective. According to personal communication with Mr. Kirpal Singh, Internet Officer with SGPC at Amritsar, and Prof. Prithipal Singh Kapur, Department of Encyclopedia of Sikhism, Punjabi University, Patiala, there is no department or section in the SGPC that is dealing with bioethical issues. However, the SGPC recognizes that such a departments is necessary to address with bioethical issues as they arise in the future.

Notes

1. The author would like to thank Dr. Parminder Singh Chahal, Biotechnology Research Institute, Montreal, Quebec, Canada for commenting on this manuscript and for his valuable suggestions to improve it. The author is also thankful to Prof. (Mrs.) Surjit Kaur Chahal, Department of Philosophy, University of Pune, Pune; Dr Harbans Singh, Principal (Retired), Ludhiana; Dr Prithipal Singh Kapur, Department of Encyclopedia of Sikhism, Punjabi University, Patiala; Dr Satnam Singh Sandhu, Liaison Officer between Institute for Understanding Sikhism, Quebec, Canada and Punjabi University, Patiala, India; and Mr Kirpal Singh, Internet Officer, Shiromani Gurdwara Parbandhak Committee, Amritsar, India for their help in seeking information about work on bioethics done by the Sikh Religious Authorities and Sikh scholars in India.
2. In references to *AGGS*, M refers to *Mahla*, the succession number of the Sikh Gurus to the House of Nanak. Jap refers to the title of the Bani in the *AGGS*.

Bibliography

Aad Guru Granth Sahib (*AGGS*). (1983 reprint). Amritsar: Shiromani Gurdwara Parbandhak Committee.

Balambal. (1997). Religion-identity-human values-Indian context. In: J. Azariah, H. Azariah, & D.R.J. Macer (Eds.), *Bioethics in India*. Proc. intl. Bioethics Workshop in the University of Madras, Madras. Christchurch, New Zealand: Eubios Ethics Institute [On-line]. Available: http://www.biol.tsukuba.ac.jp/~macer/index.html

Chahal, D.S. (2000a). The commencing verse of the Aad Guru Granth Sahib. *Understanding Sikhism Res. J. 2:1*, 8-19.

Chahal, D.S. (2000b). Sikhism: Scientific and logical religion for the third millennium. *Understanding Sikhism Res. J. 2:2*, 7-23 & 33.

Chahal, D.S. (2002). A unique concept of God in Nanakian philosophy. *Understanding Sikhism Res. J. 4:2*, 5-16.

Munro, M. (March 13, 14, 15, 2000). Book of life. *National Post* (Montreal).

Sahni, H.S. (May 1993). Religious faith and modern medicine. *The Sikh Review 41* (Calcutta), 25-27.

Sikh Rehit Maryada (in Punjabi). (1945). Amritsar: Shiromani Gurdwara Parbandhak Committee.

Singh, H. (1992-1999). *The encyclopedia of Sikhism*. Patiala, India: Punjabi University.

Singh, I.J. (April 2000). Science and religion: Bioethical issues. *The Sikh Review 48* (Calcutta), 16-21.

Singh, K. (Bhai) (1981). *Mahan Kosh* (in Punjabi). Bhasha Vibhag: Punjab, Patiala.

Singh, K. (December 16, 2000). The father Teresa of Punjab. *The Tribune* (Chandigarh). [On-line].

Daoism and Bioethics: Daode Jin's Doctrine of Naturalness and the Principle of Non-Action

Jonathan Chan

I. Does Daoism Have an Ethics?

This paper aims to reconstruct a Daoist theory of bioethics with reference to *Daode jin* (*Lao-tzu*). Before proceeding, we nevertheless need to address to the question of whether Lao-tzu Daoism has an ethics or not. Since Lao-tzu Daoism has often been construed as a philosophical movement that criticized the conventionalism of Confucian morality, one might doubt whether there is such a thing as Lao-tzu Daoist ethics at all, not to mention a Daoist bioethics. The answer to this question depends on how we understand the notion of ethics or morality. Daoism does not have an ethics in the Kantian or Confucian sense, which understands ethical action in terms of moral duty or obligation. Confucianism, for instance, holds that there are obligations that each of us should perform on the basis of the five social relationships: ruler-minister, father-son, husband-wife, elder-younger brother, friend-friend. Consider one's moral obligations in the father-son relationship. According to Confucianism, the father always should treat his son with care and concern while the son owes his father obedience and respect. As to the ruler-minister relationship, the minister should have loyalty toward the ruler while the ruler should treat the minister in accordance with the proper etiquette. For Confucianism, the aforementioned role-based moral obligations find their expression in a set of rules of *li* or ritual which, in turn, is an outward expression of an inner moral quality, *ren* or humaneness. It is only by following the rules of *li* that one could achieve humaneness. Using these cardinal Confucian moral precepts, *li* and *ren*, Confucianism distinguishes between two different categories of people – the "gentleman" and the "small man". The gentleman is the one who live by superior moral standards, i.e., by the rules of *li*, with a view to achieving his humaneness. The small man is deemed as morally inferior since he does not concern himself about his humaneness and has no intention to live by the rules of *li*.

Daoism, however, rejects all the Confucian moral precepts and, thereby, the distinction between morally superior and morally inferior people. The Daoist rejects the Confucian morals and virtues on the ground that they bury the inherent purity of the *Dao*. *Daode jin* makes this point clearly:

> Therefore, when the Great Way is rejected, it is then that we have the virtues of humanity and righteousness;
>
> When knowledge and wisdom appear, it is then that there is great hypocrisy (*Daode jin*, 18).

Then, we are told to

> Eliminate sageliness, throw away knowledge,
> And the people will benefit a hundredfold.
> Eliminate humanity, throw away righteousness,
> And the people will return to filial piety and compassion (*Daode jin*, 19).

This passage requires some explanation. One might wonder whether it is inconsistent to tell people to "eliminate humanity, throw away righteousness" and at the same time see "return to filial piety and compassion" as something recommendable, for "filial piety and compassion" is regarded as the core of morality by Confucianism. The inconsistency is, however, only apparent. To appreciate this point, we only need to make a distinction between moral goodness and non-moral goodness with respect to filial piety and compassion. It is not inconsistent to deny filial piety and compassion to have moral goodness and at the same time to hold the view that they are valuable, for they may possess non-moral goodness. For instance, Daoism may value filial piety and compassion on the basis of their naturalness, and hold the view that naturalness is the highest good in the non-moral sense. Then, Daoism may see "return to filial piety and compassion" as something good if achieved naturally and something bad if deemed as one's moral obligation. There is no inconsistency being involved.

It is clear then that from the fact that Daoism rejects the Confucian morality, it does not follow that Daoism does not have an ethics. Indeed, Daoism does have an ethics in the sense that it prescribes a certain way of life. The prescriptive verses such as "Eliminate sageliness, throw away knowledge" and "Eliminate humanity, throw away righteousness" are prescriptions for guiding one to live the Daoist way of life. They are not moral prescriptions. Acting contrary to these prescriptions is not doing something impermissible but only unadvisable. It is unadvisable because doing so would blind one to go further away from the *Dao*, and to live a Daoist way of life is to follow the course of the *Dao*.

II. Naturalness: the Core Value of the Daoist Ethics

But what is it meant by "following the course of the *Dao*"? If the Daoist way of life, on which the Daoist ethical perspective depends, is embodied in the ethical injunction of following the course of *Dao*, then it is necessary for the Daoist to specify the conditions under which one is said to be following the course of the *Dao*. To understand the above ethical injunction, we first need to capture one important aspect of the *Dao*, namely, its naturalness. In *Daode jin*, there is an important passage that expresses this important aspect:

> Man models himself on the Earth;
> The Earth models itself on Heaven;
> Heaven models itself on the Tao;
> And the Tao models itself on naturalness (*Daode jin*, 25).

The last line makes it explicit that the *Dao* models itself on the principle of naturalness. It should be noted that this reading does not imply that there exists an abstract entity called "naturalness" and the *Dao* models itself on this entity (Liu, 1998). Rather, it means only that the Dao itself exemplifies naturalness, the property which is inherent in all things, including humans, Earth, Heaven, and even the *Dao*. Along this line of interpretation, following the course of the *Dao*, then, should be understood as following the principle of naturalness. Accordingly, to live a Daoist life is to follow the principle of naturalness.

Still, we need to ask what it is meant by "following the principle of naturalness." As "naturalness" or "being natural" does not have a precise meaning in ordinary language, some clarification of these expressions is needed, if the principle of naturalness is to be used as an ethical guide to human actions. In applying the principle to bioethical issues, for instance, how do we distinguish the natural from the unnatural? Is using vaccine or carrying out a surgery unnatural? Is letting a terminally ill patient die natural and assisting that patient to kill him or herself unnatural? After all, why does naturalness matter in such cases?

III. Two Views of Naturalness in the Western History of Ethics

One account of naturalness or the natural is that to be natural is to follow the course of nature. This view of the natural can be traced back to the Stoic ethical doctrine that maxims of human conduct were the dictates of nature. This doctrine, in turn, derives from a more fundamental metaphysical doctrine that all processes are governed by cosmic reason (*logos*), and law (*nomos*) is what this universal rational principle dictates concerning the various sphere of activity. The Stoics developed an explicitly deterministic account of cosmos. According to this account, nature is a rational being that permeates the universe in the form of a divine "breath". The physical world is not an accident, but a necessary consequence of the design of this rational being. Thus, everything that happens, in the final analysis, must be considered to be determined by nature. Basing on this understanding of nature, the Stoics held that the human good consists in the perfection of human reason. The best way to achieve perfect rationality is to live "in agreement with nature", i.e., to conform to the rational order of the universe. For the Stoics, nature when considered as a whole is perfect. It is humanity's task to achieve that perfection by living in harmony with nature.

The Stoics' account of the natural as outlined above is open to objection on three scores. First, if everything that happens is determined by nature, then the injunction to conform to the laws of nature is pointless. For it is a physical impossibility for anyone not to conform. This is exactly the same argument that Mill, in his classic paper "Nature", used to argue against the aforementioned injunction as a principle by which to regulate human conduct:

> To bid people conform to the laws of nature when they have no power but what the laws of nature give them – when it is a physical impossibility for them to do the smallest thing otherwise than through some law of nature, is an absurdity (Mill, 1998, p. 16).

Second, the Stoics' account of the natural implies that the course of nature is taken as good, incapable of improvement, and that we should let nature take its course. Still, the implied views are open to objection too. Scarcity of food, floods, epidemics and droughts are all natural events. But no reasonable person would regard them as commendable. Indeed, we human beings put great effort to interrupt the course of nature, of which those natural disasters are only a part. In considering the implied views in the context of bioethics, it suffices to point out that the practice of medicine is in fact a large scale human interruption of the course of nature. In the aforementioned paper, Mill made a similar point:

> Everybody professes to approve and admire many great triumphs of Art over Nature ... But to commend these and similar feats, is to acknowledge that the ways of Nature are to be conquered, not obeyed: that her powers are often towards man in the position of enemies, from whom he must wrest, by force and ingenuity, what little he can for his own use, and deserves to be applauded when that little is rather more than might be expected from his physical weakness in comparison to those gigantic powers (Mill, 1998, p. 20).

We do not need to embrace Mill's view that nature is often hostile and an enemy to be conquered. Nor do we, however, need to accept the Stoics' view that nature is perfect and incapable of improvement. One final argument against the Stoic view of the natural is that the injunction of following the course of nature is either devoid of content or impractical. For it is unclear on what criterion an action is said not to "follow the course of nature." One even might argue that from the Stoics' point of view, no single human action is said to be not following the course of nature, for human action is also one part of the natural order.

Another influential account of the natural in the Western history of ethics was offered by Aristotle. He adopted a biological model for explaining all kinds of natural processes. According to this biological model, a thing's nature is characterized by its inner principle of change, and a change will be natural if it is the work of this inner principle. It is this inner principle that allows a plant to grow, an animal to graze, and a man to think, fully as much as it allows the sun to be eclipsed or bodies to be in motion or at rest. For instance, an oak-tree goes over different stages, from seed to seedling to an oak-tree to decaying. Since this changing process is the result of the work of the inner principle of change of the oak-tree, the process is regarded as natural. However, if the changing process involves too much human intervention, say, due to changing the genetic constitution of the oak-tree artificially, the process is unnatural. The inner principle of a thing is that which determines the thing's being what it is or is to be. Then we may distinguish what is natural from the artificial in the following manner: natural objects are that which itself contains the determination of what it is or is to be, whereas artificial objects are that which has this determination elsewhere (Woodbridge, 1983, p. 53). For instance, in a sculpture the determination is not in the sculpture but the sculptor, while in an oak-tree the determination is in the oak-tree. In other words, in the sculpture no inner principle of the sculpture is responsible for its being what it is. In the oak-tree, there is inner principle that is responsible for its being what it is or is to be.

To apply this biological account of the natural to bioethics, what we need to consider is whether an action or practice in question is in harmony with the inner principle on which human beings base for their flourishing. Consider the cases of using DNA manipulation technology. Biological scientists already have developed some techniques for inserting particular pieces of DNA into an individual's stem cell line. These techniques may be used to correct genetic disorders resulting from the deficiency in a particular gene. Also, there are somatic line manipulations techniques for removing anomalous cells. For example, if anomalous cells were detected in the early embryo, we might remove them by killing them using toxins coupled to specific monoclonal antibodies which specifically recognized those abnormal cells. Besides somatic line manipulations techniques, biological scientists also have developed techniques for manipulating the germ line of an individual. These techniques have been used on animals successfully and may be used on humans in the near future. The significance of using these technologies is that operations on the germ line of an individual alter the genome of the individual and the modifications will be passed to its offspring.

Is using these gene manipulation technologies for medical purposes such as replacing a defective gene natural? The answer is negative, if the biological account of the natural is to be considered. For the changes brought about by using the technologies would not be the results of the work of the inner principles of the individuals to whom the technologies were applied. Consider, for instance, a patient who suffers from a genetic disorder resulting from the deficiency of a particular gene. The patient's genetic disorder might be corrected by using somatic gene therapy. However, doing so would not be natural because the cure, that is, the change, was brought about by inserting a healthy gene into the patient, the cause that was not inherent in the patient. On the biological account, the cause must be inherent in the thing, if the change that occurred in it is to be counted as natural. Consider another example of using techniques of inserting genes into human beings. In this case, the purpose of using the techniques would not be to repair genetic defects but to enhance function. This would be done by inserting new type of genes that are not normally possessed by human beings. For instance, it may be possible in the near future to insert individual genes that code for genes that would retard ageing. Similarly, doing so would not be natural since the cause that brought about the change, that is, the retardation of ageing, was not a cause inherent in human beings. Along this line of reasoning, we might argue that using biotechnologies such as *in vitro* fertilization, cloning embryo by cell mass division, cloning human by nuclear substitution would not be natural. For the causes that brought about the changes occurring in the individuals were not inherent in the individuals but rather resulted from something else.

The question we need to ask is: What conclusions can be drawn from the fact that a certain use of biotechnology on an individual is unnatural? If unnaturalness is a ground for not using the biotechnology in question, then the advocate of this view needs to face the challenge that almost the whole practice of medicine is unnatural. In many cases, people would not recover from illness without medical treatment. For instance, people who suffer from severe infections might be easily cured by given some antibiotics. However, their immune system alone might not be strong enough to cure the infections. In this case, curing the infections by using antibiotics would not be counted as natural because the change was not brought about by a cause inherent in the people. The advocate might be able to meet the challenge by adding some qualification to the condition under which an action is counted as unnatural. Consider, for example, how a fruit tree is grown. Under favorable conditions, a fruit tree will grow naturally, normally going over several stages, from seed to seedling to a mature fruit-tree. However, favorable conditions do not always exist. So fruit-growers may need to do a number of things such as fertilizing the soil, spraying, pruning, keeping away fruit-fly and so on so as to provide a favorable environment for a fruit-tree to grow. In some sense, what the fruit-growers do still could be counted as natural. For we may say what they do is to help the tree grow naturally by improving its environment. The "determining cause" that makes it grow naturally is still in it. However, if the fruit-growers made the fruit tree grow bigger by using techniques in genetic engineering, say, changing the genetic constituents of the fruit tree, then what the fruit-growers did could be counted as unnatural. For what they did is not improving the external conditions but changing the "inner principle" of the fruit tree. The way that the genetically engineered fruit tree grows does not result from the determining cause inherent in the fruit tree but in something else. This distinction between improving the external conditions and changing the inner principle of a thing, despite of its vagueness, seems to have some intuitive logical force. The advocate of the biological account might use the distinction to defend his or her ethical view that unnaturalness is a ground for not acting in a certain way. For, by appealing to such a distinction, we do not need to cast, say, using antibiotics to cure people's infections as unnatural, since so doing only removes the unfavorable external conditions which hinder people live healthily and does not change their inner principle of change. On the other hand, using the techniques of somatic cell gene therapy to cure genetic disorders or diseases would not be considered natural. For doing so would not so much improve the external conditions of the patients as change their "inner principle". Still, the question that remains to ask is: what is the moral significance of making such a distinction? Why is it so bad for an action to be counted as unnatural in the sense that it is not in accordance with the inner principle of an individual? For Aristotle, naturalness, if it is to have ethical significance, must be in some way related to the good of an individual. However, it is unclear how unnaturalness in the above sense may hinder the good of an individual? We need to ask, for instance, how inserting a healthy gene into an individual, granting its unnaturalness, would hinder his or her good.

IV. The Daoist Conception of Naturalness

Now let us turn to the question of how the Daoist understands the concept of naturalness. Apparently, Daoism seems to understand the concept of naturalness in some ways similar to those of the Stoics and Aristotle. For instance, *Daode jin* has a passage that argues for the practice of non-action

> The sage manages affairs without action (*wuwei*),
> And spreads doctrines without words,
> He lets all things arise, but claims no authority.
> He creates the myriad, but claims no possession.
> He accomplishes his task, but claims no credit.
> It is precisely because he does not claim credit that his accomplishment remains with him forever (*Daode jin*, 2).

Also, it writes

> He who takes an action fails.
> He who grasps things loses them.
> For this reason the sage takes no action and therefore does not fail.
> He grasps nothing and therefore he does not lose anything...
> The sage desires to have no desire.
> He does not value rare treasures,
> He learns to be unlearned, and returns to what the multitude has missed.
> Thus he supports the naturalness of ten thousand things and dares not take any action (*Daode jin*, 63).

Daode jin's doctrine of the practice of non-action seems to imply as much a conservative ethical position as that of the Stoics. As argued above, the Stoics account of the natural implies that the course of nature is taken as good, incapable of improvement, and that we should let nature take its course. The doctrine of the practice of non-action seems to imply also the ethical injunction of letting nature take its course, although on the different ground from that of the Stoics. For Daoism, the cosmos is not so much a design of a rational being as something naturally grounded on the *Dao*, a being that has neither consciousness nor rational intention, nor is it a deterministic one. But the doctrine of non-action, if taken literally, seems to imply the view that we should do nothing and let nature take its course. Indeed, this reading of Daoism seems to be held by some interpreter of Daoism. For instance, Kirkland, when exposing the Daoist moral ideals, made the following comment

> No Taoist of any persuasion ever embraced goal-directed action as a legitimate agency for solving problems. The *Tao te ching* in fact implies that, contrary to appearances, nature is ultimately more powerful than all human endeavor, and that if humans will refrain from taking any action, however well-intentioned, nature itself will inevitably rectify any problems.

Kirkland's comment implies two things. First, Daoism holds the view that no goal-directed action can legitimately be used to solve problems. Second, the *Daode jin* holds the view that if humans will refrain from taking any action, nature itself will inevitably rectify any problem. But these readings of Daoism, and of *Daode jin* in particular, are uncharitable. First, no one could sincerely follow the injunction like this: do not attempt to solve any problem yourself but let the nature solve it. Also, no one could sincerely believe: if we refrain from taking any action to solve problems, they will be gone because nature will rectify them. How could one sincerely believe, for instance, that natural disasters such as scarcity of food, floods, epidemics and droughts will be gone by themselves, if we humans refrain from taking any action? Second, *Daode jin* never gives "nature" such an important role as Kirkland assumes. In *Daode jin*, "naturalness" does have a very important role. As the quotation occurred in section two has shown, even the *Dao* models itself on naturalness. However, "naturalness" is not the same as "nature". "Naturalness" does not even refer to an entity. Rather, it refers to a thing's being in a certain state, namely, a state of being natural or acting spontaneously, and the state of being natural "indicates the condition when a thing is what it is by itself without any external impulse or interruption" (Liu, 1998, p. 221). For *Daode jin*, all things would be in the state of being natural, should they be in their ideal condition. The sage, an ideal Daoist, is the one who exemplifies this state of naturalness, in which he not only makes himself be in such an ideal condition, but also helps all other things be in that condition – "he supports the naturalness of ten thousand things." In helping other things to keep themselves in the state of naturalness, the sage tries intervene as little as possible. But it does not mean that he would not take any action. When it is necessary, he will take action which he deems appropriate, and the action taken is deemed appropriate when it effectively helps others be in their ideal condition, even though not being realized by others. A passage in *Daode jin* which describes how the best ruler rules his subjects make this point explicitly

> The best of all rulers is but a shadowy presence to his subjects.
> Next comes the ruler they love and praise;

> Next comes one they fear;
> Next comes one with whom they take liberties...
> When his task is accomplished and his work done
> The people all say, "It happened to us naturally" (*Daode jin*, 17).

Then, it is clear that the practice of "non-action" (*wuwei*) should not be understood as refraining from taking any action. What "non-action" (*wuwei*) means is "to keep oneself in the state of naturalness and to help all other things be in that state as possible as he or she can."

Now the question remains to be answered is: What exactly is "naturalness"? The definition of "naturalness" as "the condition when a thing is what it is by itself without any external impulse or interruption" does not tell us much about what that condition is. How do we tell when a thing is in that condition? The answer lies in the concept of "*de*". There is an important passage in *Daode jin*, which makes comments about "*de*"

> The way (*Dao*) gives them life;
> Virtue (*De*) rears them;
> Things give them shape;
> Circumstances bring them to maturity.
> Therefore the myriad creatures all revere the way (*Dao*) and honor virtue (*de*). Yet the way (Dao) is revered and virtue (*de*) honored not because this is decreed by any authority but because it is natural for them to be treated so (*Daode jin*, 51).

"*De*" is often translated as "virtue" in the sense of "power," "capacities," or "potency". However, on one influential interpretation, "*de*" is understood as the virtue of a thing, in the sense of what the thing gets from the *Dao* (Lau, 1989, p.xxxiv). Then, according to this interpretation, *de* is the "inner principle" of a thing that determines the thing's being what it is or is to be. Basing on the above understanding of the concept of "*de*", we thus may define "naturalness" as the state in which a thing acts or lives in accordance with its *de*. Accordingly, to be natural is to be in accordance with one's *de*. To act naturally toward a thing is act in accordance with not only the thing's *de* but also one's *de*.

Surprisingly, *Daode jin* seems to have a conception of the natural or naturalness as much as Aristotle's. To recall, for Aristotle, what is counted as natural depends on whether a change is the result of the work of the inner principle of a thing. This understanding of the natural seems not to be very much different from that of *Daode jin*. The similarity, however, is only apparent. To appreciate this point, we only need to note that "inner principle" and "*de*" are not terms that are metaphysically neutral. We should not read them out of context. For Aristotle, the concept of the "inner principle" of a thing presupposes a teleological framework that is absent in *Daode jin*. Aristotle understood the "inner principle" of a thing in terms of its *telos*. *Daode jin* understood a thing's "*de*" in terms of the *Dao*. For *Daode jin*, the significance of living in accordance with one's *de* is that that is the only way to for one to reintegrate with the *Dao*. It is this Daoist spiritual ideal that helps shaping the content of "*de*". Thus, while there may be overlapping between the Daoist and Aristotle's account of naturalness, the two accounts, however, are essentially different.

In *Daode jin*, there is no specific content given to "*de*". One might wonder why this is so, if "*de*" is such a core concept in *Daode jin*. On my view, it is by no means an accident that *Daode jin* does not specify the content of *de*. It is because *Daode jin* has adopted an unusual approach to understanding *de*. For *Daode jin*, it is through certain practices that one understands all things' *de*. Let us call this "practical approach". This practical approach is due to one of the basic views of *Daode jin* that it is not our language but spiritual transformation that enable us to understand the deeper realities of the comos. It is, nevertheless, only through certain practices that one can attain spiritual transformation. That is why *Daode jin* puts much emphasis on how the sage, the ideal Taoist person, behaves rather than labors at explaining such core Daoist concepts as "*Dao*" and "*de*". A set of practices are often emphasized throughout *Daode jin*. Among them are the practices of "attaining emptiness" and "maintaining tranquility", which, on my view, play a central role in the Daoist ethics and through which the doctrine of non-action is understood ((*Daode jin*, 16). On one influential traditional interpretation, "attaining emptiness" means diminishing desires (Chan, 1998, p. 96). In *Daode jin*, diminishing desires is always a major theme. For instance, *Daode jin* spends a whole chapter to explain the harms caused by human desires, even though they are the most basic ones (*Daode jin*, 12). We also are told about the unfavorable consequences of having great desires and storing much and the importance of knowing contentment and when to stop (*Daode jin*, 44). Having too many desires is described as a great crime, not being content a great disaster and being covetous a great misfortune (*Daode jin*, 46). Attaining emptiness requires not only diminishing desires but also simplicity. There are two verses that may summarize this idea of attaining emptiness

> Exhibit the unadorned and embrace the uncarved block,
> Have little thought of self and as few desires as possible (*Daode jin*, 19).

Maintaining tranquility is another important theme in *Daode jin*. We are taught to "hold firmly to stillness" (*Daode jin*, 16) and to be "[c]lam like the sea" (*Daode jin*, 20). Tranquility implies harmony. If one is not in a harmonious state of mind, it is almost impossible for one to attain tranquility. However, to maintain a harmonious state of mind requires one to maintain a harmonious relationship with others. In *Daode jin*, water is used as a model that exemplifies the highest good, "[b]ecause water excels in benefiting the myriad creatures without contending with them" (*Daode jin*, 8). *Daode jin* even regards "not contend" as "the way of sage" (*Daode jin*, 81). Thus, for *Daode jin*, maintaining a harmonious relationship with all things is of utmost importance because it is a necessary condition for one to maintain a harmonious state of mind.

V. Conclusions

As we have seen in the above sections, the Daoist conception of naturalness, to a very large extent, differs from those of the Stoics and Aristotle, which are the two major views of naturalness in the Western history of ethics. The Daoist adopts what I call a "practical approach" to understanding "*de*" which, in turn, is a key concept for understanding what naturalness is. It is this practical approach that makes the Daoist conception of naturalness a distinctive one. In short, according to this approach, to understand a thing's *de* requires certain spirit-transforming practices, two of which are particularly important, namely, attaining emptiness and maintaining tranquility. The two injunctions – the injunctions of attaining emptiness and maintaining tranquility – together with the doctrine of non-action determine the ethical content of the principle of naturalness, in which the Daoist ethics is embodied.

I shall conclude this article by discussing some significant implications of the above Daoist ethical perspective for bioethics. First, at the social and political level, the Daoist will embrace a non-interventionist health care policy. This conclusion follows from the doctrine of non-action which favors a social policy that enables individuals to maintain their naturalness, a condition in which "a thing is what it is by itself without any external impulse or interruption." This, in turn, requires the government to intervene citizens as little as possible. Intervention is allowed only if it is intended for eliminating obstacles that prevents individuals from maintaining their naturalness. This non-interventionist social ideal is succinctly put in a passage in *Daode jin*

> Hence the sage says,
> I take no action and the people are transformed of themselves;
> I prefer stillness and the people are rectified of themselves;
> I am not meddlesome and the people prosper of themselves;
> I am free from desire and the people of themselves become simple like the uncarved block (*Daode jin*, 57).

Second, at the personal level, the Daoist will embrace a personal bioethical policy which is in accordance with as much as possible the doctrine of non-action as well as the injunctions of attaining emptiness and maintaining tranquility. Thus, if using a certain biotechnology, or adopting a certain medical practice, is in conflict with either the doctrine or the injunctions, the Daoist will refrain from using the technology or adopting the medical practice. For instance, a Daoist doctor would not carry out abortions for women only on demand, since it is unnatural to terminate a pregnancy without strong medical reasons. Also, a Daoist doctor would not practice assisted suicide, if he or she knows that such practice would give birth to a large scale of conflict in society. Nor a Daoist believer would use biotechnology such as human cloning only for satisfying his or her desire to produce a talented athlete. However, the Daoist would not refrain from using medicine that can help people maintain their natural life.

Hong Kong Baptist University
Hong Kong SAR, PRC

Bibliography

Algra, E., J. Barnes, J. Mansfeld, & M. Schofield (Eds.) (1999). *The Cambridge history of hellenistic philosophy*. Cambridge: Cambridge University Press.

Ames, R.T. (2001). "Taoist ethics." In: L.C. Becker & C.B. Becker (Eds.), *Encyclopedia of ethics*, 2nd ed., vol. III (pp. 1680-1684). New York: Routledge.

Bevan, E. (1965). *Stoics and sceptics*. Cambridge: W. Heffer and Sons, Ltd.

Chan, A.K.L. (1998). A tale of two commentaries: Ho-shang-kung and Wang Pi on the *Lao-tzu*. In: L. Kohn & M. LaFargue (Eds.), *Lao-tzu and the Tao-te-ching* (pp. 89-117). Albany: State University of New York Press.

Chan, W. (trans.) (1963). *A source book in Chinese philosophy*. Princeton, N.J.: Princeton University Press.

Engstrom, S. & J. Whiting (Eds.) (1996). *Aristotle, Kant and the Stoics*. Cambridge: Cambridge University Press.

Furley, D. (Ed.) (1999). *From Aristotle to Augustine*. New York: Routledge.

Henricks, R.G. (1989). *Lao-tzu: Te-tao ching*. New York: The Modern Library.

Kirkland, R. (1995). "Taoism." In: W.T. Reich (Ed.), *Encyclopedia of bioethics*, 2nd ed, vol. 5 (pp. 2463-2469). New York: Macmillan.

Kohn, L. & M. LaFargue (Eds.) (1998). *Lao-tzu and the Tao-te-ching*. Albany: State University of New York Press.

Lau, D.C. (trans.) (1989). *Tao Te Ching*, (revised ed.). Hong Kong: The Chinese University Press.

Liu, X. (1998). "Naturalness (*Tzu-jan*), the core value of Taoism: its ancient meaning and its significance today." In: L. Kohn & M. LaFargue (Eds.), *Lao-tzu and the Tao-te-ching* (pp. 211-228). Albany: State University of New York Press.

Mill, J.S. (1998). *Three essays on religion: nature, the utility of religion, theism*. New York: Prometheus Books.

Striker, G. (2001). "Stoicism." In: L.C. Becker & C.B. Becker (Eds.), *Encyclopedia of ethics*, 2nd ed, vol. III (pp. 1652-1657). New York: Routledge.

Woodbridge, F.J.E. (1983). *Aristotle's vision of nature*, J.H. Randell (Ed.). Westport: Greenwood.

Notes on Contributors

Joseph Boyle, Ph.D. is Professor of Philosophy, St. Michael's College, University of Toronto, Toronto, Ontario, Canada.

Courtney S. Campbell, Ph.D. is Professor of Philosophy and Director, Program for Ethics, Science, and the Environment, Oregon State University, Corvallis, Oregon, U.S.A.

Devinder Singh Chahal, Ph.D. is President, Institute for Understanding Sikhism – The Research Journal and former Professor of Applied Microbiology, Institut Armand-Frappier, University of Quebec, Laval, Quebec, Canada.

Jonathan Chan, Ph.D. is Research Fellow and Assistant Professor, Department of Religion and Philosophy, Hong Kong Baptist University, Kowloon Tong, Hong Kong, SAR, People's Republic of China.

Cynthia B. Cohen, Ph.D., J.D. is Faculty Affiliate, Kennedy Institute of Ethics, Georgetown University, Washington, D.C., U.S.A.

Cromwell Crawford, Ph.D. is Professor and Department Chair, Department of Religion, University of Hawaii at Manoa, Honolulu, Hawaii, U.S.A.

Corinna Delkeskamp-Hayes, Ph.D. is Director of European Programs, International Studies in Philosophy and Medicine, Freigericht, Germany.

H. Tristram Engelhardt, Jr., Ph.D., M.D. is Professor of Philosophy, Rice University, Houston, Texas, U.S.A. and Professor Emeritus, Baylor College of Medicine, Houston, Texas, U.S.A.

Harvey L. Gordon, M.D. is Clinical Professor of Urology and Medical Ethics at Baylor College of Medicine, Houston, Texas, U.S.A.

Ruth Groenhout, Ph.D. is Associate Professor of Philosophy, Calvin College, Grand Rapids, Michigan, U.S.A.

Damien Keown, D.Phil. is Senior Lecturer in Indian Religion, Goldsmith's College, University of London, London, England.

B. Andrew Lustig, Ph.D. is Director, Program on Biotechnology, Religion, and Ethics, Rice University, Houston, Texas, U.S.A.

Aaron L. Mackler, Ph.D. is Associate Professor of Theology, Duquesne University, Pittsburgh, Pennsylvania, U.S.A.

C. Ben Mitchell, Ph.D. is senior fellow at the Center for Bioethics and Human Dignity, Bannockburn, Illinois and Associate Professor of Bioethics and Contemporary Culture at Trinity International University, Deerfield, Illinois, U.S.A.

Abdulaziz Sachedina, Ph.D. is Professor of Religious Studies, University of Virginia, Charlottesville, Virginia, U.S.A.

David H. Smith, Ph.D. is Director of the Poynter Center, Indiana University, Bloomington, Indiana, U.S.A.

Christopher Tollefsen, Ph.D. is Associate Professor of Philosophy, University of South Carolina, Columbia, South Carolina.

Mark Washofsky, Ph.D. is Professor of Rabbinics, Hebrew Union College – Jewish Institute of Religion, Cincinnati, Ohio, U.S.A.

Matthias Zierenberg, Dplm. Theol., Geilnau, Germany.

Index

Abel, F., 18, 20
abortion, ix, xii, 2, 6, 8, 9, 11, 12, 17, 19, 20, 25, 27, 28, 37, 38, 43, 55, 56, 58–60, 65–67, 71, 73–77, 83, 85–88, 90–93, 101–110, 113, 114, 117, 119–122, 127, 128, 137, 138, 145, 147–150, 153, 162, 163, 179, 182, 183, 187, 188, 199, 200, 208, 211, 217, 230
  partial-birth, 102
Abraham, 80, 82, 155, 156
abstinence, 58, 73, 93, 101, 125, 190
access to health care, 49, 169
accountability, 57, 82, 85, 111, 121, 123, 125, 155
action vs. omission, 12
Adam, 7
Adams, Maldon Browning, 107
adultery, 26, 27, 99, 136, 161, 196, 213
Africa, 31, 154
afterlife, 57, 61, 62, 64, 65, 71, 74–76
agape, 48
Agapius, Saint, 30
agriculture, 92, 193
AIDS, 44, 49, 93, 170, 185
Akal Takht, 216
al-Bar, Ali, 167
alcohol, 45, 170, 193, 215
Alexandria, 30
Algra, E., 230
allocation, 2, 25, 85, 112, 143
allowing to die, 13
alms-levy, 156
Al-Shafi'i, 157, 158
altruism, 218
Alvare, H., 11, 18
Alzheimer's disease, 204, 215
America, 19, 20, 29, 31, 32, 49, 83, 97, 98, 107
America, Latin, 31
America, North, 31, 86, 168
American Fertility Society Ethics Committee, 149, 151
American Hospital Association, 180
American Medical Association, 145, 188, 212
American, North, 17, 83, 86, 88
American Revolution, 32
Ames, R.T., 230
Amman, 168
Ammerman, Nancy Tatom, 104, 108
amniocentesis, 120
Amritsar, 213, 218–220
Amundsen, D.W., 50
Anabaptist, 79
analgesics, 12, 25
Anas, Malik b., 158
anatomy, 157, 159, 191
Anderson, D., 30
anencephaly, 90
anesthesia, 198
Anglican, 31–37, 41, 47–49, 79
Anglican clergy, 49
Anglican Communion, 31, 33, 36, 47–49
animal husbandry, 92
Anscombe, Elizabeth, 4
Antiochian Orthodox Christian Archdiocese, 25, 29
Apartheid, 80
Apostles, 23–25
Appleyard, B., 102, 108
Aquinas, Thomas, 1, 2, 4, 5, 8, 37
Arabia, 154, 158
Archbishop of Canterbury, 31
Aristotle, 37, 50, 173, 186, 224, 226, 228, 229, 231
artificial insemination, 6, 26, 39, 114, 136, 161, 162
  by donor, 39
asceticism, 22, 157
Ash'arites, 159
Ashley, Benedict, 3, 4, 18
Asia, 31, 154, 174, 176, 177, 182, 211
Asoka, 177, 178, 188
Assaad, M.D., 153, 170
astrology, 159
Atharva, 189
Atlanta, 105, 106
atomic weapons, 58
Augustine, Blessed, 1–3, 28, 35, 80, 231
Austin, ii, 101
Australia, 86
Austriaco, N., 15, 18
authority, x–xiii, 1–3, 5–7, 16, 22, 80, 83, 87, 89, 93, 98, 109, 110, 112, 114, 123, 126, 128, 132, 133, 135, 136, 145, 147, 154, 158, 162, 166, 173–175, 179, 193, 197, 204, 226, 228
authority, ecclesiastical, 21
autonomy, 6, 12, 34, 38, 73, 81, 85, 93, 97, 98, 101, 125, 131, 134, 181, 186, 198, 202, 204, 205
autopsy, 117, 123, 126, 155
Avis, P., 31, 50
Avraham, A.S., 135, 137, 145
Ayurveda, 189–191, 195, 197, 205, 208

Baby Doe, 90
Babylonia, 132
Bakar, O., 153, 170
Baker, R.A., 98, 108
Bakr, Abu, 154
Balambal, 211, 220
Bangkok, 178, 188

Baptist Faith and Message 2000, 99
Barnes, J., 230
Barth, Karl, 81, 83, 86, 94
Bartholomew, Patriarch, 24, 29
Basham, A.L., 190, 195, 208
Basil the Great, Saint, 25, 27, 29, 30
Beauchamp, Tom L., 124, 129, 192, 208
Bentinck, Lord, 212
bereavement, 48
Beza, Theodore, 80, 85
Bhagavad Gita, 192
Bible, x, 1, 31, 33, 57, 58, 60, 72, 73, 99, 110, 146, 147
biotechnology, 109, 111, 129, 213, 225, 230
Birnbaum, R., 177, 187
birth, 11, 38, 53, 56, 66, 71, 74, 86, 87, 94, 102, 103, 112, 114–116, 120, 124, 128, 135–138, 145, 148, 156, 171, 176, 182, 191, 201, 215, 216, 218, 230
birth control, 38, 87, 103, 114, 115, 136, 137, 145, 182, 218
see also: contraception
blastocyst, 139, 150
Bleich, J. David, 135, 136, 141, 145, 146, 149, 151, 152
blood, 89
Board for Social Responsibility, 33, 36, 48, 50
Boer, T., 87, 88, 94
Bole, Thomas, 14, 18
Bombay, 213
bone-setting, 189
Bood, A., 94
Book of Common Prayer, 31, 33, 36, 46
Book of Mormon, 110, 127, 129
Booty, J., 33, 46, 49–51
Bouma, H., 84–86, 91, 92, 94
Bowsorth, C.E., 171
Boyle, J., v, vii, xii, 1, 4–7, 11, 15, 17–19
Boyle, P., 20
Boyle, Robert, 91, 94
Brahm Samaj, 212
Brahman, 200–202
Brahmana, 193
Brahmanism, 177
breast cancer, 49
Breck, John, 29, 30
Britain, 31
Brody, Baruch, 18
Brusatti, Louis T., vii
Buddha, 173, 174, 177, 178, 182, 184, 186
Buddhism, v, viii, ix, 173–188, 190, 211, 213
Buddhism, Theravada, 174
Buddhism, Tibetan, 174
burdensome treatment, 13
Burgel, J.C., 153, 170, 171
burial, 46, 116, 122, 159, 164
Burma, 174
Bush, Lester E., 111, 112, 120, 126, 129
Butler, J., 31, 32, 50
Butler, P., 50
Byzantine, 30, 154

cadavers, 155, 159, 164, 184
Cairo, 153
Calcutta, 218
caliph, 154
Callahan, J.D., 209
Calvin Center for Christian Scholarship, 86
Calvin, John, 80–82
Cameron, Nigel, 95, 101
Campbell, Alastair, iv, xi, 84, 85, 94
Campbell, Courtney, ix, xi, 112, 129
Campbell, Edward, 171
Canada, 151, 219
Canon (al-Qanun) of Avicenna, 159
canon law, 17, 32, 33
capital punishment, 104
Caraka, x, 190, 195, 197, 198, 200, 205, 206
Caraka Samhita, x, 190, 195, 197, 200, 206, 209
Caribbean, 31, 97
Casti Conubii, 10, 20
castration, 26, 27
casuistry, xi, xii, 1, 2, 4, 5, 16, 17, 19, 22, 32, 51, 86, 132, 133
Catholic Health Association, 4, 18
Catholic hierarchy, xii
CCAR Responsum, 139
Center for Bioethics and Human Dignity, 102
Chadwick, H., 32, 50
Chahal, D.S., 220
Chahal, Parminder Singh, 219
Chahal, Surjit Kaur, vi, 211, 213, 214, 219
Chan, A.K.L., 230
Chan, W., 231
charity, 59, 63, 80, 91
Charleston Baptist Association, 98
Charter of Rights and Freedoms of the Canadian Constitution, 86
chastity, 58, 59, 66, 71, 73, 74, 125
childbirth, 45, 137, 138
children, 9, 10, 26, 34–36, 38–40, 42, 43, 46, 57, 59, 63, 76, 86, 87, 114, 115, 125–127, 136, 139, 158, 161, 182, 183, 199, 212
Childress, James, xiii, 51, 124, 129
China, 37, 174
cholesterol, 215
Christ, xi, 7, 12, 15, 23, 25, 29, 30, 33, 46, 54, 56, 57, 62, 66, 74–77, 82, 91, 99, 100, 102, 109, 112, 118, 129, 130, 176
Christian, v, ix, x–xii, 3, 7, 14, 19–26, 28–35, 37, 38, 40, 41, 46, 48, 50, 54, 55, 60–64, 66–70, 72–74, 76, 77, 80, 81, 84–87, 89, 91, 99–102, 107, 109, 148, 150, 177, 190
Baptist, ix, 97–101, 103–105, 107, 108, 230
Episcopalian, v, ix, 31–33, 35–37, 38–44, 47, 48, 50, 51
Evangelical, 72–77, 79
Lutheran, ix, xi, 31, 72, 79
Orthodox, ix, xi, 21–30
Presbyterian, 83
Radical Reformation, xi
Reformed, v, ix–xi, 31, 79–94
Roman Catholic, v, ix–xii, 1–5, 9, 11, 12, 14, 15, 17–19, 21, 25–28, 30, 32, 53, 72, 99, 115, 128, 150, 193
Christian Legal Society on pro-life speech, 102
Christian Reformed Church, 86, 87, 94
Christianity, ix, 22, 25, 27, 31, 53, 56, 60, 66, 67, 71, 77, 176, 207, 211, 218
Chrysostom, St. John, 26, 30
Church Fathers, 22, 33, 37
Church Handbook of Instructions, 111, 129
Church of England, 31, 36, 48
circumcision, 144, 158, 212, 213
circumcision, female, 158
Clement of Alexandria, 28, 30
Clement, Pope, 31

clergy, x, 1, 14, 32, 34, 38, 45, 49, 104, 111, 158, 174
Clinton, Hillary, 101
Clinton, William J., 104
cloning, ix, 10, 24–26, 40, 69, 73, 92, 105, 112, 123, 129, 139, 145, 225, 230
Clough, V., 207, 208
Cohen, C.B., v, 31, 34–36, 38–40, 42, 43, 46–48, 50, 51
Cole, B., 15, 18
Collins, Francis, 101
Committee on Medical Ethics, 36, 42, 43, 46–48, 50
commodification, 105, 106, 151
Common Word on Dying, 74
communal discernment, xi
communism, 174
conception, 2, 5, 8, 11, 37, 43, 55, 68, 71, 81, 86, 100, 104, 107, 128, 136, 139, 151, 182, 184, 200, 228, 229
Confucianism, 184, 186, 221, 222
Congregation for the Doctrine of the Faith, 8–10, 14, 19, 151, 152
Connery, J., 2, 19
conscience, 32, 38, 57, 64, 77, 106, 107, 118, 156, 157, 160, 165, 180, 194, 216
consciousness, 14, 15, 56, 75, 92, 155, 160, 180, 184, 191, 200, 201, 206, 216, 227
consensus, v, xii, xiii, 53, 65–67, 70–72, 88, 90, 105, 123, 132, 133, 143, 144, 147, 151, 157, 162–164, 175, 179, 185
consent, informed, 34, 38, 41, 55, 74, 107, 116, 117, 119, 123, 167, 181, 183, 204
Constantelos, D.J., 25, 30
Constantinople, 25
contraception, ix, 3, 5, 6, 9–11, 26, 36, 37, 49, 83, 87, 91, 107, 110, 114, 115, 126, 127, 137, 199
  natural family planning, 11
conversion, 29, 65, 178
Corsi, P., 175, 188
Council in Ancyra, 27, 30
Council of Europe, 78
Council of Islamic Jurisprudence, 167, 168
coup de grâce, 90
covenant, ix, 80–84, 87–89, 94, 95, 134, 155
Coward, H.G., 208
Cranmer, Thomas, 31
Crawford, Cromwell, vi, x, 208
Creation/Fall/Redemption narrative, 82
cremation, 116
Cronin, Daniel, 3, 19
Crum, Gary, 101
cryopreservation, 8
culture of death, 11, 12
culture of life, 2
culture, secular, 23
Cummings, D., 30
Cunningham, A., 94
Cuomo, M., 11, 19

Daniels, E., 101
Dao, 221–223, 227–229
Daode jin, 221, 222, 226–230
Daoism, vi, ix, 221–223, 226–230
Dasgupta, 191, 206, 208
death, ix, 6, 7, 12–15, 20, 25–29, 43, 45–48, 50, 56, 57, 63–65, 67, 73, 75, 76, 84, 86, 89, 90, 100, 104, 105, 107, 110, 117–121, 123, 134, 139–141, 145, 152–155, 157, 163–170, 174, 177, 184, 185, 191–196, 198, 201–207, 215
  brain death, 145, 164, 165, 168, 184
  Declaration on Procured Abortion, 8
  deism, 62, 76
  dementia, 168
  democracy, liberal, 11
  dental care, 49
  depravity, 83
  Desai, P., 201, 206, 208
  Dharma, 173, 194
  diakonia, 65
  Diamond Sangha, 183
  Didache, 27
  Diekema, D., 84–86, 92, 94
  dignity, xi, 7, 9, 10, 34–36, 46, 55, 57, 69, 78, 85, 103, 117, 118, 147, 179, 197, 209
  discrimination, 42, 44, 105
  discrimination, genetic, 105
  disorientation, 61
  divine life, 3
  doctor-patient relationship, ix, 180, 198
  Doctrine and Covenants, 110, 129
  doctrine of double effect, 5, 17, 18, 27
doctrine of nonaction, 227, 230
Doe v. Bolton, 102, 108
Dolly the sheep, 104
domestic violence, 49
Donald, Charles, 171
Donaldson, J., 30
Donne, John, 35, 50
donor cards, 106
Donum Vitae, 6, 8, 10, 20
Dorff, E.N., 136–143, 145, 150, 152
Dorotheos of Gaza, 28, 30
Down Syndrome, 90
Dr. Falk Schlesinger Institute for Medical-Halakhic Research, 144
drowning, 205
dueling, 107
Duncan, A.S., 176, 187
Dunstan, G.R., 38, 50, 176, 187
Durant, Jean Henri, 219
Dutch Lutheran church, 87
dying, ix, 12, 14, 15, 25, 46–48, 55–57, 64, 69, 72–74, 80, 84, 85, 89, 90, 105, 110, 118, 127, 128, 139, 140, 153, 185, 201–203, 205–207, 218
Dyson, Anthony, 38, 40, 50

Ebrahim, A.F.M., 162, 171
ecclesiology, xiii, 23
economics, 211
education, medical, 195
egalitarianism, 91
ego, 192, 200, 217
Egypt, 153, 158, 164, 170
Eisenberg, D., 139, 145
Elgood, C., 159, 171
Eliyahu, Mordechai, 149, 152
Elizabeth I, Queen, 31
Elkins, Thomas, 101
Elon, M., 144, 145
embryo, 6, 8, 9, 11, 12, 15, 20, 26, 27, 37–41, 42, 50, 58, 69, 71, 73, 87, 88, 92, 101, 105, 119, 135, 137–139, 147–151, 162, 163, 182, 183, 199–201, 218, 224, 225
embryo research, 105
embryo stem cell research, 24, 41, 105, 150
  see also: stem cell research
embryology, 162, 191
end-of-life care, ix, 48
End-of-Life Task Force, 46–48
endometrial cancer, 49
Engelhardt, H. Tristram Jr., v, vii, 18, 19, 21, 29, 30

England, 4, 31–33, 39, 49, 50, 101
English colonial expansion, 31
Engstrom, S., 231
Enlightenment, 21
Enlightenment Project, 21, 22, 176
ensoulment, 8, 27, 127, 162, 163, 182, 200
Ephesians, 26, 35, 100
Episcopal Board for Social Responsibility, 40, 41
Episcopal Committee on Medical Ethics, 41, 47
Episcopal General Convention of 1985, 44, 45
Episcopal General Convention of 1991, 34
Episcopal General Convention of 2000, 48
Episcopal General Convention of 2003, 40, 42, 45
Episcopal Standing Commission on Human Affairs and Health, 39, 40, 43
Episcopal Standing Commission on Human Affairs and Health of 1988, 39
Episcopal Standing Commission on National Concerns, 45, 49
epistemology, xii, 22, 99
eproduction, assisted, 6, 26
equity, 2
eschatology, xi
esophageal blockage, 90
Ethics & Medicine: An International Journal of Bioethics, 101
Ethics & Religious Liberty Commission, 100, 101, 108
Ethics and New Genetics Task Force, 42
ethics committees, ix, 16, 186
Eucharist, 14
eugenics, 37, 43, 55, 65, 67, 73–75, 87
Europe, 31, 79, 174, 176
European Bioethics Convention, 56
euthanasia, xii, 12, 14, 18, 20, 25, 48, 71, 73, 76, 89, 90, 93, 94, 101, 103, 105, 106, 108–110, 117, 121, 122, 127–129, 139, 140, 184, 185, 187, 203–206, 212, 213, 218
Evagrios the Solitary, 22, 30
Evangelical Alliance, 72–74, 76, 77
evangelical faith, 99
Evangelical Lutheran Church of America, 99
Evangelische Kirche in Deutschland, v, 53, 54, 64, 65, 71, 72, 76–78
Evangelium Vitae, 6–9, 18–20
Evans, A., 82, 94
Eve, 7
evil, 5, 14, 26–28, 46, 54, 56, 57, 59, 61–63, 76, 77, 80, 86, 94, 124, 159, 165, 186, 191, 194, 200, 202
extraordinary care, 2, 13, 18, 26, 185, 202, 206
see also: ordinary care

Fagot-Largeault, Anne M., vii
faith, xiii, 3, 32, 46, 54, 57, 62, 65–68, 76, 77, 80, 98, 99, 101, 108, 117, 120, 154, 156, 158, 189, 190, 192, 198, 206, 211
faithfulness, 55, 57, 67, 82, 84, 88
fall of man, 63
family, xii, 6, 11, 14, 18, 30, 36, 38–40, 42, 43, 45–48, 59, 80, 110, 113, 114, 116–118, 122–127, 136–138, 155, 157, 158, 165, 166, 168, 170, 179, 184–186, 195, 198, 199, 202, 205, 206, 217, 218
family planning, 36, 38, 59
Family Research Council, 102
famine, 147
Federation Internationale des Associations Medical Catholique, 213
Feldman, D.M., 137, 138, 145, 147–149, 151, 152
fertilization, 8, 10, 37–39, 68, 69, 104, 105, 119, 139, 150, 182, 218
fetal tissue, 43, 105, 106
feticide, 137, 148, 163, 213
fetus, 5, 15, 37, 43, 44, 56, 58–60, 68, 73, 88, 113, 120, 137–139, 148–150, 162, 163, 183, 200, 201, 211, 217
filial piety, 222
Finnis, John, 9, 19
Firdawsi, Mas'ud, 155, 171
First-and-Second Council held in Constantinople, 26
First International Congress of Anesthesiologists, 13
Five Pillars of Islam, 154
Fletcher, Joseph, 32, 33, 50
Florida, 106, 107, 182
Foltz, Bruce, 22, 30
Ford, N., 8, 12, 19
fornication, 27, 73
Foster, Henry, 104
Fox, R., 112, 119, 129
Frankena, W.K., 108
fratricide, 192
Furley, D., 231

gamete intrafallopian transfer, 10
gametes, 26, 39, 87, 122, 126, 199
Gautama, 203
Gearhart, J., 150, 152
gene therapy, 41, 42, 55, 73, 110, 119, 120, 215, 225, 226
generic religiosity, 72
gene-therapy, 59
genetic couseling, 42
genetic disorder, 43, 225, 226
genetic engineering, 24, 41, 92, 101, 110, 139, 216, 225
genetic manipulation, 42, 92
genetic technology, 92, 104, 106, 123
genetic testing, 42, 105, 110, 113
genetic therapy, 129
genetics, ix, 101, 123
gene-transfer, 55
genital mutilation, 211, 212
genome mapping, 129
gentleness, 57, 63
Georgetown University, 4, 18, 19, 29
Georgia, 97, 105, 106
Gereformeerde Kerken in Nederland, 83
German constitutional court, 70
German Protestantism, 53, 70, 72
Germany, 53, 55, 58, 70–72, 77, 212
gezerot, 132
gift of life, 7, 19
Gillette, A.D., 98, 108
Giorgis, B.W., 153, 171
God, ix, xi, xii, 2, 7–9, 14, 21–29, 33, 34, 36, 38, 41–43, 46, 48, 54, 56–77, 81, 82, 84, 85, 87–89, 92, 93, 99, 102, 104–111, 115, 117, 118, 124–128, 131, 133, 135, 142, 144, 145, 147, 153–157, 159, 161, 162, 170, 214, 216, 218
God, image of, 106, 107

God's honor, 54
goodness, 57, 63, 82, 85, 222
Gormally, L., 19
Gospel, v, 7, 53, 54, 63, 65, 67, 72, 73, 76
Gospel of Life, 7
Gospels, xi, 24
Gott ist ein Freund des Lebens, 53, 66, 70, 78
Gottleib, R., 94
grace, 21–24, 27, 28, 66, 99, 109
Granrose, J.T., 108
Great Litany, 45
Gregory, John, 80
Grell, O., 94
Griffin, Leslie, 11, 18, 19
Griffiths, J., 89, 94
Grisez, Germain, 4, 9, 11, 12, 14, 19
Groenhout, Ruth, v, vii, x
Guam, 97
Guevin, Benedict, 18
guidance counselor, 38
Gupta period, 190
Guroian, V., 29, 30
Guru Ram Das Institute of Dental Sciences, 219
Guru Ram Das Medical Educational and Research Hospital, 219
Gustafson, James x, xi, xiii, 81, 83, 84, 86, 94
gynecology, 101

Habermas, H., 209
Habgood, J., 38, 50
hajj, 156
hakim, 159, 166, 194
halakhah, 131–137, 139, 141, 144, 145
halakhot, 132
halal, 213
Halevi, Hayyim David, 149, 152
Hanbal, Ahmad b., 158
handicapped, 55–57, 63, 74–77, 90, 205, 218
Hanifa, Abu, 158
Harakas, S., 29, 30
Harappa culture, 189
Hardacre, H., 183, 187
Harita, 203
Harley, David, 80, 89, 90, 94
harming the vulnerable, 3
Harris, Abbott, D., 130
Harris, J., 50
Harris, Thomas, 101
Hart, Oliver, 98
Harvard Medical School, 184
Harvey, John, v, 18, 20
Harvey, Peter, 187
Haugaard, W.P., 31, 50
health care, access to, ix, 90, 123, 129, 134, 170, 185, 219
health care, delivery, ix, 91, 92, 102
health care, distribution, 2
health care professionals, 5, 6, 16, 34, 84, 113, 179
health care system, single-tier, 16
health care system, two-tier, 16, 67, 185
health clinics, 49
Health Security Act, 101, 107
heart disease, 49
heaven, 50, 193, 212
Hefley, J., 100, 107, 108
Heller, J.C., 50
Henricks, R.G., 231
Henry, C.F.H., 31, 99, 108
Herod, James T., 102
Hessel, Dieter, 92, 94
heterological insemination, 73
heterosexuality, 88
hikmat, 194
Hillerbrand, H.J., 50
Hindu, vi, x, 189–194, 198–209, 213
Hinduism, ix, 176, 189, 190, 192–194, 202–205, 211, 218
Hinnells, J.R., 171
Hippocratic Oath, 153, 180, 195, 207, 212
Hiriyanna, M., 194, 208
history, xi, 2, 3, 19, 24, 31, 34, 42, 43, 83, 94, 100, 107, 131, 155, 159, 171, 174, 176, 177, 183, 191, 194, 207, 224, 229, 230
HIV, 44, 93
Hodgson, M.G.S., 154, 171
holiness, 22, 25, 27
Holland, S., 152
Holy Fathers of the First Six Ecumenical Councils, 24
Holy Spirit, 22, 25, 29
Holy Tradition, 29
homeless, 44, 45, 49, 127
homicide, 27, 28, 138, 148, 155, 162, 163
homosexuality, 87, 88, 93, 99
Hooker, Richard, 34, 35, 50
hormone therapy, 198
Horner, S., 50
Hoshino, Kazumasa, vii
hospice, 47, 48, 90, 105, 141, 185, 205, 218
hospices, 49, 177, 190
hospitals, 3, 4, 25, 49, 185, 213
House of Bishops, 32, 33
House of Deputies, 32
Howsepian, A.A., 19
Hugh, A., 208
Hughes, James J., 183, 187
human finitude, 71, 89
human life, 6–10, 12, 14, 19, 26, 30, 33, 37, 38, 53, 55–62, 64, 67–69, 74, 76, 82, 86, 92, 103, 104, 107, 108, 122, 127, 128, 133, 142, 149–151, 155, 158, 160, 164, 179, 182, 183, 207, 211, 215
human nature, 84, 93
Humanae Vitae, 6, 9, 10, 20
humanness, 60, 70, 128
Hume, R.E., 208
Hunter, M., 94
hydration, 14, 19, 20, 46, 140, 141, 184
hydrotherapy, 189

icon, 22, 23
'Id al-fitr, 156
identity, human, 5, 20, 26, 31, 36, 37, 39, 40, 88, 136, 162, 211, 213
ideology, 54, 64
idolatry, 22, 28, 144
ignorance, 56, 58, 173, 201–203
Im Geist der Liebe mit dem Leben umgehen, 53, 66
Imam, 154, 158
immolation, 205
in vitro embryos, 148
in vitro fertilization, 6, 8, 10, 26, 39, 41, 42, 50, 68, 71, 73, 77, 78, 87, 88, 119, 122, 136, 138, 139, 183, 198, 199, 218, 225
incest, 103, 104, 163
India, iv, 154, 173, 177, 178, 189–191, 196, 206, 209, 211–213, 218, 219
Indian caste system, 176
infanticide, 27, 103, 104, 106, 211, 213, 217
infectious diseases, 58, 60
infertility, 36, 39, 87, 101, 136
infibulation, 158
innocent life, 25, 192
insemination, 10, 74, 122, 136, 161, 162
Institute of Medicine, 101
insurance, 42, 45, 90, 91, 102, 161
integrity, professional, 85
intercourse, 9, 10, 26, 36, 114, 162, 182, 199
International Congress on Medical Ethics, 155, 171

intolerance, 66
intrauterine contraceptive device, 137
Iran, 153, 158, 164, 169
Ireland, 4
Islam, ix, x, 153, 154, 156, 158–162, 164–167, 169–171, 176, 211, 218
Islam and Family Planning, 161, 171
Islamic law, 153, 155, 156, 159, 161, 164–166, 168, 169
Islamic Medical Wisdom, 153, 171

Jacksonville, 107
Jacob, Walter, 146
Jainism, 211
Jamestown, 31
Japan, 174, 176, 182–184, 187
Jathedar Sadhu Singh Bhaura, 216
Jennings, B., 50
Jerusalem, 144, 145
Jesus, 7, 19, 29, 54, 72, 78, 99, 102, 109, 112, 118, 129, 130, 155
Jewish casuistry, xii
Jewish law, 131–139, 141, 142, 145, 148, 150
John Paul II, Pope, 1, 2, 4, 5, 7–12, 15–17, 20
John the Faster, Saint, 27, 30
John XXIII, Pope, 15
Johnson, Mark, 12, 19, 20
Jonas, Hans, 65
Jonsen, Albert, 18, 19, 80, 81, 94
Jordan, 168
Jotterand, Fabrice, vii
Judaism, ix, x, 131, 133, 135, 136, 143, 148, 176, 207, 211
Judism, 213
justice, ix, 22, 49, 57, 60, 63, 72, 73, 81–85, 87, 90, 91, 142, 150, 151, 154, 155, 158–160, 169, 170, 180

Kane, P., 202, 208
Kanhaiya, Bhai, 219
Kant, Immaneul, 11, 28, 76, 221, 231
Kapur, Prithipal Singh, 219
karma, 174, 179, 186, 191, 195, 200, 201, 205
Kauffman, C.J., 3, 19
Kausika, 192, 193
Kausikasutra, 189
Kaviratna, A.C., 208
Keenan, James, 7, 19
Keown, Damien, vi, x, 173, 179, 184, 187
Kevorkian, Jack, 105, 205
killing, 2, 3, 5–8, 12–15, 25, 48, 58, 64, 71, 73, 113, 117, 127–129, 139, 140, 162, 179, 182, 184, 185, 213, 218, 224
killing of innocent human life, 5, 6, 55
Kilner, John, 95, 102
King Fahad National Guard Hospital, 167
King Henry VIII, 31
King Hezekiah, 145
Kingdom of God, 82, 107
Kirk, Kenneth, 32, 51
Kirkland, R., 227, 231
Knight, J., 50, 51
Kohn, L., 230, 231
Kopelman, Loretta, vii
Korea, 174, 183
kosher, 213, 216
Krsna, 192
Kuyper, Abraham, 80, 82, 94

LaFargue, M., 230, 231
LaFleur, William, 183, 187
Lake, K., 30
Lambeth Conference, 33, 36, 46–48, 51
Lammers, S., 94, 95
Land, Richard, 101, 108
Lao-tzu, 221, 230, 231
Latter-day Saints, ix–xii, 109–129
Lau, D.C., 228, 231
Lebacqz, Karen, 152
Lee, P., 19
Lesch Nyhan, 90
letting die, 12
liberty, religious, 101
license, 81, 85, 134, 159, 183, 198
Ligouri, Alphonsus, 4, 16
Linacre Centre, 4, 18
Lipner, J., 201, 208
Liu, X., 222, 227, 231
living will, 50, 101, 106, 141, 164, 166, 204
Loike, J.D., 139, 145
Lomanno, Jessica, vi
Lomanno, Matthew, vii
loneliness, 61, 156
longevity, 191
long-term care, 49
lottery, 143
Louisiana, 101, 105
Louisiana State University, 101
love, 9, 10, 21, 28, 32–36, 38, 44, 46, 48, 57, 60, 62, 63, 67, 68, 72, 75, 77, 85, 88, 100, 115, 117, 126, 148, 194, 202, 227
Lustig, B. Andrew, v, ix, 18, 19, 94, 95, 129, 208
Luther, Martin, xi, 79–81, 85
lying, 2, 28, 66, 181, 193

ma'asim, 132
Macer, D.R.J., 220
Mackler, Aaron, vi, xii, 148, 152
Macquarrie, J., xiii, 51
Madsen v. Women's Health Center, 102, 108
magisterium, 1, 97
Mahabharata, 192, 193, 209
Mahoney, J., 18, 19
Mainetti, José Alberto, vii
Malta, conjoined twins of, 5, 18
Manichean, 75
Mansfeld, J., 230
manslaughter, 155
Manu, 193, 199, 200, 202, 208, 209
marital love, 10, 11
Markt der Möglichkeiten, 70
marriage, 6, 9, 11, 20, 25, 26, 30, 31, 35, 36, 40, 59, 73, 74, 87, 88, 114, 125, 126, 139, 161, 176
Masoom, S.H.F., 153, 171
masturbation, 161
Matilal, Bimal K., 192, 209
matrimony, 35, 122
May, William E., 9, 14, 15, 18, 19, 84, 94
maya b'alma, 149
Mazzarella, P., 175, 188
McCarthy, D., 18
McCormick, S.J., Richard, 4, 11, 19, 151, 152
McIlhaney, Jr., Joe S., 101
Mecca, 156
Medical College of Georgia, 101
Medical Institute for Sexual Health, 101
medicine, 16, 22, 25, 29, 30, 49, 64, 67, 69, 74, 80, 92, 95, 101, 102, 111, 118, 120, 129, 131, 134, 139–147, 153, 157, 159–161, 168, 170, 171, 175–178, 180, 181, 185, 188–191, 194, 195, 197, 206–207, 209, 211, 224, 225, 230
medicine, Indian, 190
medicine, Vedic, 189
medieval canonists, 3
Menon, A., 209
menopause, 49
mental health professional, 38

mental health services, 49
mentally handicapped, 55
mercy, 5, 22, 28, 90, 145, 154, 155
mercy killing, 117
Mettanando, Venerable, 179, 184, 188
Michael, B., 51
midrash, 133
midrashim, 132
Mill, J.S., 223, 224, 231
Millard, D.W., 188
Mirkes, R., 9, 20
miscarriage, 28, 148, 162, 183
Mishnah, 132, 137, 144, 145, 148
missionary, 54, 55, 65, 72
Mitchell, A., v, 18, 19
mitzvah, 133–145
mizuko kuyo, 182, 183
Mohrmann, M., 34, 51
Monk of St. Tikhon's Monastery, 28, 30
Montreal, 219, 220
Moore, L., 101, 108
Moracezewski, A., 18
moral absolute, 2, 7
moral agency, xi, 111, 115, 116, 118, 121–127
moral consciousness, 25
moral disorder, 8
moral knowledge, xii, 29
moral life, 1, 3, 17, 21, 23, 32, 159, 160
moral philosophy, 22
moral pluralism, 22
moral realism, 153
moral reasoning, xii, 2, 19, 93, 194
moral theology, xii, 1, 3–5, 18, 19, 21, 25, 29, 32
morality, ix, xiii, 2, 3, 9, 11, 21–23, 84, 107, 117, 193, 194, 221, 222
Morgan, E.F.M., 50
Mori, Maurizio, vii
Mormons, 109, 111, 193
Moses, 75, 109, 131, 132, 155
Mother Teresa, 218
Mouw, R., 82, 94
Mu'tazilites, 159
Muhammad, 153–156, 159, 168
Muller, F.M., 208
Munro, M., 215, 220
murder, 27, 71, 137, 138, 140, 144, 168, 212
Murthy, Srikantha K., 196, 209
Musallam, B.F., 171
Muslims, 153–159, 161, 164, 213
Myogak, Venerable, 183

Najafi, Mustafa, 155, 171
Nanak, Guru, 211, 213–217, 219
Nanakian philosophy, 213–219
narcotics, 15, 47, 141, 185
Nashville, 101, 108
Nassar, S., 24, 30
National Alliance for the Mentally Ill, 45
National Bioethics Advisory Commission, 50, 150, 152
National Catholic Bioethics Center, 4, 18
National Center for Human Genome Research, 101
National Conference of Catholic Bishops, 4, 16, 17, 20
National Institutes of Health, 106
National Socialism, 77
natural family planning, 26
natural law, xi, xii, 2–4, 7, 22, 26, 135, 139
naturalness, 222, 223, 226–230
Nazism, 65, 212
Nederlandse Hervormde Kerk, 83
Neihbur, H. Richard, 81, 83
neonates, 15
Netherlands, iv, 83, 86, 88, 89, 129
Netherlands Reformed Church, 83
New Orleans, 101, 105
New World, 31
New Zealand, 86
Newman, A.J., 171
Nicea I, 23, 26, 27
Nicodemus, Saint, 30
Nile, 154
Nizamuddin, Nabil, 167
Noah, 155
Nobel Peace Prize, 219
Noonan, J., 3, 20
Numbers, R.L., 50
Nuremberg Code, 212
nurse, 47, 84, 85, 177
nutrition, 14, 19, 20, 46, 64, 109, 140, 141, 184
nutrition, artificial, 141
Nyaya, 189, 191

O'Donovan, K., 36, 37, 41, 51
O'Rourke, Kevin, 3, 5, 6, 15, 17, 18, 20
obedience, xi, 63, 66–68, 70, 76, 77, 81, 84, 195, 197, 221
obedience to God, 66, 76, 81
obstetrics, 101
Ohio Department of Health, 101
omissions, 12, 119
On Dying Well, 48
oocyte, 37
ordinary care, 2, 13, 81, 153, 199, 202, 205, 207, 223
organ donation, 73, 106, 118, 126, 167
organ donors, deceased, 43
organ donors, living, 43
organ vending, 106
Organspende, 73
Orlando, 106, 107
orphans, 100
ova donation, 74
ovarian cancer, 49
ovum, 8, 162, 200
Oxus, 154

Pacific, 31
pain, iii, 12, 14, 15, 25, 29, 47, 48, 73, 84, 90, 105, 141, 144, 145, 184, 185, 194, 205–207
pain management, 90
Pakistan, 218
palliative care, 47
Palmer, G.E.H., 30
Panteleimon, St., 29
paradise, 75, 174
parents, 34–36, 38–40, 59, 63, 71, 74, 76, 90, 116, 139, 161, 162, 200, 218
paternalism, 5, 127, 134, 181, 186, 198
Pathways to Promise, 92, 95
Patient Bill of Rights, 180
patient's right to know, 134
patricide, 192
Paul VI, Pope, 9, 20
Paul, Saint, 19, 20, 23, 29
Payne, Franklin E., 101
peace, 57, 63, 81, 82, 118, 124, 154, 191
Pearl of Great Price, 110, 130
Pellegrino, Edmund D., vii, 4, 175, 188
Pentecost, 23
Percival, Thomas, 80, 212
permanent vegative state, 14, 15, 64, 76, 141, 165, 168, 184
permanently unconscious, 14, 15, 19, 20, 55
Persian, 153, 154
personhood, 8, 14, 35, 101, 148, 161–164, 200, 201
Peter, Saint, 30
Philadelphia Baptist Association, 98

physician, x, 6, 18, 28, 47, 71, 80, 81, 84, 85, 89, 90, 111, 128, 134, 135, 140, 142, 145, 147, 153, 160, 161, 167, 168, 178, 181, 184–186, 194, 196–198, 204, 206–208, 212
physician-patient relationship, 135, 181, 197
physiology, 157, 167, 191
piety, 48, 95, 160, 222
Pius XII, Pope, 5, 13–15, 20
plague, 45
Planned Parenthood v.Casey, 102, 108
Plessner, M., 153, 171
pluralism, ix, x, xii, 19, 70, 72, 78, 175
pluripotent cells, 9
Pohl, C., 87, 95
poisoning, 205
Pontifical Academy *Pro Vita*, 4
pornography, 100
Porter, Jean, 12, 20
Porter, Roy, 171
posek, 133
post-modernism, 22
prayer, 14, 22, 89, 116, 118
pregnancy, 3, 5, 38, 49, 58, 59, 63, 75, 86, 113, 136–138, 148, 162, 163, 183, 230
pregnancy, termination, 5
prenatal diagnosis, 9, 88
Presbyterian Church (USA), 79, 83, 84, 86, 90, 91, 95
prescription drugs, 49
priesthood of all believers, 100
Pritchard, R., 31, 32, 51
Proclamation on the Family, 130
procreation, 6, 9, 10, 35–37, 39, 40, 42, 115, 126, 135–137, 139, 145, 161, 199
professional conduct, 29
professionalism, ix, 5, 17, 33–35, 47, 84, 85, 110, 111, 129, 134, 140–142, 153, 160, 166, 179, 194, 197
pro-life, 2, 4, 55–57, 60–63, 73, 76, 89, 104
pro-life politics, 2
promise-keeping, 192
proportionalism, 11, 13
Protestant, v, 21, 28, 31, 32, 50, 53–56, 64–66, 68–72, 74, 76–79, 81, 89, 95, 97, 193
Protestant Church in Germany, v, 53, 54, 66
Protestant Reformation, 79
providence, 80, 94, 147
psychic illness, 62
psychological illness, 156
psychology, 211
Punjab, 212, 213, 217, 218
Punjabi University, 219, 220
purification, 22

Qiu, Ren Zong, vii
Quebec, 219
Quill, Timothy E., 207, 209
Quinisext Council or Council in Trullo, 27, 30
Quinlan, 112, 117, 118
Qumm, 153
Quorum of Twelve Apostles, 110
Qur'an, x, 154–162, 164–166, 168, 170

racism, 44, 87, 99
Rahman, F., 158, 160, 171
Raja Ram Mohan Rai, 212
Rajputana, 212
Ramadan, 156
Ramayana, 192
Ramsey, Paul, 81, 83, 84, 87, 89, 90, 95
Rao, Seshagiri, 199, 209
rape, 103, 104, 113, 163, 217
Rasmussen, Lisa, vii
Ratanakul, Pinit, 178, 180, 181, 187, 188
Ratzinger, Cardinal Josef, 72
rebirth, 174, 179, 182, 185, 186, 201, 202, 215
Red Cross, 219
redemption, xi
Reformation, 21, 79, 99
Reformed Church in America, 86, 90, 95
Reformed Church of America, 84
Reformed Churches in the Netherlands, 87
refusal of treatment, 13, 181
rehabilitation, 49
Reich, Warren T., 231
religious superstition, 54
Renaissance, 21
repentance, 22, 27–29, 64, 65, 74
Report of the Ad Hoc Committee of the Harvard Medical School to Examine the Definition of Brain Death, 188
reproduction, 7, 9, 10, 25, 26, 87, 104, 135, 153, 161
reproduction, assisted, 39
reproduction, non-sexual, 6, 10
reproductive ethics, 6, 11, 12, 14
reproductive technology, 6, 8, 9–11, 39, 40, 50, 110, 114, 119, 122, 212
research, 110
research on human subjects, 119
researcher, 84, 214
responsibility, iv, 7, 13, 16, 18, 34, 35, 39, 54, 58, 59, 65, 68, 73, 77, 83, 85, 87, 91, 100, 102, 103, 110, 114, 119, 128, 134, 142, 147, 151, 155, 159, 161, 166, 169, 170, 176, 180, 191, 197, 208
retardation, 90, 225
revelation, 4, 7, 11, 21, 23, 99, 121, 131, 154, 159, 192, 193
Revelation, xii
Rg Veda, 189
rights
  basic, 11
  liberty, 15, 33, 81, 100, 101, 118, 134
  to life, 55, 59, 74, 95, 163
  to self determination, 74
  to health care, 2, 15, 16
  welfare, 15, 16
Rispler-Chaim, V., 161, 171
Riyadh, 167
Roanoke, 31
Roberts, T.A., 30, 50
Roe v. Wade, 102, 108, 112
Romans, 29, 31, 77, 99, 100
Rosenthal, F., 171
Rosner, Fred, 137–146, 149, 151, 152
Roth, C., 30

Sabbath, 144, 149
Sachedina, A.A., 153, 161, 165, 170, 171
Sachedina, Abdulaziz, vi, x
Sacred Congregation for the Doctrine of the Faith, 6, 20
Sadiq, Ja'far al, 158
Sahni, H.S., 211, 220
Saint Edward's University, vii
Saint Louis University, iii, vii
saintly perfection, 22
salat, 156
Salihi, Mas'ud, 155, 171
salvation, 26, 28, 57, 58, 64, 65, 67, 75, 99, 109, 120, 212
Samkhya, 189, 191
San Antonio, 106
sanctification, xi
sanctity of human life, 85, 86, 100, 103, 104, 111, 128

Sass, Hans-Martin, vii
Saudi Arabia, 167
Saunders, Dame Cicely, 47
Saxons, 31
scarcity, 223
Schacht, J., 171
Schaff, P., 23, 29, 30
Schiedermayer, D., 95
Schmelzer, Jerome, vii
Schmitt, Kurt, 72
Schofield, M., 230
scholasticism, 3, 4, 21, 22
Schroten, E., 87, 94
Schweitzer, Albert, 65
science, xi, 8, 19, 24, 32, 80, 81, 101, 105, 111, 117, 129, 143, 176, 182, 190, 191, 211, 214, 217
Scotland, 4, 32, 86
Scott, D.A., 38, 50, 51, 101
Scripture, x, 23, 29, 99, 132, 134
Sedgwick, T.F., 32, 50, 51
self-defense, 5, 104
self-determination, 37
self-immolation, 202, 211
self-love, 83
senescence, 125
Seventh Ecumenical Council, 23
sex, 36, 38, 44, 58, 170, 190, 217
sex preference, 73
sexual activity, 26, 37
sexual fidelity within marriage, 93
sexual immorality, 99
sexual impurity, 28
sexual intercourse, 6, 9, 10, 35, 37, 38, 156, 157
sexual orientation, 88
sexuality, 9, 11, 25, 27, 35, 40, 59, 85, 87, 88, 92, 93, 115, 125, 126, 135, 199
sexually transmitted diseases, 101
shahada, 154
Shalom, 82
Shannon, T., 12, 20
Shari'a, 157, 158, 161, 164, 168, 170
Sharma, P., 208
Sherrard, P., 30
Shi'a, 154
Shilo, Shmuel, 145
Shiromani Gurdwara Parbandhak Committee, 213, 220
Sikh Rehit Maryada, 213, 218, 220
Sikhism, ix, 211–214, 218–220
sin, 3, 22, 28, 45, 56, 58, 59, 63–65, 71, 73, 75–77, 80, 82, 84, 89, 104, 150, 199, 217
  involuntary, 28
  voluntary, 28
Sinai, 131, 135
Singh, V., 211, 212, 214, 218, 219
Singh, Guru Gobind, 219
Singh, Harbans, 219, 220
Singh, I.J., 220
Singh, Kirpal, 219, 220
Singh, Puran, 218
slavery, 107
Smedes, Lewis, 82, 84
Smith, D.H., v, 10, 20, 34–39, 40, 42, 43, 46, 20–51, 83, 95
Smith, H., 51
Smith, J., 18, 20
Smith, Joseph Jr., 109
smoking, 156, 170, 213
social environment, 71, 161
social justice, 3, 19
Society of Christian Ethics, 151
Society of Jewish Ethics, 151
society, secular, 29, 53, 55–66, 70–72
Socrates, 192
sodomy, 27
solidarity, 14, 56, 60, 66, 73, 76, 127
Solomon, W. David, vii
somatic cell therapy, 120
Soni, R.L., 176, 188
Sorgenkind, Aktion, 75
soul, 8, 21, 28, 35, 37, 59, 109, 120, 125, 156, 160, 162, 164, 168, 174, 196, 199, 200, 203
Southern Baptist Convention, 97, 99, 100, 102, 105, 106
sperm, 8, 37, 39, 40, 42, 69, 73, 114, 119, 122, 136, 162, 199, 200
sperm donation, 74
spiritual goods, 14
spiritual healers, 34
spiritual needs, 48
Sri Lanka, 174, 182
Steinberg, A., 139, 144, 145
stem cell research, 108, 119, 147, 149–151
stem cells, 6, 9, 41, 73, 139, 150–152
Stenberg v. Carhart, 102, 108
sterilization, 36, 37, 73, 115, 116, 122
sterilization, compulsory, 37
sterilization, eugenic, 37
stewardship, ix, 36, 85, 106, 128, 129
stillbirth, 114
Stoicism, 223, 224
Striker, G., 231
suffering, 12, 14, 15, 20, 25, 26, 29, 41, 42, 44, 47–49, 55–58, 61–63, 67, 71, 75, 84, 85, 90, 92, 105, 106, 117, 120, 134, 147, 148, 153, 166, 169, 170, 184, 191, 201, 202, 205–207
suicide, x, 6, 12, 18, 25, 48, 50, 71, 101, 105, 109, 117, 122, 127, 128, 139, 140, 155, 184, 185, 202–205, 217, 218, 230
suicide, physician-assisted, 89, 90, 93, 95, 102, 105, 117, 129, 204, 205
Sullivan, James, 97, 99, 108
Sunna, x, 154, 157, 158, 161
Sunni, 154, 155, 158, 162
supernatural therapy, 190
Surgeon General of the United States, 104
surgery, 26, 49, 137, 140, 143, 189, 223
surrogate decision-makers, 166
surrogate motherhood, 10, 40, 73, 119, 122, 161
Susruta Samhita, 200
Swazey, J., 112, 119, 129
Sykes, S., 50, 51

Tabrizi, Ayatollah, 168
takanot, 132
Talmud, 132, 133, 135, 137, 144–146, 149, 151
Talmudic Sages, 132
Talmuds, 132
Tao te ching, 227
Taoist, 227, 229, 230
taxation, 16
Tay Sachs, 90
Taylor, Jeremy, 32, 46, 51
teacher, 38, 158, 195, 196
technology, 6, 10, 39, 40, 46, 58, 62, 72, 74, 84, 112, 114, 119, 139, 143, 150, 163, 165, 166, 169, 178, 185, 206–208, 211, 214, 217, 224, 230
  biomedical, 109
Tedesco, F., 183, 188
Tehran, 155, 168, 171
Temple, William, 34
ten Have, Henk, vii
Tendler, Moshe, 137, 146, 150, 152

Tennessee, 101
Testament, New, 99, 106
Testament, Old, 99, 106
Texas, iii, 14, 20, 101, 104, 106
Thailand, 174, 182
theodicy, 147
theology
  as an experience of God, 22
  dogmatic, 21
  orthodox, 21, 24
Therrien, Michel, 18
Third World, 83, 167
Thompson, Phillip M., vii
thou shalt not kill, 56, 69
tobacco, 109, 215
toleration, 54
Tollefsen, Christopher, v, xii
Torah, 131–135, 143–145
Torbet, R.G., 98, 108
Toulmin, Stephen, 18, 19
transplantation, 15, 43, 106, 110, 118, 126, 143, 155, 164, 167, 169, 184
Trinity, 21, 23, 95
truth-telling, 28, 181, 192, 193
tubal ligation, 137
Tunisia, 158
turban, 213
Turkey, 158
Turner, P., 51
twinning, 11
Tzitz Eliezer, 144

unborn, 19, 28, 42, 55, 57, 65, 86, 100, 102, 104, 106, 127, 200, 208
United Churches, 79
United Methodist Church, 99
United States, 4, 14, 18–20, 31, 32, 49, 83, 84, 86, 90, 91, 95, 97, 102, 105, 107, 114, 149, 174, 182, 206
  House of Representatives, 102
United States Patent Office, 106
University of Pune, 213, 219
University of Utah, 119
utilitarianism, 70, 179, 183, 186

Vacco v. Quill, 102, 108
Vaisesika, 189, 191
Vancouver, 151
Vanderbilt University, 101
vasectomy, 115, 116, 137
Vatican, 2–5, 14, 17, 20, 151
Vatican Council II, 2, 3, 17, 20
Vaux, K., 81, 84, 87, 90, 95
Veatch, Robert, 197, 207, 209
Vedanta, 189
Verhey, Allen, x, xiii, 81, 82, 84, 85, 89, 90, 94, 95
Veritatis Splendor, 5, 17, 20
vibratory stimuli, 162
violence, denial of, 54
Virginia, 31
Vlachos, H., 21, 30
vocation, 13, 80, 81, 84, 85, 91

Wace, H., 23, 29, 30
Wagner, Sister M., 29
Waldenberg, Eliezer Yehudah, 144
Wales, 4
Walters, Leroy, 208
war, 27, 31, 58, 104, 212
Ware, K., 30
Washington v. Glucksberg, 102, 108
Washington, D.C., 101
Washofsky, M., v, 131, 134–143, 145, 146
Wassmer, T., 207, 208
Watt, W.M., 158, 171
Wawrytko, S.A., 188
Welbourn, R.B., 176, 187
Weltanschauung, 80
Wensinck, A.J., 158, 171
Weyers, H., 89, 94
Wheeler, E., 30
Whitehill, J., 179, 188
Whiting, J., 231
Wildes S.J., Kevin, 14, 18–20
witchcraft, 107, 189
withdrawing of care, 12, 14
withholding care, 12
Wolter, A., 12, 20
Wood, T., 32, 51
Woodbridge, F.J.E., 224, 231
Word of Wisdom, 109, 125, 130
World Alliance of Reformed Churches, 79
World War II, 212
Wright, J.R., 31, 51

Yisrael, Eretz, 132
Yoga, 189, 191
Yoga, Hatha, 191
Yom Kippur, 134, 144
Young, K.K., 208

zakat, 156
Zanardi, William J., vii
Zemer, Moshe, 146
Zimmer, H.R., 189, 196, 209
Zoloth, Laurie, 150–152
Zoroastrianism, 211, 213
zygote, 139, 200
Zysk, Kenneth, 176–178, 188, 190, 209